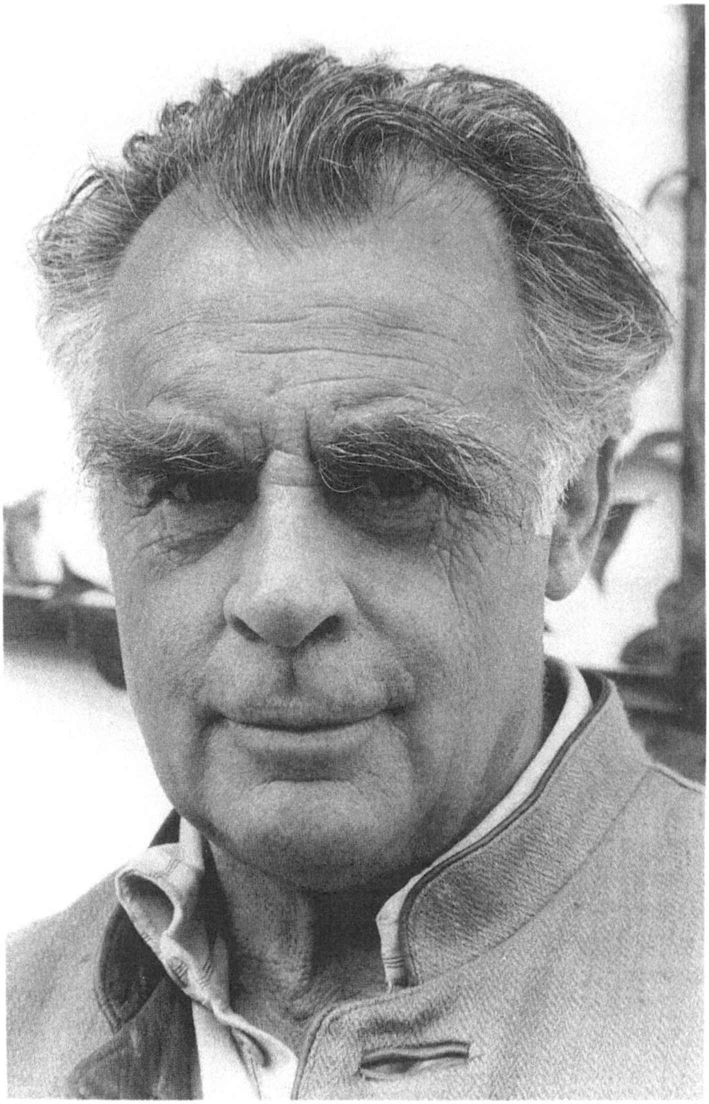

Foto: Herlinde Koelbl

A. Baethmann K. Messmer (Eds.)

Surgical Research: Recent Concepts and Results

Festschrift Dedicated to Walter Brendel
on Occasion of his 65th Birthday

Springer-Verlag
Berlin Heidelberg New York
London Paris Tokyo

Alexander Baethmann, MD
Institute for Surgical Research
Klinikum Großhadern
Ludwig-Maximilians-University

Munich, FRG

Konrad Messmer, MD
Department of Experimental Surgery
Surgical University Clinic
Ruprecht-Karls-University

Heidelberg, FRG

ISBN-13:978-3-642-73099-3 e-ISBN-13:978-3-642-73097-9
DOI: 10.1007/978-3-642-73097-9

2119-3140-543210

Preface

Since surgery became a method of treating patients, progress in the field has been intimately associated with experimentation and serendipitous research. As in other clinical specialties advances in surgery can be considered to result from experimental attempts to increase basic knowledge and to improve technical skills. However, virtually in no other area do concepts and approaches of experimental research enter clinical routine as fast as in surgery. There are numerous examples of this. Thus, allocation of manpower and resources for surgical research can be considered particularly profitable as convincingly shown, for instance, in renal transplantation by comparison of the long-term burden of hemodialysis vs. kidney grafting, apart from the relief of suffering and misery.

Surgery is a continuously spreading field, and so is surgical research. This volume is a case in point. Its spectrum reaches from basic molecular biological aspects of immune mechanisms to the current state of the art of pulmonary surgery of cancer metastases, and from the molecular processes of cell swelling in ischemic brain edema and blood-brain barrier damage to novel forms of resuscitation or of treatment of insulin-dependent diabetes mellitus. Surgical research faithfully reflects a constant reorientation of medical disciplines. Treatment of renal or gallbladder concrements was a major domain of surgery, where the introduction of extracorporeal shock wave treatment now supplies noninvasive, virtually conservative alternatives. On the other hand, insulin-dependent diabetes mellitus, until now largely a challenge for internal medicine, may evolve as a surgical modality according to recent accomplishments in islet or segmental pancreas grafting. Both examples illustrate the merits of surgical research.

The current collection of reviews and articles draws attention to the topics in surgery that are the subject of particularly active research raising expectations for progress in clinical applications. These concern, among others, discussions of the pathophysiology of ischemia and reperfusion damage and of microvascular function, the still evolving field of organ transplantation, and transplantation immunology impressively reflecting the close interaction between clinicians and immunologists. Moreover, surgery with the remaining challenges posed by gastroenterology could establish a functional association of immunology and gastrointestinal physiology as a basis for research resulting in completely new insights into the control of digestive and resorptive mechanisms by the immune system. The studies on the genetic relationships of, for example, chronic arthritis in childhood can be viewed as a pertinent spin-off from respective activities in tissue typing for the matching of donors and recipients in transplantation. As to the latter, i.e., the significance of tissue typing for clinical outcome of organ grafting, this volume provides a timely analysis of the problem, which might lead surgical centers involved in the procedure to reconsider current attitudes.

Finally, surgical research is a discipline where new technologies are conceived and developed until clinical implementation. This is perfectly illustrated in the chapters on shock wave treatment and computer applications. In renal and, lately, gallbladder concrements, shock wave treatment is in the process of becoming clinical routine, whereas future applications are under close experimental scrutiny. Those who were skeptical (including ourselves) about the feasibility of renal and, more recently, of gallbladder concrement fragmentation by shock wave exposure might be surprised again in the future by achievements of this method as a weapon in cancer treatment.

As in other dynamically evolving clinical and experimental fields, progress is always associated with personal ties and sacrifices. An exceptional case in point is Walter Brendel. The authors and editors wish to dedicate this review on the state of the art of surgical research, current accomplishments, and future perspectives to him on the occasion of his 65th birthday. The opportunity is particularly appropriate since it was Walter Brendel who opened laboratories for surgical research at the Ludwig Maximilians University in Munich 25 years ago. These laboratories have been fruitfully developed into the current activities of the Institute of Surgical Research, where Walter Brendel always was and still remains the central motor providing impulses and stimuli to unconventional thinking and approaches.

Surgeons still disagree about how surgical research should be conducted. Many maintain that it must be retained in the proper realm of clinical surgery, and that it can not be carried on by institutions and scientists who are not clinical surgeons. Fortunately, the example given by Walter Brendel and the results reported in this volume demonstrate that alternatives to this view are viable, even more, that formally independent – yet not independent as clinical targets are concerned – surgical research may probably thrive better under these circumstances than if pursued by clinicians only.

A major barrier for the clinical surgeon to exercise his obligations for surgical research is the heavy routine in the hospital and university departments. This is probably the most important reason preventing surgeons from doing surgical research as actively and as vigorously as in former times. Besides, the requirements for specialization and practical training to refine surgical skills take their toll. Although this is certainly beneficial for clinical results in patients, the price paid is a shift from the responsibility for competent surgical research to administration of clinical care.

Being particularly aware of this problem, Walter Brendel, a former physiologist, grew perfectly in his role as a partner of clinicians, producing ideas and energies in never ending supply for the benefit and progress of clinical surgery. For surgical research to remain innovative and successful, it must cross the borders not only between the surgical specialties but also to the nonsurgical fields in medicine and biology. Furthermore, surgical research requires an open mind and readiness to share and adopt new knowledge, expertise, and ideas. Walter Brendel has always been successful in unselfishly creating a fruitful environment for these endeavors as Editor-in-Chief of *European Surgical Research,* as president of the European Society for Surgical Research, and as organizer and chairman of the renowned Round Table

Symposia on Applied Immunology in Axams, Tyrolia. The current reports of friends, colleagues, and former students around the world by no means provide a comprehensive summary of the potential and achievements so effectively initiated and cultivated by Walter Brendel.

We would like to take the opportunity to thank all the authors who have contributed to this volume, and Dr. T. Graf Baumann and Dr. M. Wilson of Springer-Verlag, Heidelberg, who made it possible to publish this Festschrift in time.

Munich, Heidelberg 1987

A. BAETHMANN
K. MESSMER

Contents

II. Novel Technologies in Surgery and Medicine

III. Intestinal Immunology

IV. Transplantation Immunology

V. General Immunology

Contributors

E. D. Albert, Prof. Dr. med.
Dept. Pediatr., Ludwig-Maximilians-Univ., 8000 München 2, FRG

Anne-Marie Allmeling, Res. Assoc.,
Inst. Surg. Res., Ludwig-Maximilians-Univ., 8000 München 70, FRG

A. Baethmann, Prof. Dr. med.,
Inst. Surg. Res., Ludwig-Maximilians-Univ., 8000 München 70, FRG

F. H. Bach, Prof., M. D.,
Immunol. Biol. Res. Ctr., Dept. Lab. Med. Pathol., Minneapolis, Minn., 55455 USA

H. G. Beger, Prof. Dr. med.,
Dept. Surgery, University Ulm, 7900 Ulm, FRG

L. Brent, Prof., Ph. D., B. Sc.,
Dept. Immunol., St. Mary's Hospital, Med. School, London, W2 1PG, England

D. Burkhardt,
Inst. Surg. Res., Ludwig-Maximilians-Univ., 8000 München 70, FRG

Sir Roy Y. Calne, Prof., FRCS, M. D.,
Dept. Surg., Univ. Cambridge, Addenbrooke's Hosp., Cambridge CB 2QG, England

P. Conzen, Dr. med.,
Inst. Surg. Res., Ludwig-Maximilians-Univ., 8000 München 70, FRG

M. Delius, Dr. med.,
Inst. Surg. Res., Ludwig-Maximilians-Univ., 8000 München 70, FRG

A. Dibelius, Dr. med.,
Div. Surg. Res., Dept. Surg., Univ. Freiburg, 7800 Freiburg, FRG

H. Dienemann, Priv. Doz. Dr. med.,
Dept. Surgery, Klinikum Großhadern, Ludwig-Maximilians-Univ.,
8000 München 70, FRG

G. Enders, Dr. med.,
Inst. Surg. Res., Ludwig-Maximilians-Univ., 8000 München 70, FRG

J. Feyh, M. D.
Inst. Surg. Res., Ludwig-Maximilians-Univ., 8000 München 70, FRG

E. Fiehl,
Inst. Surg. Res., Ludwig-Maximilians-Univ., 8000 München 70, FRG

H. Forst, Dr. med.,
Inst. Anaesthesiol., Ludwig-Maximilians-Univ., Klinikum Großhadern,
8000 München 70, FRG

A. E. Goetz, M. D.,
Inst. Surg. Res., Ludwig-Maximilians-Univ., 8000 München 70, FRG

W. Gross, Dipl.-Math.,
Dept. Exp. Surg., Univ. Heidelberg, 6900 Heidelberg 1, FRG

C. Hammer, Prof. Dr. med., Dr. med. vet.,
Inst. Surg. Res., Ludwig-Maximilians-Univ., 8000 München 70, FRG

G. Heberer, Prof. Dr. med.,
Dept. Surgery, Klinikum Großhadern, Ludwig-Maximilians-Univ.,
8000 München 70, FRG

K. Heeg, Dr. med.,
Dept. Med. Microbiol. Immunol., Univ. Ulm, 7900 Ulm, FRG

S. Hildemann,
Inst. Surg. Res., Ludwig-Maximilians-Univ., 8000 München 70, FRG

J. Hobbhahn, Dr. med.,
Dept. Anaesthesiol., Ludwig-Maximilians-Univ., 8000 München 70, FRG

D. Kabelitz, Dr. med.,
Dept. Med. Microbiol. Immunol., Univ. Ulm, 7900 Ulm, FRG

O. Kempski, Priv. Doz., Dr. med.,
Inst. Surg. Res., Ludwig-Maximilians-Univ., 8000 München 70, FRG

R. Königsberger,
Inst. Surg. Res., Ludwig-Maximilians-Univ., 8000 München 70, FRG

H. Königsberger, Dr. med.,
Div. Surg. Res., Dept. Surg., Univ. Freiburg, 7800 Freiburg, FRG

H. H. Krämling, Dr. med.,
Dept. Surgery, Klinikum Großhadern, Ludwig-Maximilians-Univ., 8000 München 70, FRG

U. Kreimeier, Dr. med.,
Dept. Exp. Surg., Univ. Heidelberg, 6900 Heidelberg 1, FRG

F. Krombach, Dr. med. vet.,
Inst. Surg. Res., Ludwig-Maximilians-Univ., 8000 München 70, FRG

C. Lersch, Dr. med.,
Dept. Med., Technical Univ., 8000 München 80, FRG

H. G. Liebich, Prof. Dr. med. vet.,
Dept. Vet. Anatomy II, Ludwig-Maximilians-Univ., 8000 München 40, FRG

W. Lumper,
Inst. Surg. Res., Ludwig-Maximilians-Univ., 8000 München 70, FRG

A. Marmarou, Prof., Ph. D.,
Div. Neurol. Surg., Med. Coll., Virginia Commonwealth University, Richmond, Virginia, 23298 USA

K. Messmer, Prof. Dr. med.,
Dept. Exp. Surg., Univ. Heidelberg, 6900 Heidelberg 1, FRG

W. Oettinger, Priv. Doz., Dr. med.,
Dept. Surg., Univ. Ulm, 7900 Ulm, FRG

K. Peter, Prof. Dr. med.,
Inst. Anaesthesiol., Ludwig-Maximilians-Univ., 8000 München 70, FRG

P. Peterson, Prof., Ph. D.,
Scripps Clinic Res. Found., La Jolla, Ca., 92037 USA

I. Pichlmayer,
Zentrum Anästhesiologie Abt. IV, Krankenhaus Oststadt, Prodbielskistraße 380, 3000 Hannover 51

E. Pratschke, Priv. Doz., Dr. med.,
Dept. Surgery, Klinikum Großhadern, Ludwig-Maximilians-Univ., 8000 München 70, FRG

J. Ring, Prof. Dr. med. Dr. phil.,
Dept. Dermatol., Ludwig-Maximilians-Univ., 8000 München 2, FRG

R. Ronge,
Inst. Surg. Res., Ludwig-Maximilians-Univ., 8000 München 70, FRG

J. J. van Rood, Prof. Dr. med.,
Dept. Immunol., Univ. Leiden, N-2300 RC Leiden, Netherlands

F. A. Sanguinetti, Prof. Dr. med.,
Hospit. Clinicas, Facultad de Medicina, Univ. Buenos Aires, Buenos Aires, Argentina

W. Sass, Dr. med.,
Div. Exp. Surg., Dept. Surg., Univ. Kiel, 2300 Kiel, FRG

G. H. Schneider,
Inst. Surg. Res., Ludwig-Maximilians-Univ., 8000 München 70, FRG

S. Scholz, Dr. med.,
Dept. Pediatr., Ludwig-Maximilians-Univ., 8000 München 2, FRG

R. Schosser, Dr. med.,
Dept. Exp. Surg., Univ. Heidelberg, 6900 Heidelberg 1, FRG

L. Schürer, Dr. med., Inst.
Surg. Res., Ludwig-Maximilians-Univ., 8000 München 70, FRG

J. Seifert, Prof. Dr. med.,
Div. Exp. Surg., Dept. Surg., Univ. Kiel, 2300 Kiel, FRG

Rosemary A. Sherwood, Ph. D.,
Dept. Immunol., St. Mary's Hospital Med. School, London, W2 1PG, England

N. Silva, Dr. med.,
Hospital de Clinicas, Facultad de Medicina, Universidad de Buenos Aires, Buenos Aires, Argentina

B. U. v. Specht, Prof. Dr. med. Dr. rer. nat.,
Div. Surg. Res., Dept. Surg., Univ. Freiburg, 7800 Freiburg, FRG

F. Staub,
Inst. Surg. Res., Ludwig-Maximilians-Univ., 8000 München 70, FRG

L. Sunder-Plassmann, Prof. Dr. med.,
Dept. Surgery, Klinikum Großhadern, Ludwig-Maximilians-Univ., 8000 München 70, FRG

R.K. Teichmann, Prof. Dr. med.,
Dept. Surg., Klinikum Großhadern, Ludwig-Maximilians-Univ.,
8000 München 70, FRG

A. Unterberg, Dr. med.,
Dept. Neurosurg., Ludwig-Maximilians-Univ., 8000 München 70, FRG

M. Wahl, Prof. Dr. med.,
Physiol. Inst., Ludwig-Maximilians-Univ., 8000 München 2, FRG

H. Wagner, Prof. Dr. med.,
Dept. Med. Microbiol. Immunol., Univ. Ulm, 7900 Ulm, FRG

Christel Weiss, Dipl.-Math.,
Dept. Exp. Surg., Univ. Heidelberg, 6900 Heidelberg 1, FRG

H. Zeintl, Dr. sc. hum.,
Dept. Exp. Surg., Univ. Heidelberg, 6900 Heidelberg 1, FRG

M. Zimmer, M.D.,
Inst. Surg. Res., Ludwig-Maximilians-Univ., 8000 München 70, FRG

I. Surgical Pathophysiology: Ischemia and Reperfusion, Microcirculation, Tissue Damage and Repair

New Aspects in the Formation of Vasogenic Brain Edema*

A. Unterberg, A. Baethmann, M. Wahl, L. Schürer, and A. Marmarou

Introduction

Brain edema is frequently a major determinant of the clinical course and outcome in acute insults of the brain. Based on pathophysiological investigations, Klatzo [9] introduced more than 20 years ago the now classical distinction of brain edema into its vasogenic and cytotoxic manifestations. Although the vasogenic edema type seems to predominate, both types of brain edema occur simultaneously under clinical conditions. The availability of computer tomography and, more recently, of magnetic resonance imaging (MRI) for the first time provides a direct diagnosis of brain edema in patients [11]. Such diagnosis was formerly based on indirect measures, such as increased intracranial pressure. However, even with these new imaging techniques a differential diagnosis between vasogenic and cytotoxic edema is not yet possible.

Cytotoxic brain edema is characterized as a cerebral accumulation of fluid localized in the intracellular compartment. Failure of the cellular energy metabolism, inhibition of Na^+/K^+ -ATPase, and an uncontrollable increase in membrane permeability for Na^+ ions are considered to be mechanisms of cytotoxic brain edema [1, 7]. Brain edema from ischemia is a prominent clinical example, particularly in the early phase after onset of the blood flow disturbances. Its cytotoxic nature is concluded from the increase in brain water content inspite of an intact blood-brain barrier [4, 5, 10]. Further details regarding the significance of cytotoxic brain edema are given by Kempski et al. (this volume).

The vasogenic component of ischemic brain edema evolves secondarily with a delay of hours, when the blood-brain barrier becomes permeable. *Vasogenic brain edema* in cerebral infarction could become a major factor for the acute clinical course and outcome [17]. Formation of *vasogenic brain edema* from acute cerebral insults, such as infarction or severe head injury, appears to be closely associated with the formation of a focal brain tissue necrosis. A mere opening of the blood-brain barrier without damage of the cerebral parenchyma might not suffice to induce this process. The necrotic focus is the port of entry for the plasma-like edema fluid, which preferentially spreads through the extracellular compartment of the perifocal white matter [9]. Propagation of the vasogenic edema fluid is maintained by a hydrostatic pressure gradient from the necrotic focus, where the blood-brain barrier is broken, and the peripheral brain tissue areas [16].

* Supported by Deutsche Forschungsgemeinschaft: BA 452 and Un 56/1-1.

Surgical Research:
Recent Concepts and Results
Baethmann/Messmer (Eds.)

The most important neurological disorders associated with vasogenic brain edema are brain tumors, abscess, malignant arterial hypertension, cerebral and subarachnoidal hemorrhages, and – as mentioned above – severe head injury and cerebral infarction. The failure of the blood-brain barrier is attributable either to gross structural damage of the endothelial lining of the cerebral vasculature (see [1]) and/or, as in the case of severe hypertension, overextension of the vascular elements. A merely mechanistic interpretation may not suffice, however, to explain maintenance of blood-brain barrier failure under various conditions. In this context, the involvement of pathophysiologically active mediator substances which support and enhance formation of vasogenic and cytotoxic brain edema provides interesting perspectives. Information on this issue is not only of scientific value but also useful as a basis for the development of more specific methods of brain edema treatment.

Mediators of Vasogenic Brain Edema

It is possible in cerebral ischemia or head injury to envisage an unlimited number of chemical factors which are formed or released in damaged brain tissue or transported from the intravascular compartment into the parenchyma with the vasogenic edema fluid, making strict guidelines for their identification necessary. We hypothesize that in acute cerebral lesions mediator substances play a major role in the development of secondary processes, such as blood-brain barrier damage, brain edema, disturbances of the microcirculation, cytotoxic cell swelling, and cell death (see [2, 20]). Ample evidence has been obtained on such a mediator function in the case of the kallikrein-kinin system, glutamate, and arachidonic acid. A requirement for identification of the mediator function is the formation or release of a mediator under the respective pathophysiological conditions. This has been demonstrated for the kallikrein-kinin system and for glutamate [12, 13]. Further, it has been shown that both induce manifestations of tissue damage if administered to the brain [2, 6,18]. Formation of arachidonic acid with its cascade metabolites has also been demonstrated in acute cerebral processes, such as ischemia, seizures, and trauma [3, 13, 24].

Our laboratory has been involved in the elucidation of the mechanisms by which damage to brain tissue is elicited by kinins and arachidonic acid. This question was experimentally approached in two different models: (a) by intravital fluorescence microscopy of the exposed cerebral cortex in vivo in order to assess blood-brain barrier function, and (b) by intracerebral injection of artificial CSF together with potential mediator substances following the brain edema infusion model according to Marmarou [14]. Intravital fluorescence microscopy to investigate changes in permeability of the microcirculation has been adapted for the brain by this laboratory [19, 23]. The surface of cerebral cortex is microsurgically exposed in vivo to carry out superfusion with a given mediator dissolved in artificial CSF while maintaining normal pH, osmolarity, and electrolyte concentrations. Na^+ fluorescein and fluorescein-labeled dextran were intravenously administered as low- and high-molecular-weight blood-brain barrier markers, respectively. Intravenous fluorescein isothiocyanate (FITC) dextran of 3000–70000 mol. wt. was studied in separate experiments. It was required that the intravenously administered markers remain strictly confined to the intravascular compartment under control conditions. Even in the case of the low-molecular-weight indicator, Na^+ fluorescein extravasation into the parenchyma was not observed in the control phase during superfusion of the brain with artificial CSF only. Experiments with leakage of indicators during the control phase were discarded.

Artificial CSF was then added with mediator substances, such as bradykinin or arachidonic acid, in rising concentrations. The potential ot these substances to induce disturbances of the blood-brain barrier was assessed by extravasation of the given fluorescence markers into the cerebral parenchyma. So far, bradykinin, arachidonic acid, leukotrienes, free oxygen derived radicals, and platelet-activating factor (PAF) have been studied in this model [21].

Superfusion of the exposed cerebral cortex with *bradykinin* led to an opening of the blood-brain barrier for Na^+ fluorescein (376 mol. wt.), whereas the high-molecular weight markers did not penetrate. The minimal effective concentrations of kinins required for Na^+ fluorescein to pass the blood-brain barrier were about 10^{-7} *M*. We therefore conclude that release of kinins under pathophysiological circumstances into cerebral tissue causes selective opening of the blood-brain barrier, thereby enhancing penetration of electrolytes and water but excluding high-molecular-weight plasma constituents. The effective concentration range of bradykinin found to induce leakage of Na^+ fluorescein corresponds to the amount of kinins released in brain tissue after an acute cerebral trauma [12].

Superfusion of the cerebral surface with *arachidonic acid* led to gross disruption of the blood-brain barrier with extravasation of FITC dextran 70000 mol. wt. The degree of barrier permeability, specifically the degree to which extravasation of low- versus high-molecular-weight markers was induced, seemed to correlate with the amount of arachidonic acid in the superfusion medium. Concentrations of 10^{-5} *M* of archidonic acid sufficed to open the blood-brain barrier for Na^+ fluorescein, whereas levels of approximately 10^{-3} *M* opened the blood-brain barrier also to intravenously administered FITC dextran [22]. Electron-microscopical studies conducted in parallel revealed marked structural alterations of the cerebrovascular endothelium affecting predominantly the venous segments. Interactions of polymorphonuclear leukocytes with the endothelial wall of small veins were seen, for example, adhesion, penetration, and extravascular migration [22]. The latter findings suggest that white blood cells have a specific function in the damage to the blood-brain barrier elicited by arachidonic acid.

In contrast to bradykinin or arachidonic acid, superfusion of the pia-arachnoid with an enzyme-substrate mixture producing free oxygen-derived radicals had no significant effect on the blood-brain barrier. Hypoxanthin and xanthinoxidase were employed to generate free radicals in pathophysiologically relevant concentrations [21]. Corresponding experiments with leukotrienes (LTC_4, LTD_4, and LTE_4) again had no effect at all, not even in pharmacologically active concentrations of up to 2 μ*M*/l. Extravasation of neither Na^+ fluorescein nor FITC dextran was observed.

It should be noted, however, that opening of the blood-brain barrier per se may not suffice to induce vasogenic brain edema. This is experimentally supported by studies of Rapoport, et al. [15], who showed that transient opening of the blood-brain barrier by administration of a hyperosmolar solution into the internal carotid artery was not associated with a measurable increase in cerebral water content. Therefore, the research on cerebral superfusion of intact brain in vivo was extended by a study using the brain edema infusion model according to Marmarou [14]. In this model, artificial

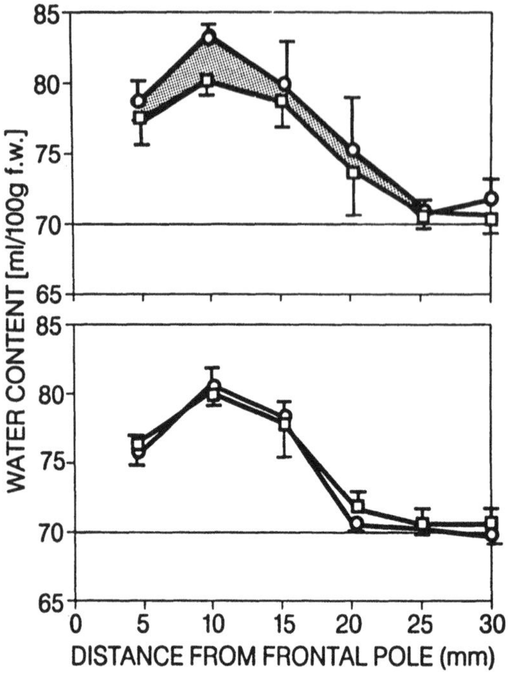

Fig. 1. Water content of cerebral white matter (ml/100 g WW) after infusion with artificial CSF (□), arachidonic acid (*upper panel,* ○), or leukotriene C_4 (*lower panel,* ○). The edema induced by slow infusion of artificial CSF was markedly enhanced by addition of arachidonic acid (3 m*M*/1) to the infusate. On the other hand, infusion of LTC_4 (15 μ*M*/l) did not increase the water content above that of controls infused with mock CSF only

CSF is slowly infused in small amounts into the white matter of cat brain. The distribution and subsequent disappearance of this fluid is studied microgravimetrically in serial sections of gray and white matter. In the present experiments 400 μl of an artificial CSF was infused into the right hemisphere (control); the same fluid but containing additionally bradykinin, arachidonic acid, or leukotrienes was infused into the left hemisphere.

Addition of bradykinin to the infusate in a concentration of 40 μ*M*/l led to marked enhancement of the infusion edema as demonstrated by an increase in the cerebral water content in the white matter by approximately 1% over that in the control hemisphere infused with mock CSF only. Intracerebral infusion with arachidonic acid was even more effective. The water content of white matter was 80–83 ml/100 g wet weight (WW) in experiments with arachidonic acid, and 75–79 ml/100 g WW in the controls receiving mock CSF only (Fig. 1, top panel). Arachidonic acid led to extravasation of intravenously administered Evans blue, in addition indicative of gross damage to the blood-brain barrier. On the other hand, infusion of leukotrienes (LTB_4 or LTC_4) in a concentration of 15 μ*M*/l did not enhance infusion-induced brain edema (Fig. 1, lower panel).

Summary and Conclusions

These findings support our hypothesis that biochemical factors formed during or after acute cerebral lesions contribute to the opening of the blood-brain barrier, thereby enhancing vasogenic brain edema. The observations provide further evidence for the role of bradykinin and arachidonic acid as mediators of secondary brain damage such as brain edema. We conclude that gross opening of the blood-brain barrier by arachidonic acid is a major mechanism for enhancement of vasogenic edema in acute cerebral lesions. The fact that neither leukotrienes nor free oxygen-derived radicals led to a failure of the blood-brain barrier or to an enhancement of the tissue water content in the infusion edema model suggests that the fatty acid itself is actively involved, not its cascade metabolites. Although cerebral administration of bradykinin, either by superfusion of the exposed cerebral cortex or by direct infusion into the parenchyma, did not result in gross but rather selective opening of the blood-brain barrier, enhancement of edema can nevertheless be surmised. Selective opening of the blood-brain barrier would facilitate influx of electrolytes and water into affected cerebral tissues. Exploration of mechanisms of mediator compounds in secondary brain damage, such as vasogenic brain edema, can be considered a rationale for the development of specific and, hence, more effective methods of treatment of acute cerebral lesions, where the development of secondary brain damage must still be viewed as a major determinant of the as yet unacceptable clinical outcome. First experimental results on specific antagonization of mediator compounds and their mechanisms appear promising.

Acknowledgements. The excellent technical assistance of Ulrike Goerke and Timothy Polk is gratefully acknowledged as well as the secretarial help for the typing of the manuscript by Isolde Juna and Angelika Sperlein.

References

1. Baethmann A (1978) Pathophysiological and pathochemical aspects of cerebral edema. Neurosurg Rev 1: 85–100
2. Baethmann A, Oettinger W, Rothenfußer W, Kempski O, Unterberg A, Geiger R (1980) Brain edema factors: current state with particular reference to plasma constituents and glutamate. In: Cervos-Navarro J, Ferszt R (eds) Advances in Neurology, vol 28. Raven, New York, pp 171–195
3. Bazan NG (1971) Changes in free fatty acids of brain by drug-induced convulsions, electroshock and anesthesia. J Neurochem 18: 1379–1385
4. Gotoh O, Asano T, Koide T, Takakura K (1985) Ischemic brain edema following occlusion of the middle cerebral artery in the rat: I: The time courses of the brain water, sodium and potassium contents and blood-brain barrier permeability to 125-I-albumin. Stroke 16: 101–109
5. Ito U, Go KG, Walker JT, Spatz M, Klatzo I (1976) Experimental cerebral ischemia in mongolian gerbils. III. Behaviour of the blood-brain barrier. Acta Neuropath (Berl) 34: 1–6
6. Kempski O (1982) Die Lokalisation des Glutamat-induzierten Hirnödems. Thesis, Ludwig Maximilians University, Munich
7. Kempski O, (1986) Cell swelling mechanisms in brain. In: Baethmann A, Go KG, Unterberg A (eds) Mechanisms of secondary brain damage. Plenum, New York, pp 203–220
8. Kempski O, Staub F, Zimmer M, Schneider GH, Baethmann A (1987) Neurosurgical research in vitro: contradiction or promise? Surgical Research: Recent Concepts and results. Baethmann, Messmer (Eds) Springer Verlag, Berlin Heidelberg New York, pp 9–17
9. Klatzo I, Wisniewski H, Smith DE (1965) Observations on penetration of serumproteins into the central nervous system. In: De Robertis EPD, Carrea R (eds) Biology of neuroglia. Progr Brain Res 15: 73–88
10. Kuroiwa T, Ting P, Martinez H, Klatzo I (1985) The biphasic opening of the blood-brain barrier to proteins following temporary middle cerebral artery occlusion. Acta Neuropathol (Berl) 68: 122–129

11. Lanksch W, Baethmann A, Kazner E (1981) Computed tomography of brain edema. In: De Vlieger M, De Lange SA, Beks JWD (eds) Brain edema. Wiley, New York, pp 67–98
12. Maier-Hauff K, Baethmann A, Lange M, Schürer L, Unterberg A (1984) The kalikrein-kinin system as mediator in vasogenic brain edema. Part 2: Studies on kinin formation in focal and perifocal brain tissue. J Neurosurg 61: 97–106
13. Maier-Hauff K, Lange M, Schürer L, Guggenbichler C, Vogt W, Jacob K, Baethmann A (1984) Glutamate and free fatty acid concentrations in extracellular vasogenic edema fluid. In: Go KG, Baethmann A (eds) Recent progress in the study and therapy of brain edema. Plenum, New York, pp 183–192
14. Marmarou A, Tanaka K, Shulman K (1982) The brain response to infusion edema: dynamics of fluid resolution. In: Hartmann A, Brock M (eds) Treatment of cerebral edema. Springer, Berlin Heidelberg New York, pp 11–35
15. Rapoport SI, Matthews K, Thompson HK (1976) Absence of brain edema after reversible osmotic opening of the blood-brain barrier. In: Pappius HM, Feindel W (eds) Dynamics of brain edema. Springer, Berlin Heidelberg New York pp 18–22
16. Reulen HJ, Graham R, Spatz M, Klatzo I (1977) Role of pressure gradients and bulk flow in dynamics of vasogenic brain edema. J Neurosurg 46: 24–35
17. Shaw CM, Alvord EC, Berry RG (1959) Swelling of the brain following ischemic infarction with arterial occlusion. Arch Neurol 1: 161–177
18. Unterberg A, Baethmann A (1984) The kallikrein-kinin system as mediator in vasogenic brain edema. Part 1: Cerebral exposure to bradykinin and plasma. J Neurosurg 61: 87–96
19. Unterberg A, Wahl M, Baethmann A (1984) Effects of bradykinin on permeability and diameter of pial vessels in vivo. J Cereb Blood Flow Metabol 4: 574–585
20. Unterberg A, Maier-Hauff K, Dautermann C, Hack U, Schürer L, Baethmann A (1986) Role of mediator compounds in secondary brain damage – current evidence. In: Baethmann A, Go KG, Unterberg A (eds) Mechanisms of secondary brain damage. Plenum, New York, pp 139–150
21. Unterberg A (1987) Veränderungen der Blut-Hirn-Schrankenfunktion und der zerebralen Vasomotorik durch Mediatoren des sekundären Hirnschadens. Habilitationsch, Ludwig Maximilians University, Munich
22. Unterberg A, Wahl M, Hammersen F, Baethmann A (1987) Permeability and vasomotor response of cerebral vessels during exposure to arachidonic acid. Acta Neuropathol (Berl) 73: 209–219
23. Wahl M, Unterberg A, Baethmann A (1985) Intravital fluorescence microscopy for the study of blood-brain barrier function. Int J Microcirc Clin Exp 4: 3–18
24. Yoshida S, Abe K, Busto R, Watson BD, Kogure K, Ginsberg MD (1982) Influence of transient ischemia on lipid-soluble antioxidants, free fatty acids and energy metabolites in rat brain. Brain Res 245: 307–316

Neurosurgical Research In Vitro: Contradiction or Promise?

O. Kempski, F. Staub, M. Zimmer, G. H. Schneider, and A. Baethmann

Introduction

For many years attempts have been made by animal protectionists all over the world to abolish the use of animals in experimental medicine. As a result, new laws and regulations make it increasingly more complicated to perform in vivo experiments. For the same reason, expenses for laboratory animals have considerably increased. We should therefore reconsider the anti-vivisectionists' argument that animal experiments can be replaced by other techniques, even in those disciplines traditionally using the whole living animal in research. In vitro tests may indeed offer alternatives for some forms of animal studies. Biochemists and cell biologists have long preferred in vitro systems in order to avoid complex in vivo conditions. Surgeons, especially neurosurgeons, often stress the necessity of in vivo studies, since they consider the in vitro approach too remote from the practical situation of the patient. The argument for in vivo study certainly holds for many lines of research, e.g., the establishment of new surgical techniques, study of diagnostic or therapeutic methods, and investigations that depend on the integrated function of whole organs. On the other hand, however, many problems met daily by the neurosurgeon are not understood in their basic pathophysiology.

These questions should be considered by neuroscientists employing in vitro systems which allow close control of the experimental environment. The purpose of this article is to evaluate some of the available in vitro techniques for research on the pathophysiology of cerebral ischemia as an example of the potential of this approach for the neurosciences.

Research on Cerebral Ischemia in vivo: Limitations

In stroke treatment we cannot avoid the fact that therapy reaches most patients too late. Five minutes of normothermic ischemia is considered the maximum which patients can tolerate without damage. In gerbils 5 min of ischemia suffices to selectively destroy the CA1 sector of the hippocampus [63]. Already 1–3 min after onset of complete cerebral ischemia, cell volume control is lost. The extracellular concentrations of Na^+ and K^+ change inversely [41, 52, 53], intra- and extracellular pH decreases [45], and cytotoxic edema develops. Cell swelling has been attributed to a failure of active transport after breakdown of the cerebral energy supply. This

Surgical Research:
Recent Concepts and Results
Baethmann/Messmer (Eds.)

interpretation, however, leaves many questions open; for instance, the early onset of ischemic cell swelling, compared to other organs, is not explained. It is conceivable that brain cells are more sensitive than other tissues to anoxia and to other factors accompanying ischemia or reperfusion. On the other hand, it has been shown that brain tissue survives prolonged periods of ischemia with good recovery, provided the experimental conditions during reperfusion are optimal.

Research devoted to these problems is being carried out in many laboratories. Scientific journals such as *Stroke* or the *Journal of Cerebral Blood Flow and Metabolism* are devoted solely to this subject. Nevertheless, up to now the underlying molecular mechanisms of cerebral ischemia are not fully understood. In part this may be due to the fact that in vivo research has its limits. A multitude of events occur simultaneously in the affected brain tissue after onset of ischemia. Causative mechanisms often cannot be discriminated from epiphenomena. In addition, manipulations such as insertion of electrodes, may influence the experimental conditions. In recent years a new understanding has emerged concerning the mechanisms of cerebral damage after an ischemic insult, based on the idea that substances released or activated in or around an ischemic focus promote nerve cell damage and glial swelling. Such mediators of secondary brain damage [7, 8, 57, 62] are acidosis [60, 86], glutamate [8, 21, 24, 55, 67, 73], free fatty acids [9, 22, 23], and free radicals [86]. An inactivation of these factors by therapeutic intervention may improve the outcome after an ischemic or traumatic insult to the brain.

The excitatory neurotransmitter glutamate is of special significance as an excitotoxin [24, 67, 73]. Swelling and destruction of brain tissue in vivo by glutamate was first described by van Harreveld [91]. In recent years the significance of glutamate and other excitotoxins in secondary brain damage has been increasingly recognized [13, 75, 80, 87]. The pathogenetic mechanisms of excitotoxins are discussed in detail below. Interestingly enough, these mediators were identified already in the late 1960s, in large measure by in vitro research. In the following paragraphs some of these experiments serve as a guideline to review the most important in vitro techniques.

Tissue Explants

A possibility for increased control in experimental conditions lies in the use of tissue explants. The advantages of this "ex-vivo" approach are evident. More than one tissue sample can generally be obtained from a single animal. Although the animal must be killed, suffering is minimal. The use of tissue explants offers experimental advantages. The extracellular environment can be accurately controlled, and tissues from the same animal can be used for control and for various treatment studies. The amount of radioactivity, if necessary, is lower. Certainly, general guidelines, e.g., regarding size of the tissue to allow optimal supply of oxygen and substrates, must be followed.

A good example for the successful use of tissue explants are the experiments of Ames et al. [2, 3]. The authors used isolated retinas to study the effects of anoxia and substrate deprivation on nervous tissue. To assess the damaging effect of anoxia these authors tested (a) tissue swelling and (b) the incorporation of radioactive leucine as a measure of protein synthesis and, hence, viability. The retinas tolerated anoxia plus substrate deprivation for 40 min *without swelling or irreversible damage* provided the extracellular compartment was large. On the other hand, the retinal water content increased in anoxia if the volume of the extracellular medium was restricted to an extra- to intracellular volume ratio of 4:1 or 1:1. Metabolic depression and a decreased protein synthesis then accompanied tissue swelling.

The retinal response to anoxia was significantly enhanced if the tissue was exposed to conditioned media from other retinas undergoing a period of anoxia. These phenomena support the concept of mediator mechanisms mentioned above, i. e., that factors are released from anoxic tissue which accelerate swelling and degeneration processes in the central nervous system. Glutamate, which is a likely candidate (see above), was also studied in isolated retinas by van Harreveld [92]. In this system glutamate caused spreading depression and a transparency change indicative of cell swelling, which could be antagonized by proline. In a more recent study, a reduced protein synthesis and subsequent degeneration of the inner retinal cells has been observed in isolated retinas [4].

Another widely used ex vivo approach is the employment of brain tissue slices. Neurochemists have used cortical brain slices for many years [1, 6, 15, 16, 17, 19, 46, 64]. Some of the early work on the effects of glutamate [6, 15, 19, 21, 46, 64, 78] and other substances [17, 22] causing brain swelling was performed in brain slices. Hippocampal slices are used for the study of physiological [36] as well as pathophysiological [14, 99] characteristics of brain tissue. Using standard procedures, hippocampal or cortical tissue remains functional in vitro for several hours.

Established cell lines

Another possibility for studing problems related to cellular pathophysiology is the use of established cell lines. The cell lines are often derived from tumors, i. e., gliomas or neuroblastomas [11, 71, 74, 94]. The tumorous origin certainly limits the use of such cell lines, since results must be verified with nontumor cells or in vivo. Nevertheless, cell lines can give answers of general value to basic questions. It is important, however, to be aware of the intrinsic properties of a given cell line, such as expression of specific proteins, receptors, and uptake systems. An extensively studied glial line whose properties are similar to those of glial cells in primary culture is C6 glioma. C6 glial cells were cloned from a chemically induced tumor in 1968 by Benda [11].

In our own experiments suspended C6 cells were incubated in a closely controlled environment to monitor and modify extracellular fluid composition [55, 56, 58]. In order to assess cell swelling, cell volume was determined by flow cytometry which may recognize volume changes of less than 1% [54]. When glial cells were exposed to anoxia (with or without inhibition of anaerobic metabolism by iodoacetate) or to ouabain, *cell swelling was never seen* during observation periods of up to 150 min – although intracellular potassium was lost [58]. The experiments confirm the results of Ames [2, 3] that anoxia per se does not suffice to induce cytotoxic edema. The findings support our view that additional mechanisms, such as release and accumulation of mediator substances, or the development of acidosis is required.

Some potential mediators have been tested using the C6 glioma model. Evidence is now available that glial swelling occurs rapidly in acidosis [60] and during exposure to glutamate [55]. In acidosis, buffering by extracellular bicarbonate generates CO_2, which then diffuses into the cells. Here carbonic anhydrase catalyzes production of carbonic acid, which immediately dissociates into bicarbonate and protons. Both products are then extruded from the glial cells by Na^+/H^+ and HCO^-/Cl^- exchangers in order to maintain a normal intracellular pH; this is a powerful mechanism of cell swelling due to the resultant intracellular accumulation of Na^+ and Cl^-. The exchangers are activated below a pH threshold of 7.0–6.8. The extra-intracellular CO_2 gradient fuels this vicious circle as long as bicarbonate is available. Replacement of bicarbonate or Na^+ in the extracellular medium, employment of Na^+/H^+ antiport antagonists such as amiloride, or employment of acetazolamide to inhibit carbonic anhydrase consequently interfere with glial swelling in acidosis. A second mechanism of glial swelling under pathological conditions is attributable to the flooding of the extracellular compartment with glutamate [57, 73]. Under physiological conditions glial cells accumulate glutamate by high-affinity uptake systems requiring metabolic energy [6, 12, 44, 47, 49, 77, 82]. Glutamate is then converted into glutamine, which diffuses back to the neuron [12, 15]. Energy for the glutamate uptake is provided by the simultaneous influx of sodium, which in turn must eventually be transported out of the cell. Using the C6 glioma model it was shown that exposure to glutamate causes a rise in oxygen consumption and cell swelling [55]. The cell volume increase may therefore indicate a functional uptake of glutamate rather than glial damage. Thus, maintenance of low extracellular glutamate concentrations or of a normal intracellular pH apparently is a better criteria than a stable cell volume. Most of the results cited above have meanwhile been validated by ourselves in primary cultured glial cells from rat brain.

Primary Culture

Primary cultures of glial [30, 34, 42–44, 48, 83–85] or nerve [28, 50, 76, 93] cells are most enticing for neuroscientists. Considerable interest is also focused on cultivation of cerebrovascular endothelium [18, 25–27, 38, 89, 98] as the cellular constituent of the blood-brain barrier. Many methods and techniques to establish primary cultures of brain cells have been published. This subject cannot be discussed comprehensively in this short review. In brief, most techniques employ fetal, newborn, or weanling rats, whose brains are freed from meninges, homogenized, centrifuged, and sieved or enzymatically dissociated. The resulting cell suspension is then plated on Petri dishes. For the culture of neural cells the dishes are usually coated with a hydrophobic substrate such as polylysine [72]. For the culture of endothelium the use of fibronectin-coated [18] or gelatin-coated [38] dishes is suggested.

In recent years many growth factors have been discovered allowing the composition of specific growth media to support propagation of a desired cell type by suppressing others [69, 70, 88, 96]. The methodology of primary culture has its own specific requirements. Cells obtained from immature animals must develop until they are fully differentiated in order to simulate the in vivo situation. This can be verified by assessment of several specific proteins or enzymes used as markers for the individual cell types. Unlike astroblasts, differentiated glial cells express, for example, glial fibrillary acidic protein (GFAP) [5, 31, 49], carbonic anhydrase II [61], and glutamine synthetase [66]. Addition of dB-cAMP to the cultures can be used to induce "differentiation" [32]. Various antibodies have been raised to identify neurons in culture [33]. Endothelial cells synthesize alkaline phosphatase [89] and can be labeled with antibodies against factor VIII [18].

Primary cultures have also been used in studies on ischemia mechanisms and neural damage, such as the effect of acidosis [60] and potassium ions [95] on cell volume and ion fluxes of glial cells. The metabolism of neurotransmitters, especially that of glutamate, has been examined in glial cultures [29, 44, 49, 77]. All these studies stress the pathophysiological significance of mediators. Rothman [79] has demonstrated in hippocampal cultures that excitatory transmitters mediate neuronal death and that anoxic damage can be prevented if synaptic activity is inhibited. The current understanding of excitotoxins is based on experiments with nerve cells cultivated in vitro [20, 51, 67, 80]. Findings suggest that excitotoxins such as glutamate act by two different mechanisms: (a) osmotic swelling due to influx of Na^+ and Cl^- and (b) influx of Ca^{2+} through opening of respective channels. Both processes involve an interaction of glutamate with specific receptors [67].

In general the use of primary cultures from nervous tissue is just in its beginnings. Neuronal cell cultures are useful for neurotoxicological or neuropharmacological studies [28, 39, 84], and for research on transmitter interactions [44, 72, 77] and immunological problems [68]. Mechanisms of vasogenic and cytotoxic edema formation are being studied in endothelial and glial cultures [18, 40, 55–60]. Last but not least, cell cultures may eventually provide insights for the development and treatment of brain tumors and viral diseases.

An "Artificial Brain" in Culture?

Up to now the value of in vitro experiments has been limited regarding problems which require an interaction of various cell types in an organ-like environment, especially those involving the effects of the microcirculation. Such problems may, however, be studied in vitro provided that artificial organs can be established. First steps toward this goal have already been made. Research on the function of the blood-brain barrier employs endothelial cells from brain capillaries, which can be grown on special substrates as an interface between two compartments in transport studies [59]. The interactions of glia and endothelium can be investigated by cocultivation of endothelial cells, either on feeder layers of glial cells [25] or on membranes [10, 18, 35, 37]. Three-dimensional glial networks have been constructed on capillary-like hollow fibers [90].

In reaggregation cultures from fetal brain, isolated cells form cellular patterns which are histotypic for the original tissue [65], allowing electrophysiological and biochemical studies. Another approach lies in explantation of fetal brain tissue slices and their subsequent culture for several months [36]. Apart from developmental studies, such explants are useful for long-term investigations on the release of growth factors, for measurements of transmitter and substrate metabolism, and for transplantation of brain tissue. Combinations of the various techniques may yield insights into the integrated function of the central nervous system, as well as into its pathology. The necessary techniques, however, will become increasingly complicated, requiring special skills and equipment. Active cooperation between clinical and theoretical institutes providing the necessary know-how and manpower will become a prerequisite for future progress in the field. In vitro techniques not only are promising for research in neurology or neurosurgery but may become mandatory where in vivo methods reach their technical, financial, or legal limits.

References

1. Ames A, Tsukada Y, Nesbett B (1967) Intracellular Cl^-, Na^+, K^+, Ca^{++}, Mg^{++}, and P in nervous tissue, response to glutamate and to changes in extracellular Ca^{++}. J Neurochem 14: 145–159
2. Ames A, Nesbett FB (1983) Pathophysiology of ischemic cell death: I. Time of onset of irreversible damage; importance of different components of the ischemic insult. Stroke 14: 219–226
3. Ames A, Nesbett FB (1983) Pathophysiology of ischemic cell death: III. Role of extracellular factors. Stroke 14: 233–240
4. Anderson RE, Hollyfield JG, Verner GE (1981) Regional effects of sodium aspartate and sodium glutamate on protein synthesis in the retina. Invest Ophth Vis Sci 21: 554–562
5. Antanitus DS, Choi BH, Lapham LW (1975) Immunofluorescence staining of astrocytes in vitro using antiserum to glial fibrillary acidic protein. Brain Res 89: 363–367
6. Arnfred T, Hertz L (1971) Effects of potassium and glutamate on brain cortex slices: uptake and release of glutamate and other amino acids. J Neurochem 18: 259–265
7. Baethmann A (1978) Pathophysiological and pathochemical aspects of cerebral edema. Neurosurg Rev 1: 85–100
8. Baethmann A, Oettinger W, Rothenfusser W, Kempski O, Unterberg A, Geiger R (1980) Brain edema factors. Current state with particular reference to plasma constituents and glutamate. In: Cervos-Navarro J, Ferszt R (eds) Advances in neurology, vol 28. Brain edema. Raven, New York, pp 171–195
9. Bazan NG (1970) Effects of ischemia and electroconvulsive shock on free fatty acid pool in the brain. Biochim Biophys Acta 218: 1–10
10. Beck DW, Vinters HV, Hart MN, Cancilla PA (1984) Glial cells influence the polarity of the blood-brain barrier. J Neuropath Exp Neurol 43: 219–224
11. Benda P, Lightbody J, Sato G, Levine L, Sweet W (1968) Differentiated rat glial cell strain in tissue culture. Science 161: 370–371
12. Benjamin AM, Quastel JH (1974) Fate of glutamate in the brain. J Neurochem 23: 457–464
13. Benveniste H, Drejer J, Schousboe A, Diemer NH (1984) Elevation of the extracellular concentrations of glutamate and aspartate in rat hippocampus during transient cerebral ischemia monitored by intracerebral microdialysis. J Neurochem 43: 1369–1374
14. Benninger C, Kadis J, Prince DA (1980) Extracellular calcium and potassium changes in hippocampal slices. Brain Res 187: 165
15. Berl S, Nicklas WJ, Clarke DD (1968) Compartmentation of glutamic acid metabolism in brain slices. J Neurochem 15: 131–140
16. Bourke RS (1969) Studies of the development and subsequent reduction of swelling of mammalian cortex under isosmotic conditions in vitro. Exp Brain Res 8: 232–248
17. Bourke RS, Kimelberg HK, Daze M, Church G (1983) Swelling and ion uptake in cat cerebrocortical slices: control by neurotransmitters and ion transport mechanisms. Neurochem Res 8: 5–24
18. Bowman PD, Ennis SR, Rarey KE, Betz AL, Goldstein GW (1983) Brain microvessel endothelial cells in tissue culture: a model for the study of blood-brain barrier permeability. Ann Neurol 14: 396–402
19. Bracco F, Gennaro J, Lajtha A (1982) Relationship of morphologic damage and amino acid uptake in incubated slices of brain. Exp Neurol 76: 606–622
20. Brookes N (1978) Actions of glutamate on dissociated mammalian spinal neurones in vitro. Dev Neurosci 1: 203–215
21. Chan PH, Fishman RA, Lee JL, Candelise L (1979) Effects of excitatory neurotransmitter amino acids on swelling of rat brain cortical slices. J Neurochem 33: 1309–1315
22. Chan PH, Fishman RA, Lee JL, Quan SC (1980) Arachidonic acid-induced swelling in incubated rat brain cortical slices. Neurochem Res 5: 629–640

23. Chan PH, Fishman RA (1982) Alterations of membrane integrity and cellular constituents by arachidonic acid in neuroblastoma and glioma cells. Brain Res 248: 151–157
24. Collins RC (1986) Selective vulnerability of brain: new insights from the excitatory synapse. Metab Brain Dis 1: 231–240
25. DeBault LE, Cancilla PA (1980) Glutamyl transpeptidase in isolated brain endothelial cells: induction by glial cells in vitro. Science 207: 653–655
26. DeBault LE, Henriquez E, Hart MN, Cancilla PA (1981) Cerebral microvessels and derived cells in tissue culture. In Vitro 17: 480–494
27. Diglio A, Grammas P, Giacomelli F, Wiener J (1982) Primary culture of rat cerebral microvascular endothelial cells. Laborat Invest 46: 554–563
28. Dimpfel W (1980) Rat nerve cell cultures in pharmacology and toxicology. Arch Toxicol 44: 55–62
29. Drejer J, Benveniste H, Diemer NH, Schousboe A (1985) Cellular origin of ischemia-induced glutamate release of brain tissue in vivo and in vitro. J Neurochem 45: 145–151
30. Duffy PE (1983) Astrocytes: normal, reactive, and neoplastic. Raven, New York
31. Eng FL (1980) The glial fibrillary acidic (GFA) protein. In: Bradshaw RA, Schneider DM (eds) Proteins of the nervous system. Raven, New York, pp 85–117
32. Fedoroff S, McAuley WAJ, Houle JD, Devon RM (1984) Astrocyte cell lineage. V. Similarity of astrocytes that form in the presence of dBcAMP in cultures to reactive astrocytes in vivo. J Neurosci Res 12: 15–27
33. Fields K (1985) Neuronal and glial cell surface antigens on cells in culture. In: Bottenstein JE, Sato G (eds) Cell culture in the neurosciences. Plenum, New York, pp 45–93
34. Frangakis MV, Kimelberg HK (1984) Dissociation of neonatal rat brain by dispase for preparation of primary astrocyte cultures. Neurochem Res 9: 1689–1698
35. Furie MB, Cramer EB, Naprstek BL, Silverstein SC (1984) Cultured endothelial cell monolayers that restrict the transendothelial passage of macromolecules and electrical current. J Cell Biol 98: 1033–1041
36. Gähwiler BH (1984) Development of the hippocampus in vitro: cell types, synapses and receptors. Neuroscience 11: 751–760
37. Garcia JGN, Siflinger-Birnboim A, Bizios R, Del Vecchio PJ, Fenton JW, Malik AB (1986) Thrombin-induced increase in albumin permeability across the endothelium. J Cell Physiol 128: 96–104
38. Goetz IE, Warren J, Estrada C, Roberts E, Krause DN (1985) Long-term serial cultivation of arterial and capillary endothelium from adult bovine brain. In Vitro 21: 172–180
39. Goldberg AM (1980) Mechanisms of neurotoxicity as studied in tissue culture systems. Toxicology 17: 201–208
40. Goldstein GW, Betz AL (1983) Recent advances in understanding brain capillary function. Ann Neurol 14: 389–395
41. Hansen AJ (1985) Effect of anoxia on ion distribution in the brain. Physiol Rev 65: 101–148
42. Hansson E, Sellström A, Persson LI, Rönnbäck L (1980) Brain primary culture – a characterization. Brain Res 188: 233–246
43. Hansson E, Rönnbäck L, Lowenthal A, Noppe M, Alling C, Karlsson B, Sellström A (1982) Brain primary culture – a characterization (part II). Brain Res 231: 173–183
44. Hansson E (1986) Primary culture from defined brain areas. III. Effects of seeding time on ^{3}HL-glutamate transport and glutamine synthetase activity. Dev Brain Res 24: 203–209
45. v. Hanwehr R, Smith M-L, Siesjö BK (1986) Extra- and intracellular pH during near-complete forebrain ischemia in the rat. J Neurochem 46: 331–339
46. Harvey JA, McIlwain H (1968) Excitatory amino acids and cation content and Na^+-ion flux of isolated tissues from the brain. Biochem J 108: 269–274
47. Henn FA, Goldstein MN, Hamberger A (1974) Uptake of the neurotransmitter candidate glutamate by glia. Nature 249: 663–664
48. Henn FA (1989) Separation of neuronal and glial cells and subcellular constituents. In: Fedoroff S, Hertz L (eds) Advances in cellular neurobiology. Academic, New York, pp 373–403
49. Hertz L, Bock E, Schousboe A (1978) GFA content, glutamate uptake and activity of glutamate metabolizing enzymes in differentiation mouse astrocytes in primary culture. Dev Neurosci 1: 226–238
50. Hild WJ (1977) Characteristics of neurons in culture. In: Fedoroff S, Hertz L (eds) Cell, tissue and organ cultures in neurobiology. Academic, New York, pp 99–119

51. Hösli L, Andres PF, Hösli E (1976) Ionic mechanisms associated with the depolarization by glutamate and aspartate on human and rat spinal neurones in tissue culture. Pflügers Arch 363: 43–48
52. Hossmann K-A (1976) Development and resolution of ischemic brain swelling. In: Pappius H, Feindel W (eds) Dynamics of brain edema. Springer, Berlin Heidelberg New York, pp 219–227
53. Hossmann K-A, Sakaki S, Zimmermann V (1977) Cation activities in reversible ischemia of the cat brain. Stroke 8: 77–81
54. Kachel V (1976) Basic principles of electrical sizing of cells and particles and their realization in the new instrument "Metrizell". J Histochem Cytochem 24: 211–230
55. Kempski O, Gross U, Baethmann A (1982) An in-vitro model of cytotoxic brain edema: cell volume and metabolism of cultivated glial and nerve cells. In: Driesen W, Brock M, Klinger M (eds) Computerized tomography. Brain metabolism. Spinal injuries. Springer, Berlin Heidelberg New York, pp 254–258 (Advances in neurosurgery, vol 10)
56. Kempski O, Chaussy L, Gross U, Zimmer M, Baethmann A (1983) Volume regulation and metabolism of suspended C6 glioma cells: an in vitro model to study cytotoxic brain edema. Brain Res 279: 217–228
57. Kempski O (1986) Cell swelling mechanism in brain. In: Baethmann A, Go G, Unterberg A (eds) Mechanisms of secondary brain damage. Plenum, New York, pp 203–220
58. Kempski O, Zimmer M, Neu A, Rosen Fv, Jansen M, Baethmann A (1987) Control of glial cell volume in anoxia – in vitro studies on ischemic cell swelling. Stroke 18: 623–628
59. Kempski O, Spatz M (1987) Blood-brain barrier: In vitro studies of endothelial permeability. In: Cervos-Navarro I, Ferszt R (eds) Stroke and microcirulation Raven, New York, pp 223–227
60. Kempski O, Staub F, Jansen M, Schödel F, Baethmann A (1987) Glial swelling during extracellular acidosis in vitro. Stroke (in press)
61. Kimelberg HK, Biddlecome S, Narumi S, Bourke RS (1978) ATPase and carbonic anhydrase activities of bulk-isolated neuron, glia and synaptosome fractions from rat brain. Brain Res 141: 305–323
62. Kimelberg HK, Bourke RS, Stieg PE, Barron KD, Hirata H, Pelton EW, Nelson LR (1982) Swelling of astroglia after injury to the nervous system: mechanisms and consequences. In: Grossman RG, Gildenberg PL (eds) Head injury, basic and clinical aspects. Raven, New York, pp 31–44
63. Kirino T (1982) Delayed neuronal death in the gerbil hippocampus following ischemia. Brain Res 239: 57–69
64. Lund-Andersen H, Hertz L (1970) Effect of potassium and of glutamate on swelling and on sodium and potassium content in brain cortex slices from adult rats. Exp Brain Res 11: 199–212
65. Marks MJ, Seeds NW (1982) Development of ion metabolism in reaggregated brain cell cultures. J Neurochem 38: 101–111
66. Martinez-Hernandez A, Bell K, Norenberg MD (1977) Glutamine synthetase: glial localization in brain. Science 195: 1356–1358
67. Mayer ML, Westbrook GL (1987) Cellular mechanisms underlying excitotoxicity. Trends Neurosci 10: 59–61
68. McCarron R, Spatz M, Kempski O, Hogan R, Muehl L, McFarlin DE (1986) Interaction between myelin basic protein-sensitized T lymphocytes and murine cerebral vascular endothelial cells. J Immunology 137: 3428–3434
69. Michler-Stuke A, Bottenstein JE (1982) Proliferation of glial-derived cells in defined media. J Neurosci Res 7: 215–228
70. Morrison RS, deVellis J (1984) Preparation of a chemically defined medium for purified astrocytes. In: Barnes JW (ed) Methods for serum-free culture of neuronal and lymphoid cells, Liss, New York, pp 15–22
71. Nelson P (1977) Neural cell lines. In: Fedoroff S, Hertz L (eds) Cell, tissue and organ culture in neurobiology. Academic, New York, pp 347–365
72. Nicoletti F, Wroblewski T, Novelli A, Alho H, Guidotti A, Costa E (1986) The activation of inositol phopholipid metabolism as a signal transducing system for excitatory amino acids in primary cultures of cerebellar granule cells. J Neurosci 6: 1905–1911
73. Olney JW (1983) Excitotoxins: an overview. In: Fuxe K, Roberts P, Schwarcz R (eds) Excitotoxins. Plenum, New York, pp 82–96

74. Pfeiffer SE, Betschart B, Cook J, Mancini P, Morris R (1977) Glial cell lines. In: Fedoroff S, Hertz L (eds) Cell, tissue and organ culture in neurobiology. Academic, New York, pp 287–346
75. Prusiner SB (1981) Disorders of glutamate metabolism and neurological dysfunction. Annu Rev Med 32: 521–542
76. Ransom BR, Barker JL (1981) Physiology and pharmacology of mammalian central neurons in cell culture. In: Fedoroff S, Hertz L (eds) Advances in Cellular Neurobiology, vol 2. Academic, New York, pp 83–114
77. Ramaharobandro N, Borg J, Mandel P, Mark J (1982) Glutamine and glutamate transport in cultured neuronal and glial cells. Brain Res 244: 113–121
78. Ramsey RL, McIlwain H (1970) Calcium content and exchange in neocortical tissues during the cation movements induced by glutamate. J Neurochem 17: 781–787
79. Rothman SM (1983) Synaptic activity mediates death of hypoxic neurons. Science 220: 536–537
80. Rothman S (1984) Synaptic release of excitatory amino acid neurotransmitter mediates anoxic neuronal death. J Neurosci 4: 1884–1891
81. Rothman SM, Olney JW (1986) Glutamate and the pathophysiology of hypoxic-ischemic brain damage. Ann Neurol 19: 105–111
82. Schousboe A, Svenneby G, Hertz L (1977) Uptake and metabolism of glutamate in astrocytes cultured from dissociated mouse brain hemispheres. J Neurochem 29: 999–1005
83. Schousboe A, Nissen C, Bock E, Sapirstein VS, Juurlink BHJ, Hertz L (1980) Biochemical development of rodent astrocytes in primary culture. In: Giacobini E, Vernadakis A, Shahar A (eds) Tissue culture in neurobiology. Raven, New York, pp 397–409
84. Schousboe A (1980) Primary cultures of astrocytes from mammalian brain as a tool in neurochemical research. Cell Mol Biol 25: 505–513
85. Sensenbrenner M, Labourdette G, Delaunoy JP, Pettmann B, Devilliers G, Moonen G, Bock E (1980) Morphological and biochemical differentiation of glial cells in primary culture. In: Giacobini E, Vernadakis A, Shahar A (eds) Tissue culture in neurobiology. Raven, New York, pp 385–395
86. Siesjö BK (1981) Cell damage in the brain: a speculative synthesis. J Cerebr Blood Flow Metab 1: 155–185
87. Simon RP, Swan JH, Griffiths T, Meldrum BS (1984) Blockade of N-methyl-D-aspartate receptors may protect against ischemic damage in the brain. Science 226: 850–852
88. Snyder EY, Kim SU (1979) Hormonal requirements for neuronal survival in culture. Neurosci Lett 13: 225–230
89. Spatz M, Bembry J, Dodson RF, Hervonen H, Murray M (1980) Endothelial cell cultures derived from isolated cerebral microvessels. Brain Res 191: 577–582
90. Tiffany-Castiglioni E, Neck KF, Caceci T (1986) Glial culture on artificial capillaries. J Neurosci Res 16: 387–396
91. Van Harreveld A, Fifkova E (1971) Light- and electron microscopic changes in central nervous tissue after electrophoretic injection of glutamate. Exp Mol Pathol 15: 61–81
92. Van Harreveld A, Fifkova E (1971) Effects of glutamate and other amino acids on the retina. J Neurochem 18: 2145–2154
93. Varon S (1977) Neural cell isolation and identification. In: Fedoroff S, Hertz L (eds) Cell, tissue and organ cultures in neurobiology. Academic, New York, pp 237–263
94. Vernadakis A, Nidess R (1976) Biochemical characteristics of C-6 glial cells. Neurochem Res 1: 385–402
95. Walz W, Hinks E (1985) Carrier-mediated KCl accumulation accompanied by water movements is involved in control of physiological K^+ levels by astrocytes. Brain Res 343: 44–51
96. Waymouth C (1977) Nutritional requirements of cells in culture, with special reference to neural cells. In: Fedoroff S, Hertz L (eds) Cell, tissue and organ cultures in neurobiology. Academic, New York, pp 631–649
97. Weinberg C, Bell E (1986) A blood vessel model constructed from collagen and cultured vascular cells. Science 231: 397–400
98. Williams SK, Gillis JF, Matthews MA, Wagner RC, Bitensky, MW (1980) Isolation and characterization of brain endothelial cells: morphology and enzyme activity. J Neurochem 35: 374–381
99. Zanotto L, Heinemann U (1983) Aspartate and glutamate induced reductions in extracellular free calcium and sodium concentration in area CA1 of “in vitro” hippocampal slices of rats. Neurosci Lett 35: 79–84

Influence of the Inhalation Anesthetics Isoflurane and Enflurane on the Normal and Ischemic Myocardium

J. Hobbhahn, K. Peter, A. E. Goetz, and P. Conzen

Introduction

Isoflurane is a new inhalation anesthetic which for various reasons is considered to be advantageous as compared to halothane and enflurane [1]. Isoflurane has an extremely low biotransformation rate and is therefore thought to have only minimal, if any, hepatic and renal toxicity at all [2]. Its low blood-gaspartition coefficient should allow easier regulation of the depth of anesthesia [3]. In contrast to enflurane no spike-and-wave pattern is observed in the EEG at concentrations above a minimal alveolar concentration (MAC) of 1,5. At the beginning of our studies in 1984 few data on organ blood flow and on tissue oxygenation of the normally perfused or ischemic myocardium were available. Furthermore, findings concerning the influence of isoflurane on myocardial contractility were controversial.

In the first part of this paper we present our data on myocardial tissue oxygenation and left ventricular contractility at two different concentrations of isoflurane in comparison to equi-anesthetic concentrations of enflurane. Additional findings on cerebral, renal, and hepatic blood flow and tissue oxygenation have, in part, already been published [3, 5, 6].

In the second and third parts of this paper we present data on tissue oxygenation of the collateral flow dependent and poststenotic myocardium and compare them to tissue oxygenation of the unimpaired myocardium under isoflurane and enflurane. Inhalation anesthetics are almost unanimously considered to have advantageous effects on the O_2 balance in the ischemic myocardium during pronounced surgical stimulation and are considered effective in therapy and in prevention of pain-induced tachycardia and hypertension. However, their effects on O_2 balance in periods of hypotension due to lack of surgical stimulation are controversial. We consider here the question as to which effect is predominant: decreased perfusion due to the fall in coronary perfusion pressure or decreased myocardial O_2 consumption due to reduced afterload and contractility, as proposed by van Ackern [14].

In the fourth part the value of myocardial surface tissue PO_2 measurement is demonstrated. In addition, isoflurane- and enflurane-induced changes in myocardial blood flow and tissue oxygenation are discussed in a microcirculatory context.

Influence of Isoflurane and Enflurane on Myocardial O_2 Supply and Contractility

Methods

The study was performed in 15 open-chest dogs (mean body weight [mbw] 29 ± 2.6 kg) under basic anesthesia with piritramid. Catheters were introduced into the

Surgical Research:
Recent Concepts and Results
Baethmann/Messmer (Eds.)

abdominal aorta, pulmonary artery, coronary sinus, and left atrium. Additionally, a tip manometer (Millar) was advanced to the left ventricle and, finally, a highly flexible silicon caoutchouc plate was attached with atraumatic sutures on the surface of the left ventricle to hold a platinum multiwire surface electrode (PME) [8] in position.

Myocardial blood flow (MBF) was determined by left atrial injection of a well agitated suspension of $2.5-4.0 \times 10^6$ 15-μm radionuclide-labelled microspheres (^{51}Cr, ^{95}Nb, ^{85}Sr, ^{141}Ce) in randomized sequence. At the end of the experiment the heart was dissected into 51 tissue samples. Septum and left ventricular free wall were sliced into three transmural layers. Organ blood flow was calculated by comparing the corrected measurements of the tissue samples to those of the arterial reference samples by means of a multichannel autogammaspectrometer.

Data on myocardial surface tissue PO_2 (p_tO_2) was obtained by means of an eight-wire electrode for simultaneous and independent polarographic measurement of local O_2 pressures at eight different sites. Each 15-μm platinum wire had a hemispherical catchment area with a diameter of 25 μm. To obtain O_2 pressure distribution curves (pO_2 histograms) the electrode was rotated repeatedly. Before, during and after the experiments the electrode was calibrated with N_2 5% and O_2 10%.

As a measure of left ventricular contractility the maximum myocardial contractile element velocity (V_{max}) was used. To determine V_{max} the signals of the tip manometer were transferred to a PDP-11-34 computer in 5-ms intervals and corrected off-line for baseline drift. The velocity of contractile element shortening (V_{CE}) was calculated from isovolumic left ventricular pressure curves [12]. An exponential fit of the V_{CE} stress curve was used to extrapolate to V_{max} at zero level.

Baseline mearurements were performed under intravenously piritramid anesthesia. Isoflurane or enflurane were then added to the inspiratory gas mixture (O_2 in air). The end-expiratory concentrations were 0.7 and 1.4 vol.% isoflurane and 1.1 and 2.2 vol.% enflurane. These concentrations are considered to be equi-anesthetic. Left atrial pressure was kept constant throughout the experiments, primarily by transfusion of autologous blood. Arterial PO_2 was maintained between 90 and 120 mmHg.

Fisher's exact test was applied to detect significant differences between equi-anesthetic concentrations of isoflurane and enflurane. Intragroup differences were analyzed by Friedman's rank analysis of variance followed by Wilcoxon and Wilcox multiple comparisons.

Results

Our findings are presented in Table 1. Heart rate (HR) was slightly reduced in both groups. Left atrial pressure was held constant at 7 mmHg. Mean arterial pressure (MAP) and cardiac output (CO) fell in both groups, the latter significantly more with enflurane than with isoflurane. The stronger decreases in CO and stroke volume under enflurane cannot be attributed to differences in systemic vascular resistance, but result from the stronger reduction of left ventricular contractility under enflurane. Left ventricular blood flow increased with isoflurane and decreased with enflurane. The stronger coronary vasodilating capacity of isoflurane is also indicated by the more pronounced increase in coronary venous pO_2 and the more marked fall in the difference of arterial/coronary sinus O_2 content (a-CsO_2). The endocardial/epicardial

Table 1. General and coronary hemodynamics in dogs with piritramide anesthesia, isoflurane, and enflurane (means ± S.D.)

		Piritramid anesthesia	Concentrations of inhalation anesthetics 0.5 MAC	1.0 MAC
Heart rate	ISO	93 ± 12	87 ± 13	87 ± 16
(min^{-1})	ENF	94 ± 8	87 ± 5	85 ± 6
Left atrial pressure	ISO	7.0 ± 2.6	7.0 ± 2.6	7.6 ± 2.3
(mmHg)	ENF	7.4 ± 2.2	7.3 ± 1.9	8.2 ± 2.0
Mean arterial pressure	ISO	110 ± 12	73 ± 10*	60 ± 13*
(mmHg)	ENF	99 ± 9	65 ± 15*	48 ± 13*
Cardiac output	ISO	133 ± 36	117 ± 33*	106 ± 34*
($ml\ kg^{-1}\ min^{-1}$)	ENF	132 ± 25	106 ± 33*	81 ± 35*°
Stroke volume	ISO	42 ± 5	40 ± 7	36 ± 7*
(ml)	ENF	44 ± 12	36 ± 11	30 ± 11*
Systemic vascular resistance	ISO	2215 ± 447	1594 ± 177*	1382 ± 149*
($dyn\ s\ cm^{-5}$)	ENF	1908 ± 460	1525 ± 222*	1389 ± 180*
Left ventricular contractility	ISO	3.8 ± 0.8	3.5 ± 0.7*	3.4 ± 0.6*
(dl/dt)	ENF	3.9 ± 0.5	3.2 ± 0.4*	2.9 ± 0.2*°
Left ventricular blood flow	ISO	99 ± 29	119 ± 52	137 ± 50*
($ml\ 100\ g^{-1}\ min^{-1}$)	ENF	101 ± 19	82 ± 14*	66 ± 19*°
Subendocardial/sub-	ISO	1.0 ± 0.2	1.0 ± 0.2	1.0 ± 0.1
epicardial flow rate	ENF	1.0 ± 0.2	0.9 ± 0.1	0.8 ± 0.2
Left ventricular coronary vascular resistance	ISO	0.8 ± 0.2	0.4 ± 0.2*	0.3 ± 0.1*
($mmHg\ min\ ml^{-1}$)	ENF	0.7 ± 0.1	0.6 ± 0.1	0.5 ± 0.2*°
Coronary sinus pO_2	ISO	30 ± 3	37 ± 6*	38 ± 7*
(mmHg)	ENF	28 ± 3	31 ± 4*	31 ± 3*°
Arterial/coronary sinus	ISO	9.3 ± 1.2	5.5 ± 1.4*	4.6 ± 1.2*
O_2 content difference (vol. %)	ENF	8.4 ± 1.2	7.1 ± 1.3*	7.1 ± 0.6*°
O_2 availability/	ISO	1.7 ± 0.2	2.5 ± 0.8*	3.0 ± 1.0*
consumption ratio	ENF	1.7 ± 0.2	1.8 ± 0.3*	1.9 ± 0.2*°

ISO, isoflurane; ENF, enflurane
*$p < 0.05$ versus baseline (piritramid)
°$p < 0.05$ versus corresponding isoflurane concentration

perfusion ratio was maintained with isoflurane and slightly reduced with enflurane. Both inhalation anesthetics effected a marked fall in myocardial O_2 consumption als calculated from left ventricular blood flow and a-CsO_2. The availability/consumption ratio for O_2 (O_2A/O_2C) improved to a greater extent with isoflurane than with enflurane. However, the increase of the O_2A/O_2C ratio was not associated with an improvement in myocardial surface p_tO_2, which remained essentially unchanged with both concentrations of isoflurane and deteriorated under the higher enflurane concentration (Fig. 1).

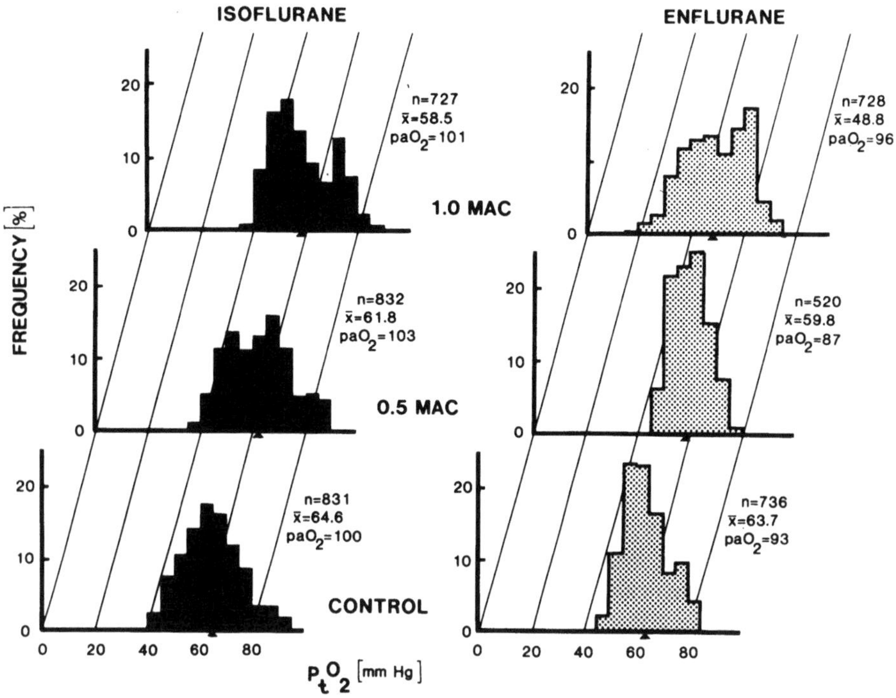

Fig. 1. Left ventricular surface pO_2 (pO_2 histograms) in dogs with piritramide anesthesia control, (*lower panels*), 0.5 MAC (*middle panels*), and 1.0 MAC (*upper panels*), isoflurane, and enflurane. $\bar{x}$, mean p_tO_2 values; *n*, number of single measurements; *paO_2*, arterial pO_2 values. A leftwardshift is observed with 1.0 MAC enflurane

In summary, both anaesthetics:

- depress left ventricular contractility in a dose-related fashion – isoflurane less than enflurane.
- improve the left ventricular O_2 availability consumption ratio – isoflurane more than enflurane; this, however, is not associated with an improvement of myocardial surface p_tO_2.

Influence of Isoflurane on the Collateral flow dependent Myocardium

Methods

In our second study on dogs (mbw 30–40 kg) a ring constrictor made from ameroid was implanted around the left anterior descending coronary artery (LAD). By swelling of the ameroid the constrictor leads to complete occlusion of the vessel within 1–2 weeks. The myocardium distal to the constrictor is then assumed to be exclusively dependent on quantity and quality of the collateral blood flow (MBF_{COL}).

Six dogs were studied 3–4 weeks after surgery. Anesthetic and operative procedures were the same as in the first study. Myocardial surface p_tO_2 was determined in the normally perfused myocardium (CX area) as well as, using a second PME, in the collateral flow dependent region distal to the constrictor (LAD area). Measurements were performed under baseline conditions and with 1.4–2.1 vol.% isoflurane. To compare flow distribution in the LAD area to that in the CX area the Wilcoxon test was applied; statistical significance was considered at $p < 0.05$.

Results

Under baseline conditions MBF_{col} was significantly lower than MBF_{cx} (Table 2). Additionally, the endocardial/epicardial flow ratio (Table 2) and the surface p_tO_2 (Fig. 2) were somewhat lower in the LAD area than in the CX area. With an unchanged left ventricular filling pressure and an unchanged HR, isoflurane led to a marked fall of MAP and to a slight decrease in CO (Table 2). Isoflurane led to a reduction in collateral blood flow by about 40%, whereas blood flow in the normally perfused myocardium was unchanged (Table 2). Myocardial left ventricular strokework/sec and myocardial O_2 consumption were reduced by about 50%. Figure 2 shows the cumulative histograms of the four animals, in which the PME had, in fact,

Table 2. Collateral flow dependent and normally perfused myocardium of dogs under piritramid anesthesia and isoflurane (means ± S.D.)

	Piritramid anaesthesia	Isoflurane
Mean arterial pressure (mmHg)	112 ± 14	60 ± 9*
Heart rate (min^{-1})	91 ± 9	95 ± 22
Cardiac output ($ml\ kg^{-1}\ min^{-1}$)	106 ± 14	83 ± 24*
Left atrial pressure (mmHg)	6.8 ± 2.7	7.3 ± 2.2
Left ventricular stroke work/sec (Watt/s)	0.78 ± 0.19	0.32 ± 0.11*
Arterial/coronary sinus O_2 content difference (vol. %)	8.1 ± 1.1	4.7 ± 0.9*
Left ventricular O_2 consumption ($ml\ 100\ g^{-1}\ min^{-1}$)	7.9 ± 1.8	3.9 ± 1.0*
Regional blood flow in normally perfused myocardium ($ml\ 100\ g^{-1}\ min^{-1}$)	98 ± 20	93 ± 26
Regional blood flow in collateral flow dependent myocardium ($ml\ 100\ g^{-1}\ min^{-1}$)	75 ± 20°	47 ± 20*°
Subendocardial/subepicardial flow rate in normally perfused myocardium	1.0 ± 0.1	1.0 ± 0.1
Subendocardial/subepicardial flow rate in collateral flow dependent myocardium	0.8 ± 0.2	0.7 ± 0.4°

* < 0.05 versus baseline (piritramid)
° < 0.05 versus normally perfused myocardium

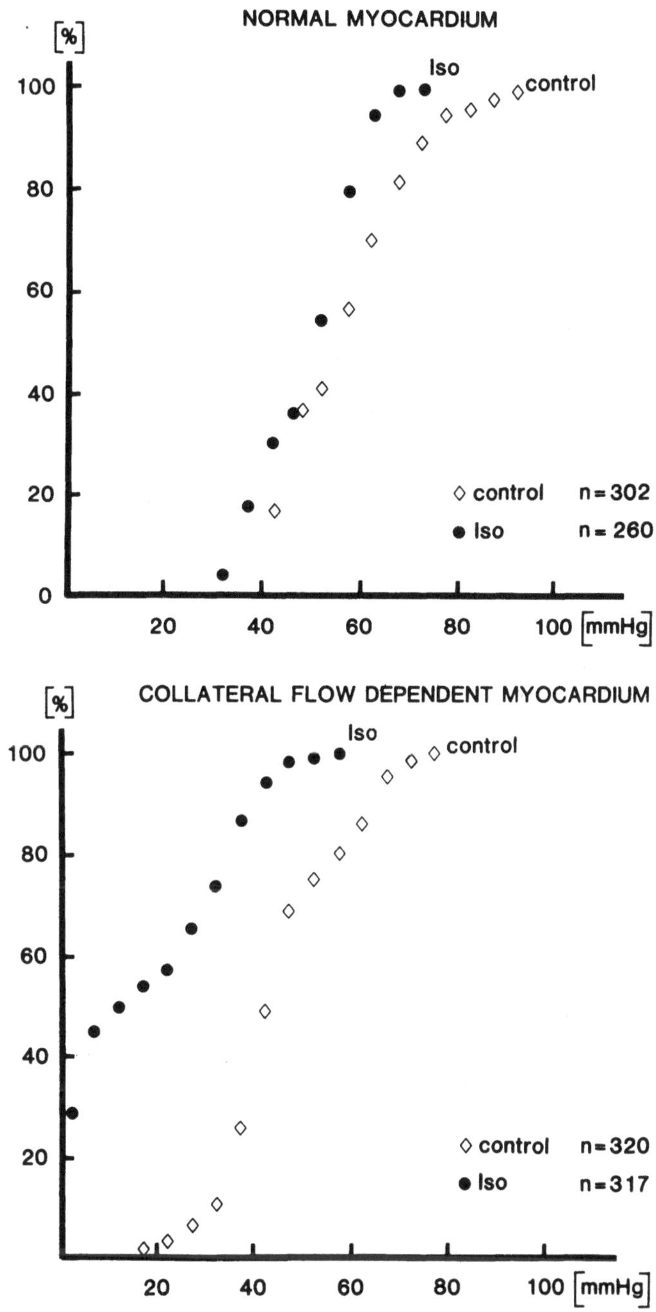

Fig. 2. Left ventricular surface p_tO_2 of the normally supplied and of the collateral flow dependent myocardium under baseline conditions (◇) and under isoflurane (●). Surface p_tO_2 of the collateral flow dependent myocardium is lower even under baseline conditions (lowest p_tO_2 values about 15 mmHg) compared to the normally supplied myocardium (lowest p_tO_2 values about 40 mmHg). Isoflurane leads to a pronounced fall in surface p_tO_2 of the collateral flow dependent myocardium (30% of all values between 0 and 5 mmHg). In contrast, surface p_tO_2 of the normal myocardium decreases only slightly with isoflurane

been placed in the centre of the collateral flow dependent myocardium. The application of isoflurane led to a marked leftward shift of the cumulative PO_2 histogram for the collateral flow dependent myocardium but not for the normally perfused myocardium.

We conclude from these data that tissue oxygenation of the collateral flow dependent myocardium is jeopardized with a moderate isoflurane-induced hypotension, in spite of a marked reduction in left ventricular O_2 consumption.

Influence of Isoflurane and Enflurane on the Poststenotic Myocardium

Methods

This study was performed in pigs, the coronary system of which is considered more similar to that of humans than is that of dogs. Additionally, poor collateralization here allows the more stable maintenance of a given stenosis than in the case of dogs. In open-chest pigs (30 kg mbw) under neurolept anesthesia a highly flexible teflon-coated copper wire was placed around the LAD to create a stenosis. To sample blood from the area predominantly supplied by the LAD a catheter was inserted into the great cardiac vein. Again, surface p_tO_2 was monitored on the LAD-supplied and on the CX-supplied myocardium.

In a first set of experiments different degrees of stenosis were performed in order to correlate changes of LAD surface p_tO_2 with lactate extraction. Increasing constriction of the LAD led to a progressive decrease in surface p_tO_2. Coronary venous lactate concentrations increased, while arterial levels remained constant. No changes in p_tO_2 values in the CX area could be observed. Linear regression analysis revealed a strong correlation between changes in surface p_tO_2 and changes in arterial/coronary venous lactate difference ($Y = -0.59 + 0.62\,X$; $R = 0.86$; $p < 0.001$). This demonstrates that myocardial surface p_tO_2 strongly correlates with transmural disturbances of O_2 supply.

Finally, a model of stenosis was established, based on creating a degree of stenosis, where a pacemaker-induced increase in HR by 40 beats/min caused a fall of myocardial tissue p_tO_2 to or near zero mmHg, a marked increase in net lactate production, and a pronounced fall in the endocardial/epicardial flow ratio of the LAD area. This degree of stenosis was reached when surface tissue p_tO_2 in the LAD area was reduced to about 50% of the baseline value, i.e., to about 20 mmHg.

Using this model we studied myocardial-tissue oxygenation of the poststenotic and the normally perfused myocardium under the influence of mild enflurane- or isoflurane-induced hypotension often observed clinically.

After baseline recordings the LAD was constricted until surface p_tO_2 in the LAD area was reduced by about 50% (Fig. 3). Following measurements under this degree of stenosis either isoflurane ($n = 7$) or enflurane ($n = 7$) was administered to reduce the MAP to 75 mmHg for a period of 30 min. All measurements were repeated at this time as well as 30 min after elimination of both inhalation anaesthetics.

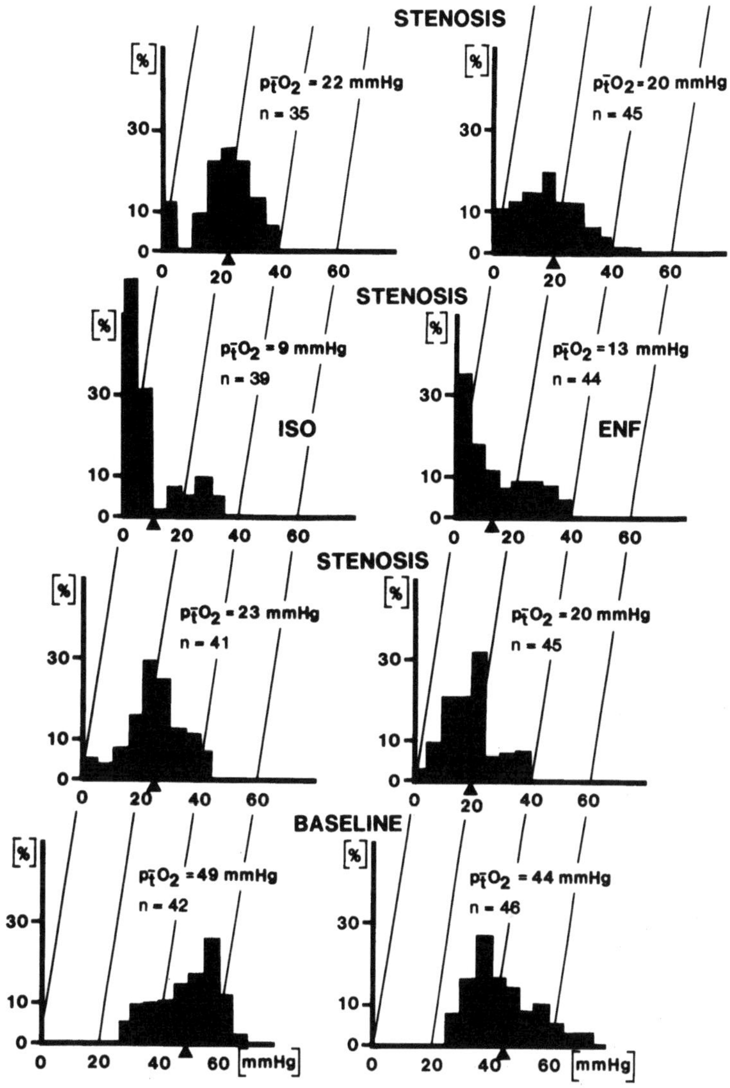

Fig. 3. The influence of isoflurane and enflurane on the poststenotic myocardium. The continous registrations are summarized as pO_2 histograms. Creation of stenosis led to a decrease in surface p_tO_2 by about 50%. Isoflurane (*left*) and enflurane (*right*) decreased the p_tO_2. After discontinuation of both inhalation anesthetics p_tO_2 returned to higher values. Surface p_tO_2 of the CX area (not shown) remained unchanged during all experiments

Results

Mean values for surface p_tO_2 were about 45 mmHg in both the LAD area (Fig. 3) and the CX area (not shown). Coronary venous PO_2 for the LAD area was 25 ± 5 mmHg. The arterial/coronary venous O_2 content difference ($AVDO_{2LAD}$) amounted to 9 vol. % and the arterial/coronary venous lactate content difference ($AVDL_{LAD}$) to 0.4 ± 0.4 mmol/l.

Table 3. Influence of isoflurane and enflurane on the poststenotic and the normally supplied myocardium of pigs under piritramide basic anesthesia (means ± S.D.)

Stenosis		Stenosis	Stenosis with inhalat. anesthetics[b]	Stenosis
Mean arterial pressure (mmHg)	ISO	101 ± 13	76 ± 3*	99 ± 13
	ENF	92 ± 10	74 ± 3*	88 ± 12
Heart rate (min^{-1})	ISO	89 ± 17	91 ± 11	90 ± 16
	ENF	99 ± 6	98 ± 11	100 ± 11
Left ventricular end-diastolic pressure (mmHg)	ISO	9 ± 3	9 ± 3	10 ± 3
	ENF	9 ± 1	10 ± 3	10 ± 1
Cardiac output (ml kg^{-1} min^{-1})	ISO	104 ± 19	92 ± 17	101 ± 15
	ENF	108 ± 21	96 ± 33	120 ± 56
Left ventricular stroke work/sec (Watt/sec)	ISO	0.67 ± 0.16	0.44 ± 0.07*	0.61 ± 0.10
	ENF	0.62 ± 0.17	0.42 ± 0.07*	0.61 ± 0.18
Regional blood flow in normally perfused myocardium (ml 100 g^{-1} min^{-1})	ISO	106 ± 23	84 ± 18*	-
	ENF	105 ± 19	86 ± 15	-
Regional blood flow (ml 100 g^{-1} min^{-1})	ISO	87 ± 18°	58 ± 20*°	-
	ENF	77 ± 8°	54 ± 10*°	-
Arterial/coronary venous lactate content difference in LAD (mMol/l))	ISO	−0.4 ± 0.4	−1.0 ± 0.7	−0.5 ± 0.5
	ENF	−0.6 ± 0.7	−0.8 ± 0.5	−0.4 ± 0.5
Arterial/coronary venous O_2 difference in LAD (vol. %)	ISO	11.2 ± 1.7	10.7 ± 1.4	10.3 ± 0.9
	ENF	10.1 ± 2.0	10.0 ± 1.6	9.8 ± 1.8

ISO, isoflurane; ENF, enflurane; LAD, left anterior descending coronary artery
* $p < 0.05$ versus baseline (piritramid)
° $p < 0.05$ versus normally supplied myocardium
[a] Before application of inhalation anesthetics
[b] 30 Min after application of inhalation anesthetics
[c] 30 Min after discontinuation of inhalation anesthetics

Under the degree of stenosis chosen, no changes in hemodynamics (Table 3) were observed. However, regional blood flow was 20% less in the LAD area than in the CX area (Table 3). This was associated with an increase in $AVDO_{2LAD}$ and a net lactate production (Table 3). Measurement of poststenotic pressure in some animals revealed a pressure gradient of 40–50 mmHg across the stenosis.

The administration of isoflurane and enflurane led to a 30% decrease in left ventricular stroke work per second (LVSW/s) for both groups (Table 3). Regional blood flow of the LAD area fell by 30%, regional blood flow of the CX area by 20%. Mean poststenotic pressure was about 30 mmHg. Surface p_tO_2 in the LAD area was reduced (Fig. 3), while surface p_tO_2 in the CX area remained constant. The lactate balance worsened in both groups, whereas $ADVO_{2LAD}$ did not change.

At 30 min after discontinuation of both inhalation anesthetics MAP, CO, LVSW/s, $AVDL_{LAD}$ and surface p_tO_2 in the LAD area returned to levels similar to these prior to isoflurane and enflurane administration.

Discussion

Methods

The essential aspect in these studies was the measurement of myocardial surface p_tO_2. This is considered to reflect the net effect between capillary O_2 availability and myocardial O_2 utilization in the most superficial layer of the subepicardium. Values of 64 mmHg were determined for p_tO_2 in the canine myocardium supplied by the left circumflex artery under piritramid anesthesia and under stable hemodynamic conditions, with arterial pO_2 values of about 100 mmHg (Figs. 1 and 2). In contrast to these high p_tO_2 values, the mean coronary sinus pO_2 was only 30 mmHg. The latter is considered a measure for global mean tissue PO_2 [1]. Using comparable anesthetic technique Vogel and coworkers found similar surface p_tO_2 values (57 mmHg), with concomittant coronary sinus pO_2 values of 30 mmHg as well [15]. No conclusive explanation for the discrepancy between surface p_tO_2 and coronary venous pO_2 exists thus far. A possible explanation may be the transmural pO_2 gradient, i.e., low pO_2 values in the deeper and higher pO_2 values in the superficial layers of the heart. High surface p_tO_2 values may be consistent with a less pronounced development of pressure in the subepicardial layer.

The lower mean p_tO_2 values found by others in the dog myocardium (48 [9] and 49 mmHg [13]) may result from lower arterial pO_2 values [9, 13], different anesthetic technique [9] and unphysiological hemodynamics [13]. In addition p_tO_2 measurements may have been influenced by additional manipulation performed at the surface as well as in deeper layers of the heart [9]. No coronary sinus pO_2 values were published by these investigators.

In the pig heart we found lower surface p_tO_2 values, with a mean of 45 mmHg; these were, however clearly associated with lower coronary venous pO_2 values. Thus, one may conclude that pigs have a distinctly lower myocardial tissue PO_2 than do dogs under similar experimental conditions.

The question as to whether the high p_tO_2 values measured on the surface of the myocardium actually reflect myocardial tissue oxygenation can be acertained in view of the clear correlation with myocardial lactate release.

Results

Our results concerning the effects of isoflurane and enflurane on the healthy dog myocardium demonstrate that it is not justified to draw conclusions from a positive supply demand ratio regarding myocardial tissue oxygenation. A marked increase in coronary sinus pO_2 with isoflurane was concomittant with an unchanged surface p_tO_2. A slight increase in coronary sinus pO_2 with enflurane was associated with a decrease in surface p_tO_2, at least with the higher concentration. A redistribution of myocardial blood flow in favor of subendocardial layers is an unlikely explanation for the lack of increase in epicardial p_tO_2 in view of the unchanged (isoflurane) or even decreased (enflurane) subendocardial/subepicardial flow ratios. Thus, shunting of blood as a possible explanation must be considered. Since no anatomic shunts in the myocardium have thus far been identified, and since no microspheres were found in the coronary sinus reference samples, we assume that functional shunting may have occurred via microvascular channels with diameters smaller than those occluded by the microspheres, i.e., on the capillary level. This hypothesis is supported by the findings of Vogel and coworkers, who discovered an increase in coronary blood flow with isoflurane concomittant with a marked increase in coronary venous pO_2, whereas capillary microflow (H_2 clearance) was increased only minimally and surface p_tO_2 remained unchanged [15]. In addition when studying the microcirculation of the striated muscle during isoflurane anesthesia, we found arteriolar vasodilation, which, however, was associated with an increase in the proportion of capillaries which were not perfused [4]; this suggests redistribution of capillary blood flow. One could therefore speculate that the increased coronary sinus pO_2 values under both inhalation anesthetics predominantly reflect the relatively higher degrees of oxygenation of the venous end of these preferentially perfused (short?) capillaries, but not myocardial tissue oxygenation.

We believe that redistribution of capillary flow also is a factor which must be taken into consideration when explaining the decrease in tissue p_tO_2 of the collateral flow dependent or the poststenotic myocardium under isoflurane and enflurane. Both inhalation anesthetics led to a marked reduction in total left ventricular O_2 consumption, the decrease in which was in relation to the decrease in the collateral flow dependent or poststenotic myocardium perfusion. LVSW/s and left ventricular O_2 consumption were reduced by 50% with isoflurane whereas collateral blood flow was decreased by 40%. This indeed suggests a well maintained O_2 balance in the compromised myocardium. Surface p_tO_2, however, worsened. LVSW/s fell by 30% under enflurane and isoflurane in the pig hearts, as did poststenotic blood flow, again suggesting a maintained O_2 balance. However, poststenotic p_tO_2 also worsened. We therefore conclude that the deterioration of the compromised myocardium under isoflurane and enflurane perhaps is not due to a decrease in perfusion alone but rather also to a redistribution of capillary flow.

Our hypothesis is that the perfusion pressure in the compromised myocardium was distinctly under 40 mmHg, and that this fall in perfusion pressure led to a shift of capillary flow from the longer, nutritive capillaries to the shorter, functionally non nutritive capillaries. This hypothesis is supported, first of all, by microcirculatory studies in vasodilated striated muscle, in which a reduction of the mean arterial pressure below 50 mmHg resulted in a significant decrease in functional capillary density [10]. Second, studies on striated dilated gastrocnemius muscle, in which a decrease of total blood flow was achieved not by stenosis as in our study, but by partial microembolization, showed a disproportionally lower capillary transport coefficient compared to the observed decrease in total flow [2]. Furthermore, an increase in muscle venous O_2 saturation despite decreasing total blood flow in the working muscle was found after this microembolization. These authors concluded that redistribution of microcirculatory flow rather than the decrease of total perfusion provides the basis for the disturbances in tissue function described under conditions of impaired microcirculation [2]. Third, our own studies showed a fall in surface p_tO_2 in the normally perfused myocardium as soon as coronary perfusion pressure fell below 40 mmHg with enflurane and isoflurane. Furthermore, this fall in p_tO_2 was associated with slightly increased coronary sinus pO_2 values [7]. Fourth, mean poststenotic coronary perfusion pressures of about 30 mmHg with enflurane and isoflurane were not associated with relevant changes in coronary venous pO_2, as evidenced by the unchanged $AVDO_2$. We do not know the pressure in the collateral dependent myocardium under isoflurane, however, in view of a mean aortic blood pressure of 60 mmHg a very low values must be assumed.

Conclusion

Our results demonstrate that it is not justified to draw conclusions on the influence of the inhalation anesthetics on myocardial tissue oxygenation from O_2 supply/demand ratios or from changes in coronary venous pO_2. This applies both for the normally perfused as well as for the critically hypoperfused myocardium. Assessments of tissue oxygenation can only be made by the direct measurement of tissue pO_2. A deterioration of myocardial surface p_tO_2 is observed when perfusion pressures are reduced below 40 mmHg. A redistribution of capillary blood flow as relevant pathophysiological substrate for the deterioration of the poststenotic and collateral flow dependent myocardial tissue pO_2 may be assumed. Assumption of protection for the ischemic heart by a slight to moderate hypotensive anesthesia ("hypodynamic anesthesia") effected with inhalation anesthetics, as postulated by some authors [11, 14], seems to be disproven, even though the decrease in oxygen supply is paralleled by a fall in myocardial O_2 consumption.

The less pronounced negative inotropic effects of isoflurane should be considered when anesthesia is performed in patients with impaired cardiac function.

References

1. Feigl EO (1983) Coronary physiology. Physiol Rev 63: 1–205
2. Gaethgens P, Benner KU, Schickendanz S (1976) Nutritive and non-nutritive blood flow in canine skeletal muscle after partial microembolization. Pflügers Arch 361: 183–189
3. Goetz AE, Conzen PFM, Hobbhahn J, Granetzny T, Peter K, Brendel W (1985) Regional cerebral blood flow with increasing doses of isoflurane and enflurane in a canine model. Anesthesiology 63: A41
4. Goetz AE, Conzen PFM, Schmidt AF, Hobbhahn J, Brendel W (1986) Microcirculatory effects of isoflurane. Anesthesiology 65: A1
5. Hobbhahn J, Conzen P, Goetz A, Habazettl H, Brendel W, Peter K (1986) Leberperfusion und -oxygenation unter Isoflurane, Anästh Intensivther Notfallmed 21: 85–89
6. Hobbhahn J, Conzen P, Goetz A, Granetzny T, Brendel W, Peter K (1986) Dose dependent reduction of renal perfusion during anesthesia with isoflurane or enflurane. Anesthesiology 65: A262
7. Hobbhahn J, Conzen P, Goetz A, Brendel W, Peter K (1986) Volatile Anästhetika - neue Aspekte. In: FW Eigler et al. (eds) Stand und Gegenstand chirurgischer Forschung. Springer, Berlin Heidelberg New York, pp 95–109
8. Kessler M, Lübbers DW (1966) Aufbau und Anwendungsmöglichkeiten verschiedener pO_2-Elektroden. Pflügers Arch Ges Physiol 291: R82
9. Klövekorn WP (1986) Das Verhalten der regionalen myokardialen Sauerstoffversorgung unter normalen und pathologischen Bedingungen: tierexperimentelle Untersuchungen am schlagenden Herzen. Habilitationsschrift, Ludwig-Maximilians-Universität Munich
10. Lindbom L, Arfors KE (1985) Mechanisms and site of control for variation in the number of perfused capillaries in skeletal muscle. Int J Microcirc Clin Exp 4: 19–30
11. Moffitt EA (1986) The coronary circulation and myocardial oxygenation in coronary artery disease: effects of anesthesia. Anesth Analg 65: 395–410

12. Sonnenblick EH, Parmely WW, Urschel CW (1969) The contractile state of the heart as expressed by force-velocity relations. Am J Cardiol 23: 488–503
13. Spiegel HU, Bergermann M, Hauss J, Wendt M, Schönleben K (1986) Die hochdosierte Piritramid-Basisanästhesie in der experimentellen Anästhesie und Chirurgie. Anesthesist 35: 36–42
14. Van Ackern K, Adler M, Brückner UB, Buell U, Haller M, Mittmann U, Ragaller M, Raithel E, Vetter H, Wöllner W (1986) Regional changes during myocardial ischemia: an animal experimental study. In: K Peter (ed) Inhalation anesthetics, new aspects. Springer, Berlin Heidelberg New York, pp 196–206
15. Vogel H, Günther H, Harrison WK, Kessler M, Peter K (1984) The influence of isoflurane and enflurane on tissue oxygenation and microcirculation of the dog myocardium. Anesthesiology 61: A5

Prostaglandin, and Thromboxane Release in Critical States

W. OETTINGER, and H.G. BEGER

Except for metabolic emergencies and intoxications, critical states in medicine generally result from ischemia, thromboembolism, various types of shock, sepsis, and severe trauma. The most common clinical entities are myocardial infarction, postoperative embolic complications, septic shock, and multiple trauma with ensuing organ failure, in particular of the lungs and kidney. The prostaglandins (PGs) and thromboxane (TX) belong to a highly complex system of mediators, which in both research and clinical practice is believed to account for the numerous aspects of acute-phase host responses, ranging from disseminated intravascular coagulation to pulmonary edema.

Vascular motor tone, endothelial integrity, and balanced blood cell rheology constitute the mainstay of normal micro- and macrocirculation, extracellular-intracellular fluid equilibrium, and finally, organ performance. It is for these reasons that among the presently known mediators, the PGs and TX are still attracting increasing attention from scientists and clinicians. Both potent vasoconstrictors and vasodilators are derived from a common source, arachidonic acid, via the cyclo-oxygenase pathway. Among the prevalent dienoic PGs, and TXs, are the vasoconstrictors $PGF_{2\alpha}$ and TXA_2 and the vasodilators PGE_2 and prostacyclin (PGI_2). In addition, TXA_2 aggregates platelets and leukocytes, and PGI_2 inhibits aggregation.

Collagen exposed after ischemic endothelial damage promotes platelet aggregation and TX formation. While the stable PGE_2 and $PGF_{2\alpha}$ are inactivated enzymatically in vivo, PGI_2 and TXA_2 are highly unstable and are transformed nonenzymatically into the stable degradation products 6-keto(k)-$PGF_{1\alpha}$ and TXB_2, respectively. Vane and coworkers [1] have shown that the lung plays a major regulative role in PG metabolism. PGE_2 and $PGF_{2\alpha}$, for instance, are inactivated by more than 90% during a single passage through the lungs. There is also evidence for pulmonary synthesis of various PGs and TXs and their release into the systemic circulation [2–4]. On top of all this, the pulmonary vasculature is an important target for PGs and TXs [2]. Another distinctive element of the PG system is that its active compounds are detectable in circulating blood only in critical states, not, however, in healthy conditions, and to a negligible extent during elective surgery. Methods of determination vary from elaborate high-performance liquid chromatography and mass spectrometry to highly sensitive radioimmunoassays. The latter method was used by our group following Peskar et al. [5] It was applied to those derivatives which represent the most active antagonists

Surgical Research:
Recent Concepts and Results
Baethmann/Messmer (Eds.)

of the system, PGI_2 and TXA_2, and to those which can be even more reliably measured and indicate the general state of metabolic activity: $PGF_{2\alpha}$ and its actively synthesized metabolite 13,14-dihydro-15-keto-$PGF_{2\alpha}$ ($KH_2PGF_{2\alpha}$). Due to the fact that only a few clinical trials have as yet been carried out, the following data are mainly the result of our own investigations on patients. The data will be discussed in the light of the few clinical findings available from other groups.

Endotoxemia is a formidable trigger of PG and TX synthesis being used experimentally and evaluated clinically. The implications of PG and TX release in endotoxemia and clinical septic shock are reported elsewhere in more detail [4, 6] and will only be summarized here. PGs and TX are enhanced during septic shock to measurable concentrations in the systemic circulation. This partly results from decreased pulmonary PG inactivation, in addition to an increased de novo PG synthesis. Data suggest that the impaired pulmonary gas exchange secondary to septic injury coincides with an impaired metabolic function of the lung.

Another finding in humans is an imbalance between plasma concentrations of PGI_2 (measured as 6-K-$PGF_{1\alpha}$) and TXA_2 (measured as TXB_2), which can be correlated to organ function and survival. Patients with a predominance of PGI_2 over TX do better than those with an inverse ratio [6]. A third result of research in patients is a good correlation between transpulmonary TXB_2 plasma concentration gradients and the development of pulmonary hypertension. So far, septic shock can be regarded as the sole clinical condition where a general stimulation of the arachidonate cascade can be detected, including all measurable derivatives of the cyclo-oxygenase pathway. This is quite in contrast to what is found in patients after severe trauma.

An isolated release of TXB_2 was found in a prospective study on 24 multiply injured patients with an injury severity score > 35 (no head injury entered) and defined criteria of pulmonary insufficiency (i.e., $PaO_2 < 75$ mmHg at $FIO_2 = 0.5$). Patients were monitored for PG and TX release on admission, 6, 12, 18, and 36 h later, and subsequently twice daily until discharge from the intensive care unit (ICU). The results are illustrated in Fig. 1, indicating TXB_2 release up to a peak of 1218 ± 354 pg/ml only a few hours after trauma and a decline to near normal levels after only 36 h, i.e., long before recovery from functional deterioration. Again, pulmonary net release of TX is part of the mechanism involved, as indicated by significant differences between central venous and arterial plasma concentrations of radioimmunoactive TXB_2 (Fig. 2). In contrast to septic patients, $PGF_{2\alpha}$, $KH_2PGF_{2\alpha}$, and 6-K-$PGF_{1\alpha}$ vary slightly above the detection limit in these 24 patients.

A release pattern similar to that seen in trauma patients was recognized locally in patients undergoing elective femoral nailing. Figure 3 shows the release pattern of TXB_2 into the femoral venous blood during the procedure. Again, no general activation of the PG system is observed in this clinical model, but there is a remarkable release of platelet-activating TX. In this group of 12, we saw one patient who developed acute respiratory distress syndrome (ARDS), 3–4 h after surgery. At the time of ICU monitoring, there were still transpulmonary TX gradients detectable in this patient, coinciding with massive pulmonary hypertension and interstitial edema. It was presumed that local TX release helped trigger the cardiopulmonary disaster. Long before the recovery of respiratory and hemodynamic function, however, the TXB_2 gradients disappeared. TXB_2 in arterial plasma remained slightly elevated until the patient was released from the ICU (Fig. 4).

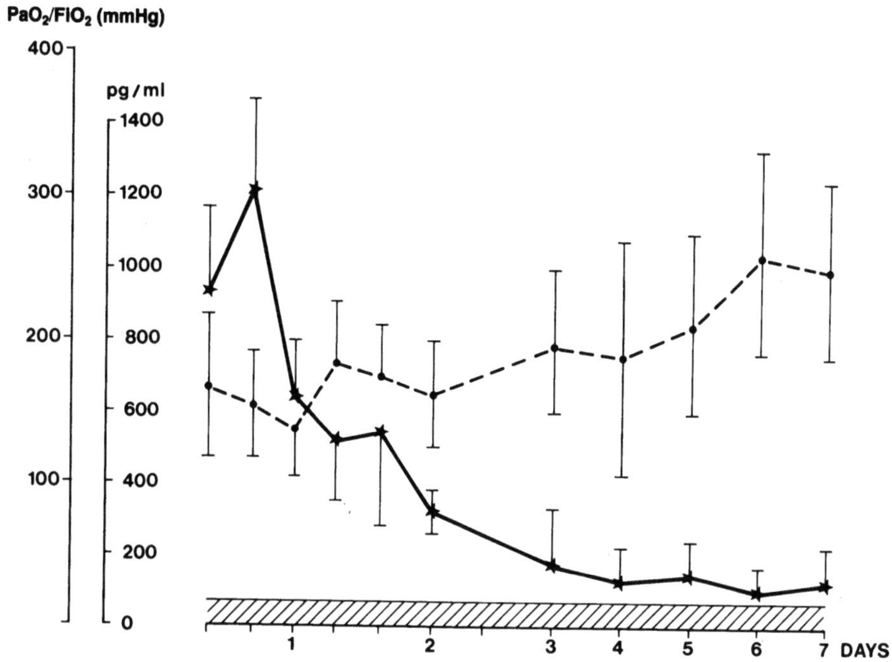

Fig. 1. Respiratory function *(broken line)* given as PaO_2/FIO_2 and TX release *(continuous line)* in arterial blood of 24 severely traumatized patients

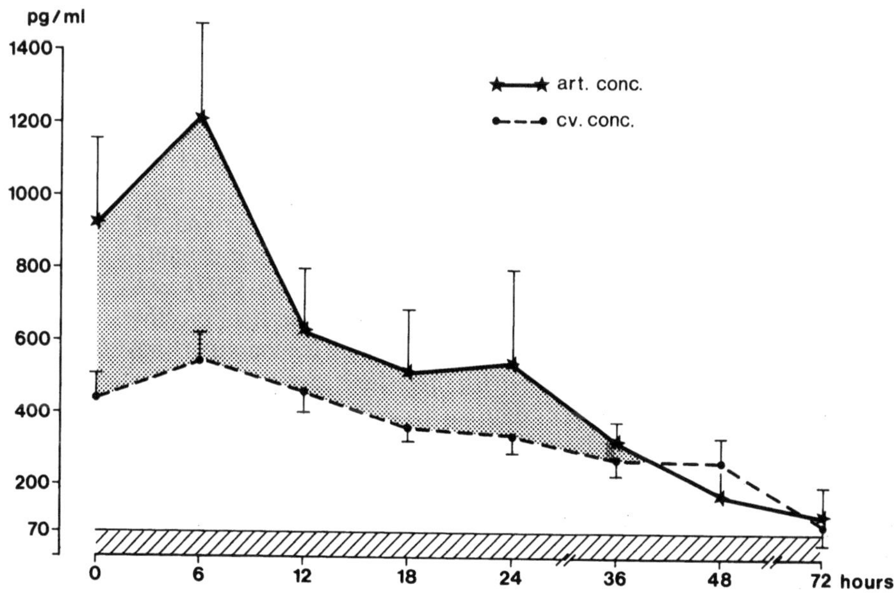

Fig. 2. Transpulmonary TXB_2 gradients in 24 severely traumatized patients early after trauma. *art. conc:* arterial plasma concentration; *cv. conc:* central venous concentration

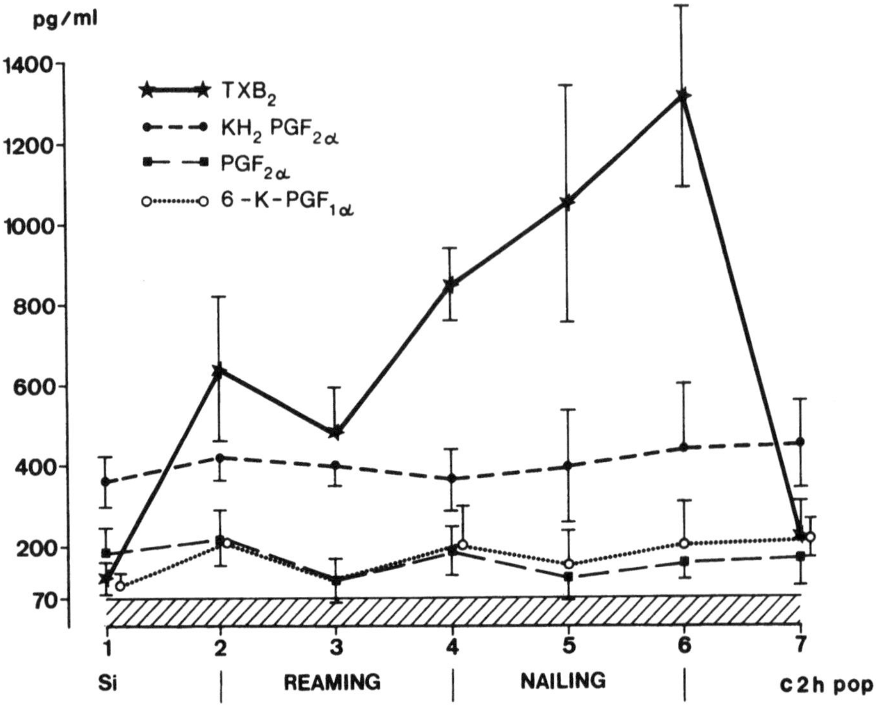

Fig. 3. PG and TX release pattern as measured in femoral venous blood of 12 patients undergoing elective femoral nailing. *Si:* skin incision; *c:* control; *pop:* postoperatively

Patients undergoing hip surgery are known to run a statistically higher than average risk of postoperative thromboembolism, particularly if cement is used [7]. We therefore investigated a total of 28 patients during surgery for total hip prosthesis. Blood samples were drawn in the sequence given in the legend of Fig. 5, and various hemodynamic data, including cardiac output and pulmonary vascular resistance, were recorded.

The results given in Figs. 5, 6 led to the following conclusions: None of the patients showed general PG stimulation, and a subgroup of 12 again exhibited a marked release of TXB_2 in central venous plasma. This coincided most significantly with a rise in central venous pressure after cement implantation and final prosthesis fixation. Another subgroup of 16 patients remained unremarkable in terms of both PG and TX release and hemodynamics throughout the procedure; they are referred to as "nonresponders." It was only retrospectively recognized that ten of these patients were receiving chronic, nonsteroidal anti-inflammatory medication of more than 200 mg indomethacin daily. They are presented in Figs. 5, 6 as separate subgroups. These findings suggest that TX might also contribute to intra- and postoperative pulmonary and thromboembolic complications in the course of hip surgery using cemented prosthetic devices.

The sensitive reaction of central venous pressure coinciding with the release of TX should encourage use of a central venous line for the perioperative monitoring of

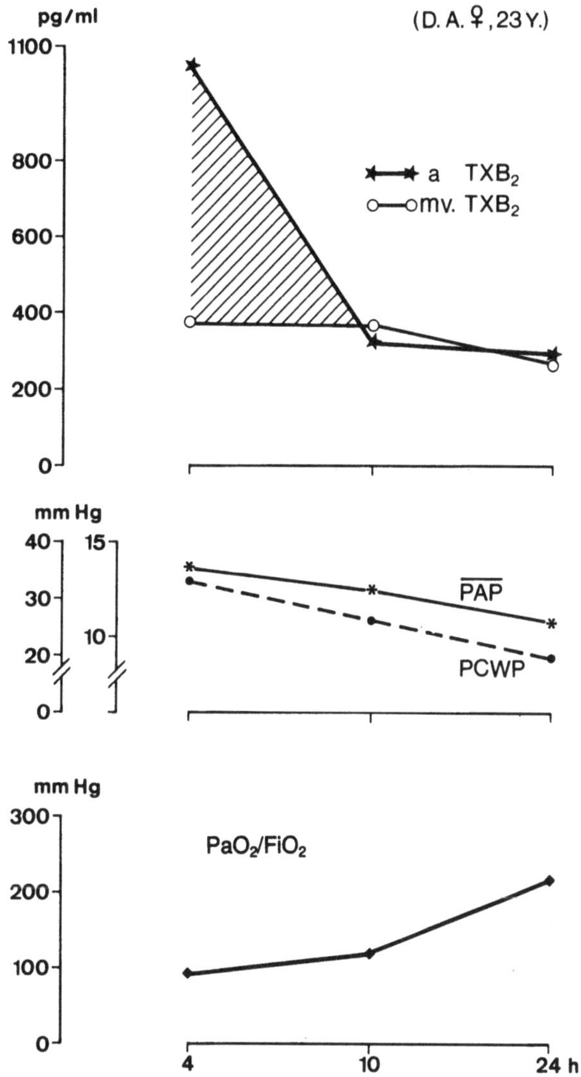

Fig. 4. Individual data of 23-year-old female patient developing ARDS 4 h after elective femoral nailing. *a:* arterial; *mv:* mixed venous; *PAP:* mean pulmonary artery pressure; *PCWP:* pulmonary capillary wedge pressure

these mostly elderly patients. TX is a potent vasoconstrictor and platelet aggregator. Once it is released systemically, it may contribute to, or at least coincide with, life-threatening septic, post-traumatic, and postoperative insults to the lung. There is evidence from the literature that TX is also involved in the pathogenesis of myocardial infarction and kidney transplant rejection.

Various groups, e.g., Hirsh et al. [8] and Lefer et al. [9], demonstrated the release of TX into coronary sinus blood of patients after myocardial infarction. Ramwell argued that TX is a mediator of sudden death in coronary disease [10].

These findings sparked ongoing therapeutic studies with various doses of anticyclo-oxygenase and antithromboxane drugs [11]. Ramwell's group was also the first to

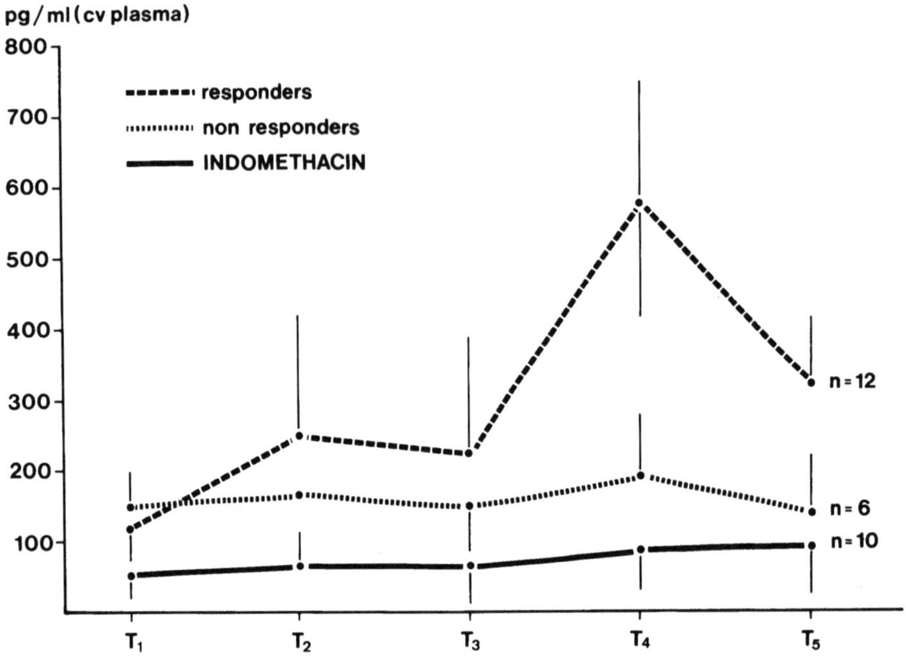

Fig. 5. TXB_2 release pattern in 28 patients undergoing hip replacement with cemented devices. *cv:* central venous; T_1: baseline value after induction of anesthesia; T_2: removal of femoral head; T_3: time before cement implantation; T_4: during prosthesis fixation under pressure and hardening of cement; T_5: control 2 h postoperatively. (For subgroups, see text)

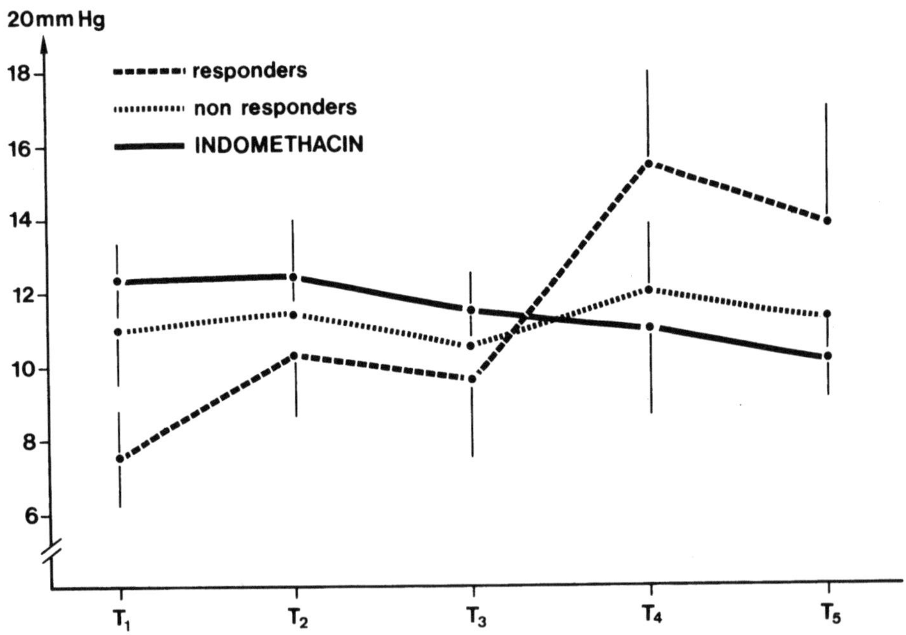

Fig. 6. Central venous pressure *(CVP)* recording of 28 patients undergoing total hip replacement with cemented prosthesis. For T_1–T_5, see legend to Fig. 5. (For subgroups, see text)

report on a series of kidney transplant patients being investigated for their daily urine TX output. TX turned out to be a very sensitive indicator of transplant rejection since elevated concentrations were found before clinical signs of rejection. In addition, there was a correlation between the severity of rejection and the urine concentration of TX metabolites [12, 13].

Summarizing the present state of knowledge of PG and TX release in clinical conditions, the following statements can be made. There is sufficient evidence that biologically active PGs and TXs which normally act only as tissue hormones reach the systemic circulation in a variety of critical clinical states. This is reliably established in sepsis and septic shock, although the interpretation of results by and large varies according to the methods used, the number and classification of patients examined, and the different PGs measured [4, 6, 14, 15].

Significant correlations exist between TX alone or in relation to other arachidonate derivatives and pulmonary and peripheral resistance, pulmonary and "peripheral" shunting (liver, kidney), bronchoconstriction, interstitial edema formation, intravascular coagulation, and selective or multiple organ failure. Systemic release of TX, however, is widely accepted as a toxic event. In addition to sepsis and septic shock, it sheds light on the pathophysiologic mechanisms of thromboembolic states including fat embolism, myocardial infarction, acute pulmonary hypertension, and organ failure after severe trauma. It is, therefore, a major challenge for the future to establish and introduce a TX antagonist with fewer side effects and more stability than those currently available.

References

1. Piper PJ, Vane JR, Wyllie JH (1970) Inactivation of prostaglandins by the lung. Nature 225: 600–604
2. Hyman AL, Spannhake EW, Kadowitz PJ (1978) Prostaglandins and the lung, state of the art. Am J Respir Dis 117: 11–136
3. Frölich JL, Ogletree M, Peskar BA, Brigham KL (1980) Pulmonary hypertension correlated to pulmonary thromboxane synthesis. In: Samuelsson B, Ramwell PW, Paoletti R (eds) Advances in prostaglandin and thromboxane research. Raven, New York, pp745–750
4. Oettinger WKE, Walter GO, Jensen UM, Beyer A, Peskar BA (1983) Endogenous prostaglandin $F_{2\alpha}$ in the hyperdynamic state of severe sepsis in man. Br J Surg 70: 237–239
5. Peskar BA, Anhut A, Kröner EE, Peskar BM (1975) Development, specificity and some applications of radioimmunoassays for prostaglandins and related compounds. In: Tillement JP (ed) Advances in pharmacology and therapeutics. Pergamon, Oxford, pp 275–286
6. Oettinger W, Peskar BA, Beger HG (1987) Profiles of endogenous prostaglandin $F_{2\alpha}$ ($PGF_{2\alpha}$), thromboxane A_2 (TXA_2) and prostacyclin (PGI_2) with regard to cardiovascular and organ functions in early septic shock in man. Eur Surg Res 19: 65–77
7. Gruber UF (1982) Prevention of fatal postoperative pulmonary embolism by heparin dihydroergotamine or dextran 70. Br J Surg 69: 54–58
8. Hirsch PD, Hillis CD, Campbell WD, Firth BG, Willerson JT (1981) Release of prostaglandins and thromboxane into the coronary circulation in patients with ischemic heart disease. N Engl J Med 304: 685–689
9. Lewy RI, Weiner L, Walinsky P, Lefer AM, Silver MJ, Smith JB (1980) Thromboxane release during pacing-induced angina pectoris: possible vasoconstrictor influence on the coronary vasculature. Circulation 61: 1165–1168
10. Myers AK, Ramwell PW (1985) Thromboxane in sudden death. In: Neri GG, McGiff JC, Paoletti R, Born GVR (eds) Advances in prostaglandin, thromboxane and leukotriene research, Raven, New York, pp 81–88

11. Preston FE, Whipps S, Jackson CA, French AJ, Wyld PJ, Stoddard J (1981) Inhibition of prostacyclin and platelet thromboxane A_2 after low-dose aspirin. N Engl J Med 304: 76–79
12. Alexander HR, Thompson WR, Ramwell PW, Fletcher JR (1985) Urinary thromboxane (TXA_2) reflects the response to tissue injury in humans. Curr Surg 42: 18–20
13. Foegh ML, Winchester JF, Zmudka M, Helfrich GB, Ramwell PW, Schreiner GE (1982) Aspirin inhibition of thromboxane release in thrombosis and renal transplant rejection. Lancet ii: 48–49
14. Reines HD, Haluschka PV, Cook JA, Wise VC, Rambo V (1982) Plasma thromboxane concentrations are raised in patients dying with septic shock. Lancet 2: 174–175
15. Hechtman HB, Huval WV, Mathieson MA, Stemp LI, Valeri CR, Shepro D (1983) Prostaglandin and thromboxane mediation of cardiopulmonary failure. Surg Clin North Am 63: 263–283

New Perspectives in Resuscitation and Prevention of Multiple Organ System Failure

U. Kreimeier, and K. Messmer

As result of improved primary care, fewer patients suffering from trauma, multiple injuries, or forms of shock will succumb within the first hours except those presenting with lethal injuries to the vital organs. One-half of the deaths among trauma victims occur within 1 h after injury and are due to rapid hemorrhage or CNS trauma [26]. As a consequence of vigorous and rapid resuscitation and volume substitution many trauma patients survive the initial critical hours and appear to be in a stable reconvalescent condition. With time, however, dysfunction of one or several of their organs becomes apparent and they are prone to die from the primary complications of trauma in sepsis and multiple organ failure [2, 6, 9]. Deterioration of organ function sequentially involves the lung, liver, and cardiovascular system, followed by blood, central nervous system, kidneys, and gastrointestinal tract [10].

Development of Multiple Organ Failure

To explain the pathogenesis of multiple organ system failure after trauma and/or shock the following hypotheses have been forwarded:

1. Patients after severe injury or major surgery suffer from reduced blood supply to the intestine, allowing microorganisms to enter the systemic circulation, which results in bacteremia, endotoxinemia, and eventually sepsis and septic shock [3].
2. Bacteria invade lung, liver, and kidneys, where they activate macrophages and monocytes to release interleukin-I, a small peptide known to have the potential to affect the function of most organs and tissues [4, 8].
3. Multiple organ failure is the result of a general activation of the immune system [10, 6].
4. Local ischemia and local reperfusion trigger the adherence of leukocytes to the endothelial surface, the release of oxygen free radicals, and the generation of mediators, which in turn activate the cascade systems, i.e., the arachidonic acid pathway, complement, and coagulation system [17, 19, 22].

According to the last hypothesis, the efficacy of primary volume therapy can not be adequately judged from the restoration of the central hemodynamic parameters, because normal macrohemodynamics do not exclude the presence of severe maldistribution of cardiac output and the persistence of shock-specific impairment of the microcirculation. Moreover, it is known that damage of tissues and organs remote

Surgical Research:
Recent Concepts and Results
Baethmann/Messmer (Eds.)

from the injury is not exclusively the result of reduced nutritional blood flow and hence lack of oxygen, but that tissue damage is enhanced by reperfusion and reoxygenation following temporary ischemia [16]. One reason for this phenomenon is the generation of oxygen free radicals, which induce lipid peroxidation and thereby have the potential to initiate irreversible denaturation of cellular proteins. Reperfusion injury may partially be prevented by means of scavenging the radicals in the moment they are produced. Although this concept is theoretically attractive and persued by many groups, a more pragmatic approach consists in the prevention of long-lasting local ischemia by restoration of microvascular blood flow at the time of primary resuscitation.

Efficacy of Primary Resuscitation from Trauma

Baker et al. [1] have demonstrated that age, severity of injury, shock with systolic pressures below 80 mmHg, and duration of the shock are the most important factors for the outcome from multiple trauma. Concerning optimal resuscitation, agreement is limited to the priorities that ventilation be reestablished by ventilatory support and the circulating blood volume rapidly restored.

With regard to the ongoing controversy whether crystalloids or colloids should be used for primary volume therapy, it is surprising that systematic comparative studies of primary treatment modalities related to cardiovascular function and survival are sparse. Modig [20] carried out a prospective randomized study on severely traumatized patients and analyzed the relative effectiveness of dextran 70 versus Ringer's acetate to treat shock and to protect from trauma-induced acute respiratory distress syndrome (ARDS). In the group receiving dextran 70 the hemodynamics improved significantly faster and the preset systolic arterial blood pressure of 100 mm Hg was achieved after 110 ± 18 min (M ± SD); in contrast, the patients treated with Ringer's acetate required three to four times the amount of volume and needed 170 ± 40 min to achieve a stable hemodynamic status. Cardiac index of the dextran-treated patients was significantly higher and rose significantly more upon challenge with 500 ml of dextran 70 as compared to the patients challenged with 2 l of Ringer's acetate. During the post-trauma period, none of the patients in the dextran group developed ARDS, while five out of 17 patients in the Ringer's acetate group presented with ARDS in the 7–8 day post-trauma period. The author concluded that early aggressive shock treatment with dextran 70, followed by continuous dextran administration in the post-trauma period might prevent late complications such as ARDS.

In 1980, De Felippe [7] reported on the surprising effect of intravenous injections of hypertonic (7.5%) sodium chloride (100–400 ml) in 12 consecutive patients in refractory hypovolemic shock, who had failed to respond to vigorous volume replacement, corticosteroid treatment, and dopamine infusions. The hypertonic sodium chloride solution promptly reversed the shock in 11 of 12 patients. The immediate effects of the injections of hypertonic saline were a moderate rise in arterial pressure, the resumption of urine flow, and recovery of consciousness. These effects tended to persist for a few hours, during which the requirements for isotonic fluids were reduced by 90%.

The clinical use of hypertonic saline by De Felippe was based on the favorable effects the same group of researchers had observed in treating anesthetized dogs in

Table 1. Use of hypertonic-hyperoncotic solutions for primary volume treatment in hemorrhagic hypotension and hemorrhagic shock

Author(s)	Year	Species	Solutions investigated
Brooks et al.	1963	dogs	1.8% NaCl
Reinert et al.	1964	rats	1.8% NaCl
Messmer	1968	rats	1.8% NaCl, 3.8% NaCl, 20% mannit, 21.6% glucose, 20% sorbit/10% rheomacrodex
De Felippe et al.	1980	humans[α]	7.5% NaCl
Velasco et al.	1980	dogs	7.5% NaCl, 0.9% NaCl
Lopes et al.	1981	dogs	7.5% NaCl
Nakayama et al.	1984	sheep	7.5% NaCl, 0.9% NaCl
Smith et al.	1985	sheep	2400 mosmol/l of: NaCl, $NaHCO_3$, NaCl/sodium acetate, NaCl/mannitol, NaCl/6% dextran 70, glucose
Rocha-e-Silva et al.	1986	dogs	7.5% NaCl, 50% glucose
Kramer et al.	1986	sheep	7.5% NaCl, 6% dextran 70
Maningas et al.	1986	pigs	7.5% NaCl/6% dextran 70, 6% dextran 70, 7.5% NaCl, 0.9% NaCl
Kreimeier et al.	1987	dogs	7.2% NaCl/10% dextran 60, 0.9% NaCl/10% dextran 60, 7.2% NaCl

[α] ICU patients in refractory hypovolemic shock

severe hemorrhagic shock [27] (see Table 1). Velasco et al. [27] investigated the effect of 7.5% hypertonic NaCl (2400 mosmol/l), given in small amounts, namely 10% of the total volume loss (shed blood volume). Blood pressure and acid base equilibrium were rapidly restored towards normal and long-term survival was 100%. These authors found also that after infusion of highly concentrated NaCl no appreciable plasma volume expansion – measured by the Evan's blue dilution technique – occurred for at least 12 h; they concluded that fluid shift into the vascular bed played no essential role in the rapid cardiovascular response. In contrast, in an animal model on sheep, Nakayama et al. [21] reported that 10 min after injection of hypertonic saline (2400 mosmol/l) the increase of plasma volume amounted to more than twice the infusion volume.

The mechanisms discussed to explain the instantaneous and pronounced hemodynamic effects of hypertonic NaCl include an action on myocardial contractility, dilatation of preferentially precapillary resistance vessels, as well as an increase in circulating blood volume as result of an osmotically driven shift of fluid into the vascular compartments. Moreover, Lopes et al. [13] reported that in comparison to intravenous administration the infusion of hypertonic NaCl into the aorta resulted in only transient recovery of arterial pressure and cardiac output without long-term survival. Intravenous infusions after bilateral blockage of the cervical vagal trunks again produced only a transient recovery of cardiac output, with no long-term survival. These authors therefore concluded that the first passage of hypertonic blood through the pulmonary circulation and concomittant release of the vagal reflex is essential to provoke the full hemodynamic-metabolic response needed for indefinite survival.

Lateron, Rocha-e-Silva et al. [24] studied the distribution of cardiac output to various organs by means of electromagnetic flowmeters. Infusion of 7.5% NaCl as well as of 50% glucose increased renal, mesenteric, total splanchnic, and coronary flows independently upon blockade of the vagal trunks. When compared to normotonic saline the hypertonic NaCl solution allowed permanent survival, which appears to be related to the ability of hypertonic solutions to elicit a pulmonary reflex, which in turn induces muscular/cutaneous precapillary constriction. The authors suggest that by this mechanism blood flow becomes redirected into the viscera, where the hypertonicity produces an unspecific vasodilatation.

Already in 1963 Brooks et al. [5] had concluded from experiments on hemorrhagic shock in dogs that the favorable hemodynamic response and the increase in survival rate observed after infusion of 1.8% NaCl solution was due to the sodium ions in the solution; according to Reinert et al. [23] the ratio between sodium ions and water determines the efficacy of hypertonic saline (1.8%) in shock. In experiments on rats, in which the mean arterial pressure was lowered by hemorrhage to 30 mmHg for a period of 240 min, Messmer demonstrated in 1968 that the favorable response of hypertonic solutions (1200 mosmol/l) was primarily dependent upon the tonicity of the solutions but not upon the sodium ions: the survival rate was uniformly increased after i.v. application of hypertonic solutions of glucose, sodium chloride, mannit and sorbit-low molecular weight dextran [18].

Smith et al. [25] compared in awake sheep the duration of the initial circulatory effect of five different solutions, each having a tonicity of 2400 mosmol/l. They found that – compared to identical amounts of the other solutions – a single bolus infusion of 7.5% NaCl with 6% dextran 70 resuscitated sheep subjected to standardized hemorrhagic shock best, mainly because cardiac output remained at significantly higher values during the 3-h observation period.

Kramer et al. [11] demonstrated that after small-volume resuscitation with hypertonic/hyperoncotic saline dextran solution (2400 mosmol/l NaCl, 6% dextran 70) of sheep, the initial volume effect was prolonged and total volume requirements during the subsequent hours were reduced when only 4 ml/kg of this solution – equivalent to 10% of the shed blood volume – were infused. Maningas et al. [14] explored the effect of 7.5% NaCl given together with 6% dextran 70 in awake pigs: 96 h after the infusion 100% of the animals treated with 7.5% NaCl in dextran 70 were alive, whereas the survival rate of pigs treated with dextran 70 alone was 69%, with 7.5% NaCl alone 53%, and 13% only when 0.9% NaCl was administered.

Present Investigations

The preceding discussion of the findings in the literature has revealed that there is general agreement regarding the circulatory efficacy of hypertonic solutions; however, the operational mechanisms have not yet been identified. Moreover, no studies are available in which the effects of hypertonic solutions on the microvasculature have been studied and in which nutritional blood flow was quantified. We have therefore analyzed the organ distribution of cardiac output as affected by the infusion of hypertonic and hyperoncotic solutions in dogs during standardized hemorrhagic hypotension by means of the radioactive microsphere technique [12].

Method

Eighteen beagles, splenectomized at least 4 months prior to the experiment, were anesthetized by pentobarbital i.v. (20 mg/kg b.w.) and ventilated by means of a respirator (FiO_2 = 0.21). Within 10 min the animals were bled to a mean arterial pressure of 40 mmHg; this value was maintained for 45 min by means of a Servo-Control System. Then 10% of the shed blood volume (on average 38 ml blood/kg b.w.) were replaced within 2 min by the intravenous infusion of either (a) HHS – 10% dextran 60 in 7.2% NaCl ($n = 6$); (b) HDS – 10% dextran 60 in 0.9% NaCl ($n = 6$); or (c) HSS – 7.2% NaCl ($n = 6$). All animals received an identical volume (avg = 3.8 ml/kg b.w.) of 6% dextran 60 (Macrodex 6%, Schiwa GmbH, Glandorf/FRG) intravenously 35 and 45 min after volume resuscitation. Measurements were performed at control, end of hypotension, as well as 5, 30, and 60 min after primary infusion, including central hemodynamics, extravascular lung water content (EVLW; thermo-dye technique), concentrations of electrolytes, lactate, total protein, osmolality, and colloid-osmotic pressure (COP) in plasma, as well as systemic arterial and pulmonary arterial blood gas analyses. Regional blood flow (RBF) was measured by means of microspheres (15 μm Tracer Microspheres, 3M Company, St. Paul, MN, USA), with ^{141}Ce, ^{51}Cr, ^{85}Sr, and ^{95}Nb as radioactive labels. Approximately 3×10^6 microspheres were suspended in 6 ml saline and well shaken on a vortex mixer for 2 min; they were then injected with 10 ml saline into the left atrium over a 50-s period. Simultaneous blood samples were withdrawn from the inferior abdominal aorta and from the pulmonary artery at a rate of 3.28 ml/min (Harvard Apparatus Infusion/Withdrawal Pump, Harvard Apparatus, Soth Natick, USA); sampling started 10 s prior to the microspheres injection and lasted for 3 min (reference arterial and total venous blood samples).

At the end of each experiment the animal was killed by 20 ml potassium chloride injected intracardially, and 271 samples were taken from the following 11 organs for analysis of RBF: brain, heart, kidneys, adrenal glands, thyroid gland – measurement of the entire organs; and liver, pancreas, gastric mucosa, small intestine, colon, and skeletal muscle (average of five to thirty samples from the organs and m. rectus abdominis, m. adductor magnus, m. psoas respectively). Depending upon the anatomical locations the weight of the samples taken varied between 1 and 4 g. The estimated number of microspheres in these specimens had been calculated in advance to exceed 384 per specimen.

Because not all values revealed normal distribution, results are given as median values. The data were analyzed for significant differences (at the 5% level) using the nonparametric one-way analysis of variance according to Kruskal and Wallis and the paired Student's t-test corrected according to Bonferroni.

Results

Five min after the infusion (3.8 ml/kg b.w.) of both hypertonic solutions (HHS, HSS) cardiac output had increased beyond the initial control values (Fig. 1); peripheral vascular resistance was significantly decreased (HHS > HSS > HDS). Mean arterial blood pressure reached only 70 mmHg, corresponding to 60% of control, and did not

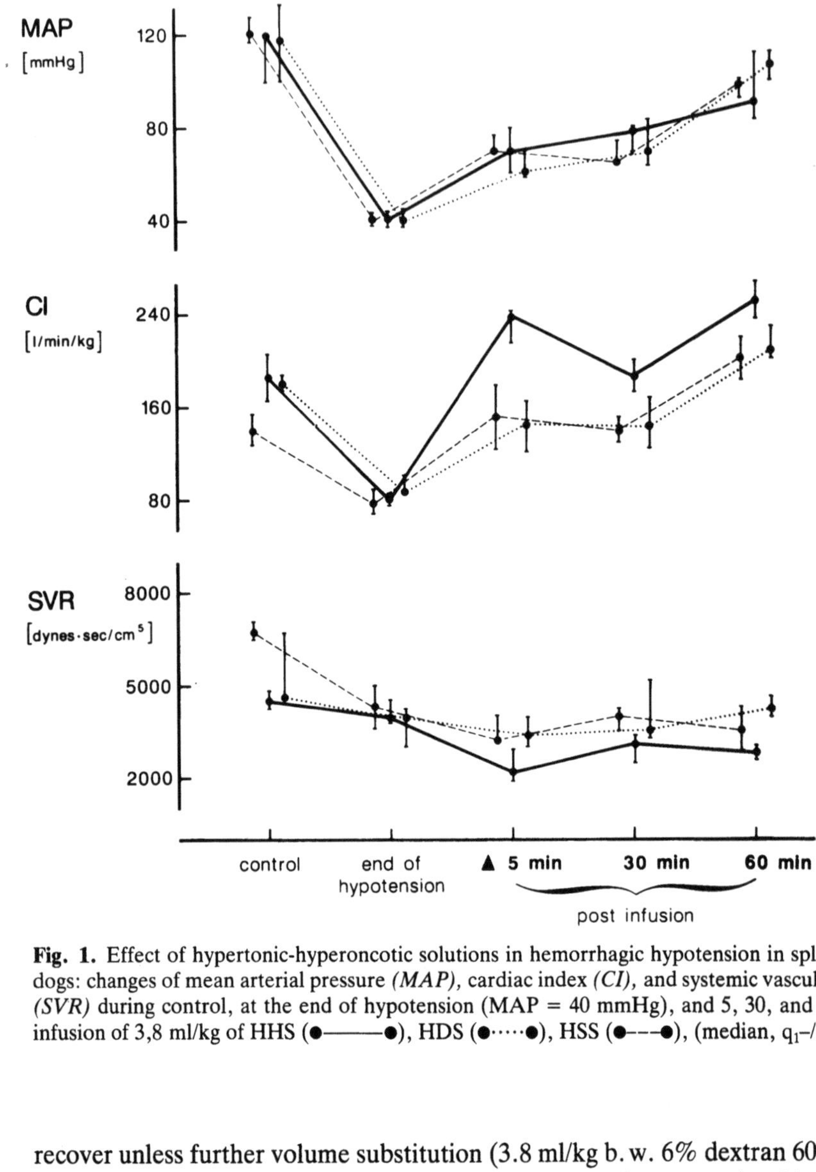

Fig. 1. Effect of hypertonic-hyperoncotic solutions in hemorrhagic hypotension in splenectomized dogs: changes of mean arterial pressure *(MAP)*, cardiac index *(CI)*, and systemic vascular resistance *(SVR)* during control, at the end of hypotension (MAP = 40 mmHg), and 5, 30, and 60 min after infusion of 3,8 ml/kg of HHS (●———●), HDS (●·····●), HSS (●---●), (median, q_1–/q_3 quartiles)

recover unless further volume substitution (3.8 ml/kg b.w. 6% dextran 60 each after 35 and 45 min) had taken place. Heart rate increased as a result of hemorrhagic hypotension and remained elevated after primary volume replacement in all groups; stroke volume index was highest in the HHS-animals (11.9 vs. 8.4 (HDS) and 7.9 ml/min/10 kg (HSS), respectively).

During the hypotension period the pulmonary vascular resistance had increased in some animals, but returned to normal upon volume resuscitation. The pulmonary capillary wedge pressure never exceeded 6 mmHg, and the extravascular lung water content remained in the control range of 6–8 ml/kg in all animals (Fig. 2). PaO_2 and the oxygenation index (PaO_2/FiO_2) did not significantly differ from control values after primary resuscitation with HHS, HDS, and HSS. At the same time the

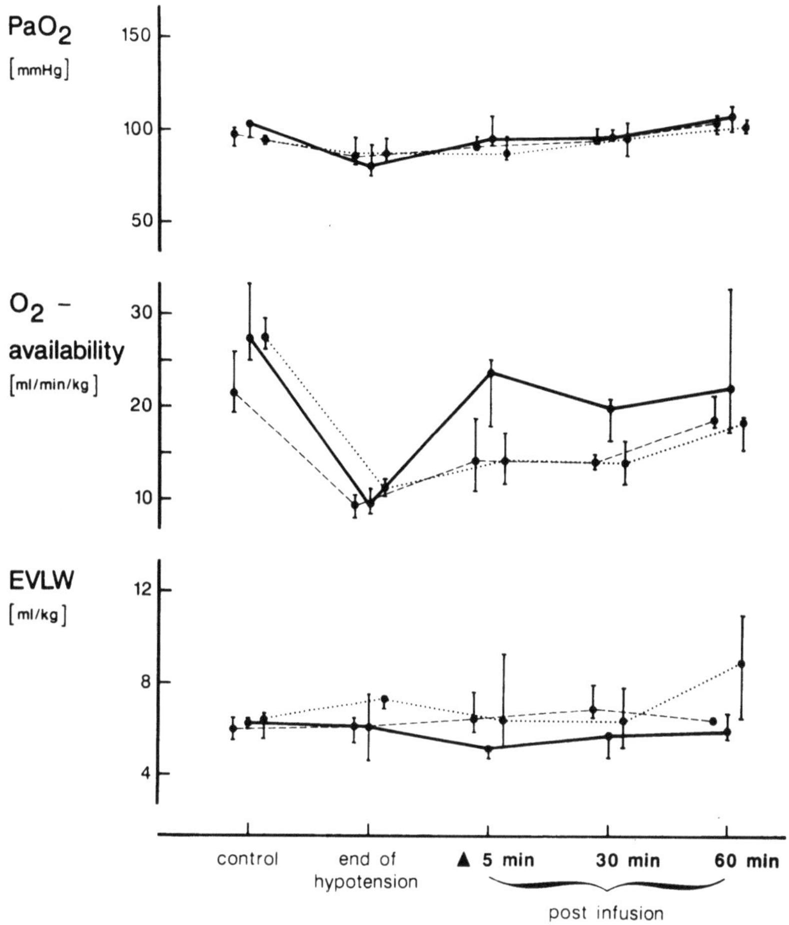

Fig. 2. Effect of hypertonic-hyperoncotic solutions in hemorrhagic hypotension in splenectomized dogs: changes of arterial oxygen tension *(PaO_2)*, oxygen availability, and extravascular lung water content *(EVLW)* during control, at the end of hypotension (MAP = 40 mmHg), and 5, 30 and 60 min after infusion of 3.8 ml/kg of HHS, HDS, HSS

peripheral oxygen availability was found highest in group HHS (24 ml/min/kg) and directly related to the high cardiac output achieved. While in these animals oxygen uptake increased after volume resuscitation, in animals receiving HSS or HDS it remained unchanged.

After primary resuscitation hematocrit in all groups had decreased by 5% and ranged between 20% and 25% for the rest of the observation period. The sodium concentration in plasma amounted to 149 (HHS) and 153 mmol/l (HSS). Colloid-osmotic pressure in group HDS was 19.5 cm H_2O and significantly higher than in animals of group HHS and HSS (15.5 and 12.0 cm H_2O, respectively). Until the end of the observation period plasma osmolality in arterial blood was significantly above control values in groups HHS and HSS (324 and 326 mosmol/kg, respectively). The concentration of lactate in venous blood ranged from 2.7 to 3.0 mmol/l, and slowly decreased after volume resuscitation without showing differences between the three groups. The concentration of total protein in plasma amounted between 2.40 and 2.95 g/dl at the end of the experiments.

At the end of the hypotension period, regional blood flow (RBF) had significantly decreased in all organs except brain, heart, and adrenal glands. However, just 5 min after infusion of the test solutions blood flow to the brain, adrenal glands, and colon had increased above control values, while the control values were reestablished in kidneys, small intestine, liver, and thyroid gland (Fig. 3). The most striking flow improving effect was found in the heart: myocardial blood flow was two to three times the control values. The highest flow values were found in the animals treated with HHS. Blood flow increased in all regions of the heart investigated.

In all three groups, blood flow to the pancreas and to the gastric mucosa remained diminished (30% –60% of control) and only slowly recovered with further infusion therapy. Upon infusion of HHS, HDS and HSS the blood flow to skeletal muscle increased and was significantly higher as compared to the control measurements (4.5–5.7 ml/min/100 g); this augmentation of muscle blood flow was most pronounced in animals receiving hypertonic saline.

After a 45-min period of systemic hypotension a redistribution of blood flow had taken place within the myocardium favoring the epicardium, as indicated by the decrease in the ratio of endo-/epicardial blood flow. Though this decrease persisted after primary volume resuscitation, blood flow to both the endocardial and the epicardial tissue was increased significantly in all groups. Cerebral blood flow was redistributed during hypotension, and the blood flow ratio of cerebral cortex/medulla remained elevated after primary volume replacement. In contrast, redistribution of intraorgan blood flow did not occur in kidneys, where the ratio of cortex/medulla blood flow did not change significantly throughout the whole observation period.

Looking at the fractional distribution of cardiac output (CO) it became evident that coronary flow was enhanced from control range of 3.1%–4.1% to 7.6%–12.0% of CO after infusion without any differences between the HHS, HDS, and HSS treated animals. At the same time, fractional cerebral blood flow significantly exceeded control values, while in kidneys, small intestine, colon, and liver the organ fraction of cardiac output returned to control values; fractional blood flow in gastric mucosa and pancreas remained significantly reduced despite volume replacement.

The total peripheral arteriovenous shunt calculated for 15-μm diameter microspheres had decreased during hypotension and remained low upon volume substitution (14%–20% of CO) without presenting significant differences between HHS, HDS and HSS.

Discussion

In our model of 45-min hemorrhagic hypotension (MAP = 40 mmHg) the cardiovascular effect of infusing hypertonic solutions (HHS, HSS) was predominantly related to the elevation in cardiac output, which exceeded control values. In contrast, after infusion of hyperosmotic solution alone, the increase in cardiac output was significantly less. Both central venous and pulmonary capillary wedge pressure (PCWP) increased only slightly after primary resuscitation; though mean arterial

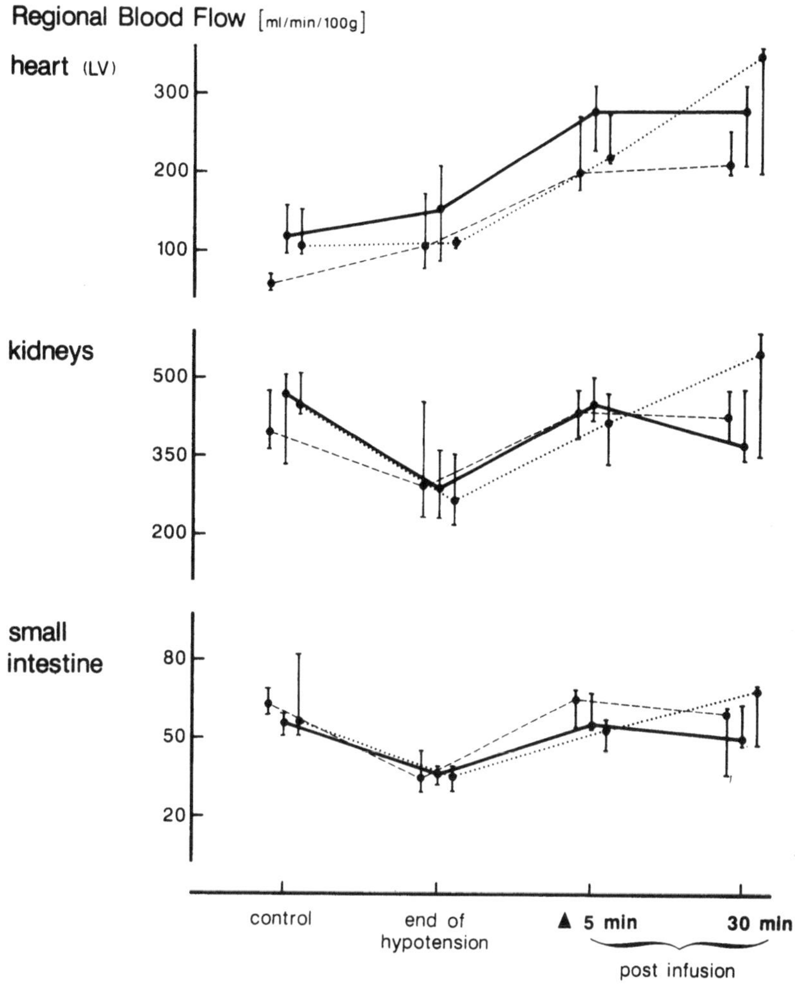

Fig. 3. Effect of hypertonic-hyperoncotic solutions in hemorrhagic hypotension in splenectomized dogs: changes of blood flow (RBF) in heart (left ventricle), kidneys, and small intestine during control, at the end of hypotension (MAP = 40 mmHg), and 5, 30 and 60 min after infusion of 3.8 ml/kg of HHS, HDS, HSS

pressure reached approximately 60% of control only, nutritional blood flow in all organs investigated – except the gastric mucosa and pancreas – returned to or even exceeded control values. Since the peripheral shunt was not significantly augmented upon infusion of hypertonic-hyperoncotic solutions, the high cardiac output became available for nutritional organ perfusion. In particular, high blood flow to the myocardium and hence high myocardial oxygen availability set conditions for high cardiac performance, a characteristic feature seen after infusion of hypertonic solutions. The immediate normalization of blood flow in both renal cortex and medulla facilitate resumption of kidney function and urine production. In contrast to Nakayama et al. [21], who found that cardiac output and heart rate increased while stroke volume remained constant, in our experiments stroke volume increased significantly without change in heart rate after infusion of hypertonic-hyperoncotic solutions. On the basis of their results obtained by means of electromagnetic flowmeters, Rocha-e-Silva et al. [24] concluded that precapillary constriction takes place in the musculocutaneous vasculature for the benefit of the perfusion of the viscera. Since we have not quantified blood flow to the skin – for methodological reasons the values for skin blood flow obtained from the microsphere technique are highly variable and lack good reproducibility – we cannot decide whether the hypertonic-hyperoncotic solutions have produced a shift of blood away from the skin in our experiments. From the pathophysiological point of view such a shift is unlikely because the skin is the first organ in which precapillary constriction takes place upon sympathetic stimulation due to hemorrhage. Consequently this mechanism should not contribute to a great extent to redistribution of cardiac output and restoration of blood volume upon infusion of hypertonic solutions.

Most strikingly, oxygen availability reached almost control values after infusion of HHS, even though the hematocrit was significantly reduced. From the estimated intravascular volume in beagles, which amounts to 82 ml blood/kg b. w., 38 ml/kg had been removed at the end of the hypotension period. Considering the decrease in protein conc. of 13% from control values until the end of the hypotension period, calculated intravascular volume amounted to 50 ml/kg b. w. As result of the infusion of 3.8 ml/kg b. w. of hypertonic-hyperoncotic solution intravascular volume would have been expected to increase to 54 ml/kg b. w. Since the protein conc., decreased by 20% of its value at the end of hypotension, an additional volume effect must have been provoked by the hypertonic-hyperoncotic infusion within 5 min. This should have resulted in an intravascular volume of 60 ml/kg b. w., i. e., 73% of control.

This calculated increase in plasma volume of 11 ml/kg b.w. is higher than that reported by Nakayama et al. [21], who found an expansion in average plasma volume of 8 ml/kg b.w. in sheep. Applying a mathematical model, Mazzoni et al. [15] described the osmotic shift of intracellular and interstitial fluid into the intravascular space following a bolus injection of a hypertonic-hyperosmotic solution. Their model predicts that blood volume is reestablished within 1 min after the addition of 7.2% NaCl/6% dextran 70 amounting to 1/7 of the lost blood volume. From these and our own findings we conclude that the cardiovascular mechanisms resulting in high cardiac output observed after small-volume infusion of hypertonic-hyperoncotic solutions involve an increase in myocardial preload following restoration of intravascular volume and augmentation of myocardial performance.

Future Aspects of Volume Therapy in Traumatic Shock

Initial volume therapy is the primary step for resuscitation of trauma patients. Apart from normalization of central hemodynamic parameters (arterial pressure, cardiac output), prevention of microcirculatory disturbances and local ischemia are the primary goals for effective treatment and prophylaxis of multiple organ system failure. Traditional solutions used for primary volume resuscitation require large volumes to achieve a stable hemodynamic status; moreover, large amounts of fluid are difficult to administer at the site of the accident and require exact monitoring of the patient to avoid the danger of fluid overload.

The excellent effect of small-volume resuscitation using hypertonic saline can be summarized as follows:

1. Rapid restoration of central hemodynamics is achieved by myocardial stimulation and an additional volume effect by fluid recruitment from extravascular compartments due to osmotic gradients.
2. The high cardiac output does not pass through arteriovenous shunts, i. e., the high flow is nutritional in nature and the blood supply to various organs is improved.
3. Simultaneously with the restoration of regional blood flow, peripheral oxygen availability is augmented despite a decrease in oxygen carrying capacity (decrease in hematocrit); it is highest after infusion of 10% dextran 60 in 7.2% saline favoring adequate cell metabolism.
4. Though only small amounts – 10% of the shed blood – are used, restoration of macro- and microhemodynamics occur within few minutes, reducing the risk of ongoing deterioration in cell function and thus the generation of oxygen free radicals and other toxic metabolites.
5. In addition to its superior effect on oxygen availability, addition of 10% dextran 60 to 7.2% saline solution will prolong the initial circulatory effect and help to stabilize the patient for transport and final clinical management.

Acknowledgement: The author thanks Mrs. Jutta Schulte, Roswitha Schwarz, and Karin Sonnenberg for skillfull technical assistance.

References

1. Baker CC, De Santis J, Degutis LD, Baue AE (1985) The impact of a trauma service on trauma care in a University Hospital. Am J Surg 149: 453–548
2. Baue AE (1975) Multiple, progressive or sequential systems failure – a syndrome of the "70"s. Arch Surg 110: 779–781
3. Baue AE, Guthrie D (1986) Moderne Aspekte des Multiorganversagens. In: Eigler FW, Peiper HJ, Schildberg FW, Witte J, Zumtobel V (eds) Stand und Gegenstand chirurgischer Forschung. Springer, Berlin Heidelberg New York, pp 66–72
4. Beisel WR (1986) Sepsis and metabolism. In: Little RA, Frayn KN (eds) The scientific basis for the care of the critically ill. Manchester University Press, Manchester, pp 103–122
5. Brooks DK, Williams WG, Manley RW, Whiteman P (1963) Osmolar and electrolyte changes in haemorrhagic shock. Lancet i: 521–527
6. Carmona R, Catalano R, Trunkey DD (1984) Septic shock. In: Shires GT (ed) Shock and related problems. Churchill Livingstone, Edinburgh, pp 156–177
7. De Felippe J, Timoner J, Velasco IT, Lopes OU, Rocha-e-Silva M (1980) Treatment of refractory hypovolaemic shock by 7.5% sodium chloride injections. Lancet ii: 1002–1004
8. Dinarello CA (1984) Interleukin I. Rev Infect Dis 6: 51–95
9. Fry DE, Pearlstein L, Fulton RL (1980) Multiple system organ failure. The role of uncontrolled infection. Arch Surg 115: 136–140
10. Goris RJA, te Boekhorst TPA, Nuytinck JKS, Gimbrère JSF (1985) Multiple-organ failure. Generalized autodestructive inflammation? Arch Surg 120: 1109–1115
11. Kramer GC, Perron PR, Lindsey DC, Ho HS, Gunther RA, Boyle WA, Holcroft JW (1986) Small-volume resuscitation with hypertonic saline dextran solution. Surgery 100: 239–247
12. Kreimeier U, Schmidt J, Brückner UB, Schoenberg M, Yang Zh, Messmer K (1987) Primary resuscitation using hypertonic saline colloid solution. Langenb Arch Chir (suppl): 329–332

13. Lopes OU, Pontieri V, Rocha-e-Silva M, Velasco IT (1981) Hyperosmotic NaCl and severe hemorrhagic shock: role of the innervated lung. Am J Physiol 241: H883–H890
14. Maningas PA, De Guzman LR, Tillman FJ, Hinson CS, Priegnitz KJ, Volk KA, Bellamy RF (1986) Small-volume infusion of 7.5% NaCl in 6% dextran 70 for the treatment of severe hemorrhagic shock in swine. Ann Emerg Med 15: 1131–1137
15. Mazzoni MC, Arfors KE, Intaglietta M (1987) Fluid shifts between endothelium, and intra- and extravascular compartments during hyperosmotic reperfusion in hemorrhage. Model analysis. Second international symposium on hypertonic saline resuscitation, Monterey Calif., Abstracts
16. McCord JM (1985) Oxygen-derived free radicals in postischemic tissue injury. New Engl J Med 312: 159–163
17. McCord JM, Fridovich I (1978) The biology and pathology of oxygen radicals. Ann Int Med 89: 122–127
18. Messmer K (1968) Die Wirkung hypertoner Lösungen bei Ratten im irreversiblen Schock. Anaesthesist 17: 295–299
19. Messmer K (1983) Traumatic shock in polytrauma: circulatory parameters, biochemistry, and resuscitation. World J Surg 7: 26–30
20. Modig J (1986) Effectiveness of dextran 70 versus Ringer's acetate in traumatic shock and adult respiratory distress syndrome. Crit Care Med 14: 454–457
21. Nakayama S, Sibley L, Gunther RA, Holcroft JW, Kramer GC (1984) Small-volume resuscitation with hypertonic saline (2.400 mosm/liter) during hemorrhagic shock. Circ Shock 13: 149–159
22. Parks DA, Bulkley GB, Granger DN (1983) Role of oxygen free radicals in shock, ischemia and organ preservation. Surgery 94: 428–432
23. Reinert M, Piroth M, Höer PW, Görsch H (1964) Morphologische Veränderungen an den inneren Organen der Ratte im standardisierten reversiblen und irreversiblen Schock. Virch Arch path Anat 338: 21–29
24. Rocha-e-Silva M, Negraes GA, Soares AM, Pontieri V, Loppnow L (1986) Hypertonic resuscitation from severe hemorrhagic shock: patterns of regional circulation. Circ Shock 19: 165–175
25. Smith GJ, Kramer GC, Perron P, Nakayama SI, Gunther RA, Holcroft JW (1985) A comparison of several hypertonic solutions for resuscitation of bled sheep. J Surg Res 39: 517–528
26. Trunkey DD (1983) Trauma. Sci Am 249: 20–27
27. Velasco IT, Pontieri V, Rocha-e-Silva M, Lopes OU (1980) Hyperosmotic NaCl and severe hemorrhagic shock. Am J Physiol 239: H664–H673

Histological, and Hemodynamic Alterations Produced by Progressive Ligation of the Pulmonary Artery Branches

F. A. SANGUINETTI, and N. SILVA

Introduction

Due to relatively low resistance, the vasculature of the lung is capable of tolerating marked increases in blood flow with virtually no pressure changes occurring in the pulmonary artery; at the same time, it maintains its capacity to carry out effective homeostasis.

Generally speaking, the lung has the capacity to tolerate a wide range of flow variations. These only lead to problems when flow values are extreme. High-flow states result in an increase in pulmonary capillary pressure, thus causing extravasation of fluid into the extravascular space, producing pulmonary edema. The latter was first described by Laennec in 1819, and later, in 1956, Visscher [15] coined the term. It was hypothesized that when a large section of the pulmonary vascular bed is occluded, pulmonary artery pressure increases, thus establishing a gradient in nonoccluded pulmonary veins with a hyperemic state and increased capillary pressure producing edema. Based on macroscopic observations, Ebert [5] in 1962 described the acute increase in pulmonary artery pressure and flow, followed by extravasation of fluid into the pulmonary parenchyma and the airway system.

The pathophysiology of pulmonary artery embolism is determined mechanically by the occlusion of the pulmonary arterial trunks. Anatomopathologic studies by Gorham and work by Sabiston [13], Broffman et al. [2], Lloyd [10], and Marshall et al. [13] support this theory.

Gibbon and Churchill [7] demonstrated that a 60% occlusion of the pulmonary artery is necessary before a decrease in systemic arterial pressure takes place. Del Guercio [4] measured the right ventricular pressure in patients with pulmonary embolism. Hyland [9] and Weidman [16] correlated large occlusions of the pulmonary bed with changes in pulmonary arterial pressure. While ligating branches of the pulmonary arteries, Ebert et al. [5] studied alterations in cardiac output and pulmonary vascular resistance, relating these to the decrease in functioning pulmonary volume.

The aim of this study was to describe the histological alterations in the pulmonary parenchyma caused by hyperperfusion of the upper left lobe as a consequence of successive ligations of the branches of the pulmonary arteries. We also wish to establish the relationship between changes occurring in systemic blood pressure, central venous pressure, and pulmonary arterial pressure while graduated degrees of occlusion are being applied to the pulmonary vascular bed.

Surgical Research:
Recent Concepts and Results
Baethmann/Messmer (Eds.)

Materials and Methods

Ten half-breed dogs weighing an average of 18 kg were anesthetized with pentobarbital sodium in alcoholic solution, and mechanically ventilated at a pressure of 15 cm H_2O with 100% O_2 at a frequency of 15 cycles per minute. Polyvinyl K-30 catheters were introduced into the carotid artery, superior vena cava, and pulmonary artery, connecting the first to a mercury manometer and the remaining two to water manometers. The right branch of the pulmonary artery, the left inferior lobar, and the middle lobar arteries were successively ligated at intervals of 15 min through a left thoracotomy. The pressure readings were made 15 min after each ligature. Biopsy samples were obtained from the left superior lobe 15 min after thoracotomy and 15 min after each of the three ligatures. These samples were studied microscopically following hematoxylin-eosin staining.

Results

Histologic Variations

The biopsy findings were grouped into four grades according to the severity of pulmonary edema present, 0 representing normal pulmonary parenchyma, and III severe edema (Fig. 1):

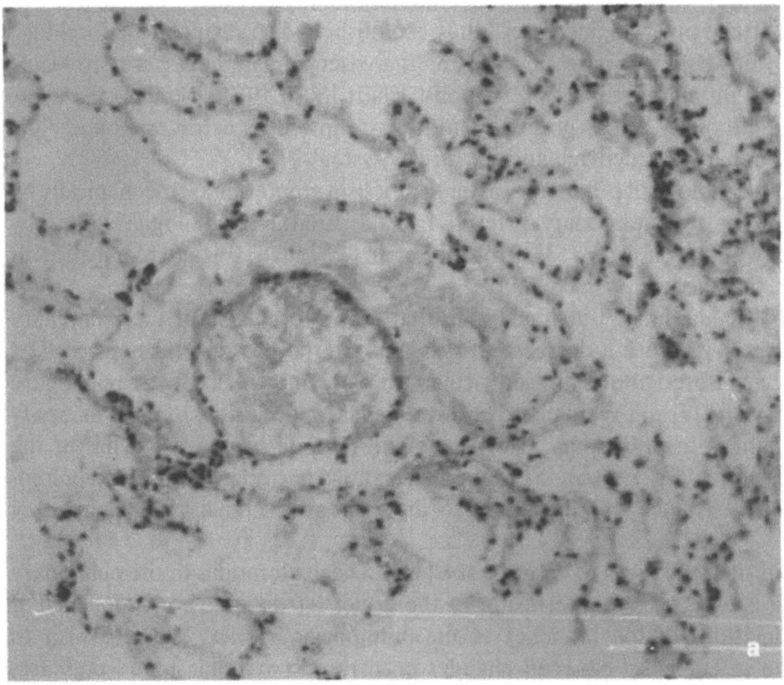

Fig. 1 a–c. Histological aspect of pulmonary edema of various degrees of severity. **a** Grade I (slight). **b** Grade II (moderate). **c** Grade III (severe). Note in particular the appearance of intraalveolar hemorrhages (hematoxylin-eosin staining)

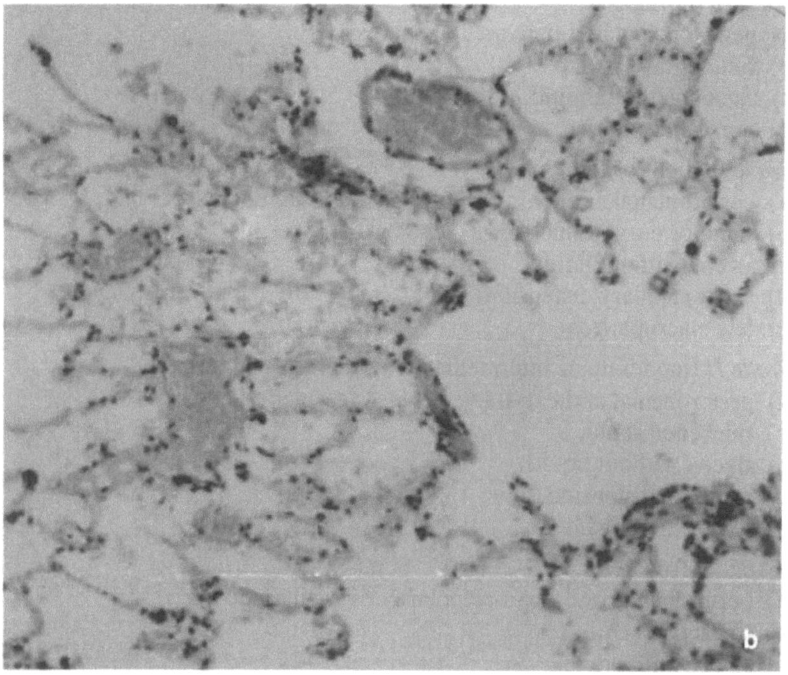

Fig. 1b

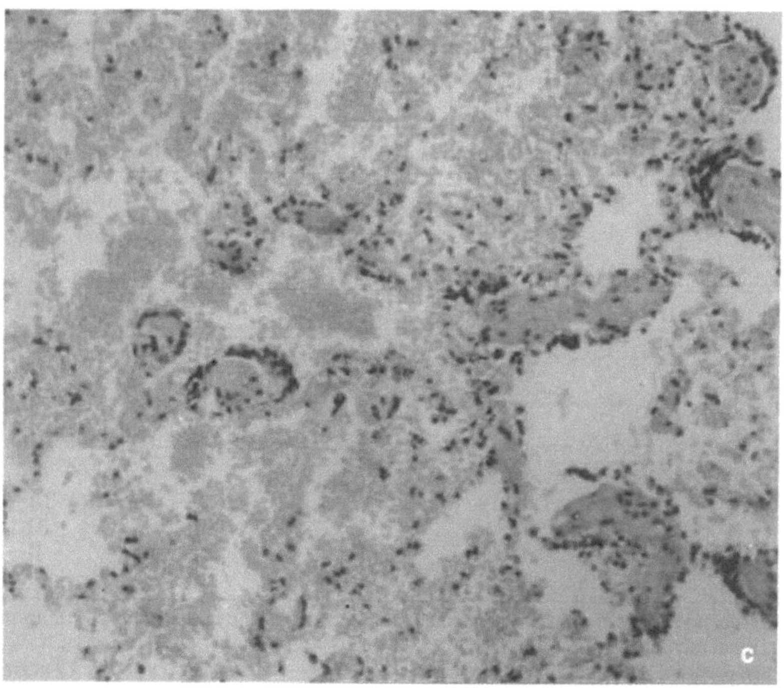

Fig. 1c

Grade 0 (normal).
(a) peribronchial and perivascular spaces,
(b) fine septa,
(c) alveoli without liquid,
(d) normal capillaries

Grade I (slight or initial).
(a) peribronchial and extra-alveolar perivascular edema,
(b) septa of normal thickness,
(c) alveoli without liquid,
(d) slight capillary distension, and
(e) few macrophages

Grade II (moderate or intermediate).
(a) peribronchial and extra-alveolar perivascular edema,
(b) thickened septa,
(c) alveoli without liquid,
(d) capillary distension, and
(e) some macrophages

Grade III (severe or final).
(a) peribronchial and extra-alveolar perivascular edema,
(b) thickened septa,
(c) alveoli with liquid,
(d) capillary distension,
(e) abundant macrophages,
(f) atelectasis, and
(g) focal hemorrhages

The degree of pulmonary edema caused by the successive ligatures in relation to the perfused pulmonary parenchyma is shown in Table 1.

Table 1. Degree of pulmonary edema caused by successive ligatures in ten half-breed dogs

Animal	No ligatures	Right pulmonary artery ligature	Left inferior lobar artery ligature	Left middle lobar artery ligature
	(PPP 100%)	(PPP 44%)	(PPP 24%)	(PPP 14%)
1	0	0	II	III
2	0	I	II	III
3	0	I	II	III
4	0	0	II	II
5	0	I	III	III
6	I	II	III	III
7	0	0	0	III
8	0	I	II	III
9	0	I	I	II
10	0	I	II	III

Degree of severity of pulmonary edema is represented by the numerals 0–III: 0, normal; I, slight; II, moderate; III, severe.
PPP, perfused pulmonary parenchyma

Table 2. Variations in pulmonary arterial pressure (PAP) with progressive occlusion of the pulmonary artery branches

Perfused parenchyma (%)	PAP ($cm\ H_2O$)	PAP (%)
100 (both lungs)	21.3	100
44 (left lung)	42.7	202
24 (middle lobe and left superior lobe)	58.6	280
14 (left superior lobe)	62.7	299

Pulmonary Arterial Pressure Variations

Table 2 shows the changes in pulmonary arterial pressure (PAP), in absolute (cm H_2O) and relative (%) values, which occur as the ligatures are applied.

In Fig. 2, the absolute values of PAP are related to the percentage of perfused pulmonary parenchyma. The relative values are used in order to eliminate the weight differences between animals: the initial PAP is regarded as 100%, and the results are expressed as percentages of this value.

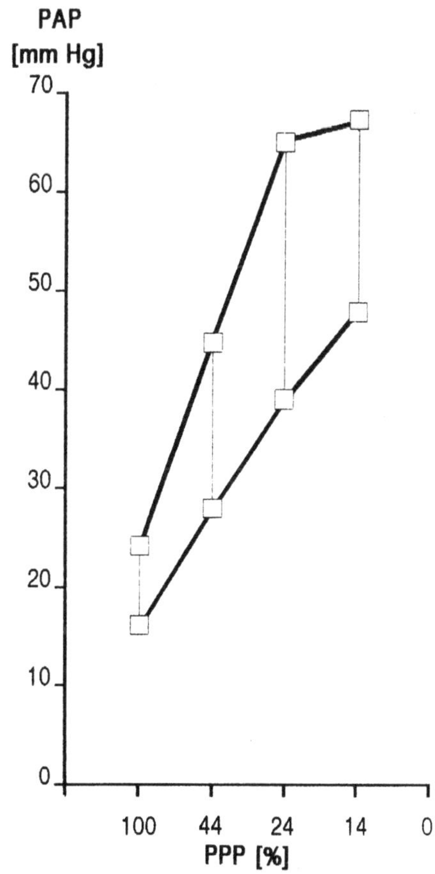

Fig. 2. Changes in systolic (*upper line*) and diastolic (*lower line*) pulmonary arterial pressure (*PAP*) as a function of the amount of perfused pulmonary parenchyma (*PPP*)

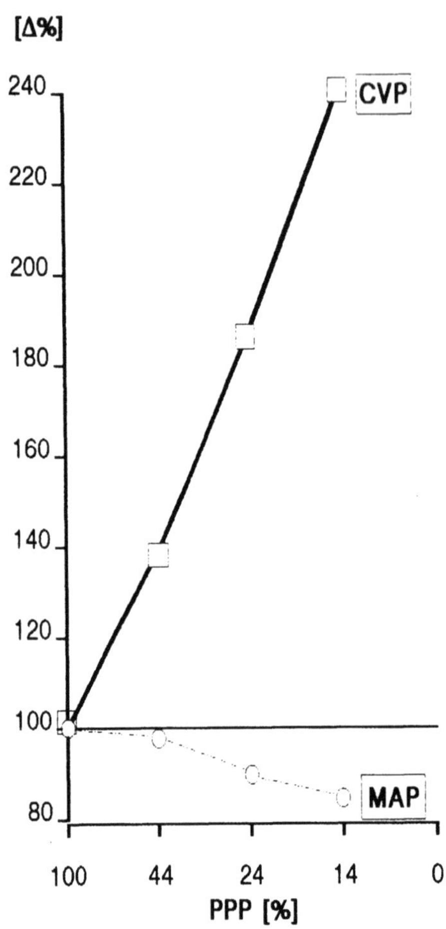

Fig. 3. Changes in arterial blood pressure (*MAP*) and central venous pressure (*CVP*), expressed as a percentage difference from control, as a function of the amount of perfused pulmonary parenchyma (*PPP*)

Variations in Systemic Arterial Pressure and Central Venous Pressure

The changes in these parameters are shown in Fig. 3, the data being presented as relative values.

Discussion

Analyzing our results, we observe that accumulation of liquid in perivascular and extra-alveolar peribronchial spaces differs in character from slight (grade I) edema and the characteristic thickening of the septa seen in moderate (grade II) edema. These two histological aspects, together with alveolar filling, comprise severe (grade III) edema. Progressing in severity from grade I to grade III, we observe capillary distension, atelectasis, macrophages, and the passage of erythrocytes into the interstitial liquid, with hemorrhagic foci. This would tend to imply that edema caused by hyperperfusion follows the same pattern as that caused by other etiologic agents.

Meticulous microscopic evaluation of carefully prepared histological preparations offers a semiquantitative measure of the edema present in the lung tissue. It is a reliable technique, particularly for detecting early accumulation of extravascular fluid, whereas other methods give little or no indication of interstitial fluid in these stages due to experimental, biological, or methodological variables. The weight of the lung is a good measure of pulmonary edema [6], and an increase of 4%–6% is observed prior to the establishment of histological alterations.

As indicated by Prichar and Herrheiser [7], although the difference between the three grades of edema is apparent in a histological section, these findings are not always uniform throughout the lobe. Actually, the edema first appears in the central regions of the lung, next to the hilum, possibly due to differences in ventilation and lymphatic flow. Therefore, the edema found in our biopsies is secondary to that in the center of the lung. However, pulmonary biopsies stand alone as an excellent example of both diagnostic and prognostic value in all aspects of pulmonary edema [1].

Ligature of the right pulmonary artery in the dog causes an increase in PAP, which in relative values reached an average of 202% ± 32.4% SD. This increase which we observed although it does not coincide with the findings of Hyland et al. [9] and Weidman et al. [16], is due to the fact that the still perfused lung tissue represents 44% of the total lung volume but receives the full output of the right ventricle. The right ventricle encounters a pulmonary vascular resistance increase by: (a) occlusion of the pulmonary artery branches in an open thorax, which diminishes the distensibility of the pulmonary capillaries due to the tendency of the parenchyma to collapse; (b) the necessity of ventilating the animal mechanically; and (c) ventilation with 100% O_2, which, according to Cropp [3], increases the pulmonary vascular resistance by venular or arteriolar constriction. Subsequent ligation of the left inferior lobar artery and the left middle lobar artery increased PAP to relative values of 280% ± 58.4% SD and 299% ± 51.9% SD, respectively.

Initially, the right ventricle maintains homeostasis through mechanisms of adaptation. Once these can no longer compensate, right ventricular insufficiency occurs, generally when PAP exceeds 40 cm H_2O. This right ventricular insufficiency manifests itself as an increase in pressure in the right cardiac cavities and central venous system.

In our experimental model, ligation of the right pulmonary artery branch resulted in an increase in central venous pressure to a relative value of 138% ± 56.8% SD. Following the ligature of the left inferior lobar artery and left middle lobar artery, the relative values were 182% ± 92.3% SD and 236% ± 108.7% SD, respectively. These figures represent a reduced ventricular adaptability to the successive increases in PAP.

We thus deduce that right ventricular insufficiency depends on: (a) the amount of vascular occlusion, (b) the stage of evolutionary development, (c) the previous condition of the cardiovascular and respiratory systems, and (d) the experimental circumstances.

According to studies by Racz [12] and Gibbon and Churchill [7], the systemic arterial pressure remains steady 15 min after ligation of the right pulmonary artery. Later, it diminishes progressively until it reaches a value of 88% ± 23% SD, when the perfused pulmonary parenchyma amounts to 14% of control. Hemodynamically the final outcome is cardiogenic shock, mainly due to right ventricular failure and impaired oxygenation.

Summary

Progressive occlusion of the pulmonary artery branches in the dog causes histologic changes as a result of hyperperfusion of the lung tissue in the nonligated lobe. Slight, moderate, and severe edema are subsequently observed, peribronchial at first, and then perivascular with thickened septa and fluid in the alveoli. Ligation of the right pulmonary artery resulted in an increase in PAP to 202% of controls. Subsequent ligation of the left inferior lobar and left middle lobar arteries led to a further increase in pressure, to 299%. The central venous pressure increased to 138%, 182%, and finally 236% following the above-mentioned ligatures. The right ventricle maintains homeostasis through mechanisms of adaptation until PAP exceeds 40 cm H_2O, at which time cardiac insufficiency finally occurs.

References

1. Ali J et al. (1983) Does increased pulmonary blood flow redistribute towards edematous lung units? J Surg Res 35: 188–194
2. Broffman B, Charms B, Kohn P, Elder J, Neuman R, Rizika M (1944) Unilateral pulmonary artery occlusion in man-control studies. Arch Int Med 73: 403–410
3. Cropp G (1965) Effect of high intra-alveolar O_2-tension on pulmonary circulation in perfused lungs of dogs. Am J Physiol 208: 130–138
4. Del Guercio L (1965) Shock and pulmonary embolism. Clin Anesth 2: 167
5. Ebert P, Algood R, Sabiston D, Jones H (1962) Hemodynamics during pulmonary artery occlusion. Surgery 62: 18–24
6. Fishman A (1972) Pulmonary edema: the water-exchanging function of the lung. Circulation 46: 390–408
7. Gibbon J, Churchill E (1932) Changes in the circulation produced by gradual occlusion of the pulmonary artery. J Clin Invest 11: 543–553
8. Gorham L (1961) A study of pulmonary embolism. Arch Intern Med 108: 8–22
9. Hyland J, Smith L, McLuire L (1963) Effect of selective embolization of various size pulmonary arteries in dogs. Amer J Physiol 204: 619–625
10. Loyd T Jr (1986) Pulmonary artery distension does not cause pulmonary vasoconstriction. J Appl Physiol 61: 745
11. Marshall R, Sabiston D, Allison P, Bosman A, Dunnill M (1963) Immediate and late effects of pulmonary embolism by large thrombi in dogs. Thorax 18: 1–9
12. Racz G (1974) Flujo sanguineo pulmonar en estados normal y anormal. Surg Clin North Am 54: 967–970
13. Sabiston D Jr (1976) Pulmonary embolism. In: Gibbon J (ed) Surgery of the chest, 3rd edn. Saunders, Philadelphia, p 595
14. Staub N (1974) Pulmonary edema. Physiol Rev 54: 755
15. Visscher M, Haddy F, Stephens G (1956) The physiology and pharmacology of lung edema. Pharmacol Rev 8: 389–434
16. Weidman W, Marshall R, Sheperd J (1983) Relation in dogs of pulmonary vascular obstruction and pulmonary vascular resistance. Lab Invest 12: 821

A Model of Experimental Silicosis in a Compressed Air Environment

F. KROMBACH, R. RONGE, S. HILDEMANN, E. FIEHL, A. WANDERS, D. BURKHARDT, A. ALLMELING, and C. HAMMER

In new tunneling technologies, compressed air is combined with shotcrete lining methods. During the construction stage, compressed air is used for the removal of ground water under certain geohydrologic conditions [1]. Since silicosis is one of the most striking occupational diseases among underground miners, the question arises whether a compressed air environment affects the development of silicosis.

Apart from oxygen, silicon is the most abundant element in the earth's crust. Silicosis, a chronic fibrosing disease of the lung, is caused by prolonged and extensive exposure to free crystalline silica (for reviews see [2, 3]). Free silica is the uncombined form of SiO_2, in contrast to silicates, which contain cations. Quartz, the most common of all minerals and a constituent of many rocks, is described as consisting of SiO_4 tetrahedra. In occupations such as mining, sandblasting, quarrying, and tunneling, workers are exposed to free silica.

The pathogenic mechanisms producing fibrosis in silicosis are poorly understood. However, serial interactions between silica particles, macrophages, and fibroblasts are the basis of current conceptions of the genesis of fibrosis (for reviews see [4, 5]). A hyperbaric environment might induce some effects on mechanical and physical factors in lung function: decrease in gas-phase diffusibility, decreased effective alveolar ventilation, high airway resistance during expiration and inspiration, and an increased tendency for lung airways to become choked during expiration [6]. These effects might lead to changes in the deposition of respirable dust particles as compared with normobaric conditions. On the other hand, the increased alveolar oxygen tension in a compressed air environment might have effects on free lung cells, e.g., the interactions between free silica and alveolar macrophages, finally leading to changes in the development of silicotic fibrosis. Thus, the aim of the project was to establish an experimental model of long-term exposure to both silicogenic and hyperbaric conditions in order to investigate the changes in relevant parameters in a longitudinal study. The parameters investigated in this study include the morphological and functional evaluation of free lung cells obtained by bronchoalveolar lavage (BAL), biochemical factors of the BAL supernate, pulmonary function, pathohistology, and radiological examinations. The present paper is a survey of the experimental design, the techniques applied, and some preliminary data concerning BAL constituents and lung function.

Surgical Research:
Recent Concepts and Results
Baethmann/Messmer (Eds.)

Material and Methods

Animals

Thirteen months prior to the start of exposure, 28 *Macaca fascicularis* monkeys (four male, 24 female) with a body weight of approximately 3–6 kg were separated into four groups. Previously, the animals had been kept in quarantine, dewormed, and tuberculin tested. In exposure-free intervals, the animals were housed in spacious stainless steel cages under natural daylight. A standard primate chop diet, additional fruit supplement, and tap water were supplied *ad libitum.*

Experimental Design

Following an acclimatization period of 6 months, control BAL was performed three times in each animal. After the start of exposure, BAL was carried out at intervals of 4 weeks. After 1 year, BAL intervals were 8 weeks [7]. Open lung biopsies were performed 12 and 18 months after the start of exposure. At various times, X-ray examinations and lung function tests were performed. After 28 months, the exposure will be terminated, and final cytological, radiological, and pathohistological investigations will be performed.

Exposure Conditions

The four groups of animals received an intermittent inhalational exposure regimen of 8 h/day and 5 days/week, except for public holidays and a 1-week rest following open lung biopsies. The animals were placed in open stainless steel cages, and the exposure took place in 7.5-m^3 capacity inhalational dust/pressure chambers. All chambers featured controlled climatic conditions (25 °C chamber temperature, 70% relative humidity). One group of animals (quartz-exposed group) received a time-weighted concentration of 5 mg DQ12 dust per cubic meter (Dörentruper quartz, particle size < 5 μm). A second group (quartz/compressed air group) was exposed to a concentration of 5 mg DQ12 per cubic meter and additional hyperbaric conditions of 2.5 atmospheres absolute (ATA). A third group (compressed air group) was exposed to 2.5 ATA. A fourth group of animals (control group) was sham exposed to clear normobaric air only. The density of airborne respirable dust was measured with a TM digital μP photometer (OEB H. Hund GmbH, Wetzlar, FRG). The photometer reading is calibrated in terms of mass concentration of respirable dust by means of a gravimetric respirable dust sampler [8]. In each chamber, the temperature, humidity, pressure, and concentration of respirable dust were monitored and controlled continuously (Fig. 1). Compression of the pressure chambers lasted 10–15 min. Decompression was initiated with a decompression step to 1.3 ATA within 10 min, followed by decompression to 1.0 ATA within 69 min.

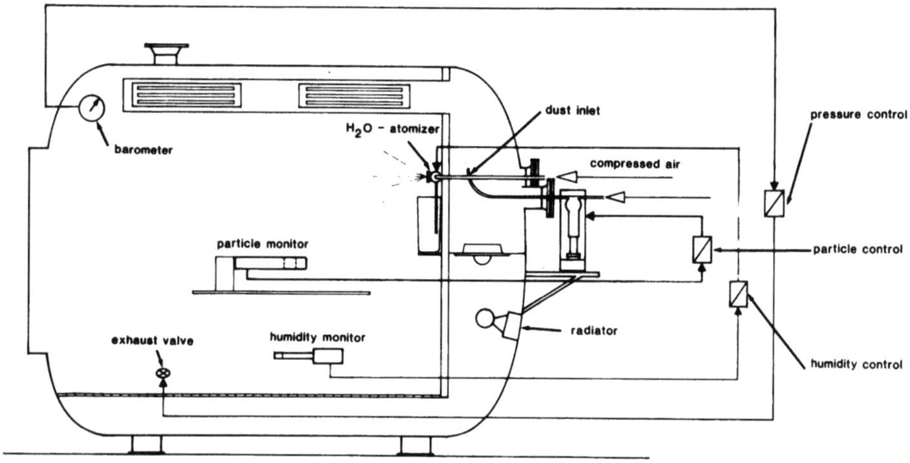

Fig. 1. Schematic illustration of the inhalational dust pressure chamber

BAL

For BAL, the animals were anesthetized with 15 mg/kg ketamine (Ketanest, Parke, Davis and Co., Munich, FRG) and 2 mg/kg xylazine (Rompun, Bayer, Leverkusen, FRG). With the animal in a supine position, a flexible fiber-optic bronchoscope (BF P10, Olympus, Munich, FRG) was wedged into the main bronchus of the left lung. Following instillation of 100 ml sterile 0,9% saline in aliquots of 20 ml, fluid was withdrawn, applying moderate suction. The lavage fluid was immediately filtered through sterile gauze, and the cells were pelleted at 300 g for 10 min. For some assays, the BAL supernate was examined in a fresh state. Otherwise, the supernate was aliquoted and stored at −70 °C for further studies. In addition, possible bacterial contamination was assessed in each BAL sample. The BAL cells were washed twice and counted with a Coulter Counter. Cell viability was determined by the trypan blue exclusion technique. Cytocentrifuge smears served to identify the cellular populations stained with May-Grünwald Giemsa, naphthyl acetate esterase, toluidine blue, and alcian blue/safranin. Three hundred cells were counted, and the percentage of macrophages, lymphocytes, neutrophils, eosinophils, and mast cells was determined (Fig. 2). In the BAL supernate, the activity of the cytoplasmatic enzyme lactate dehydrogenase (LDH) was measured with a commercially available test combination (LDH opt., Boehringer-Mannheim, FRG). Phosphatidylglycerol, the second major surface-active phospholipid, was determined with the enzymatic colorimetric PG-Numeric test (Isolab, Akron, USA).

Phagocytosis Assay

Using a modified assay originally described by Steinkamp et al. [9], alveolar macrophage phagocytosis was measured with a FACS analyzer flow cytometer equipped

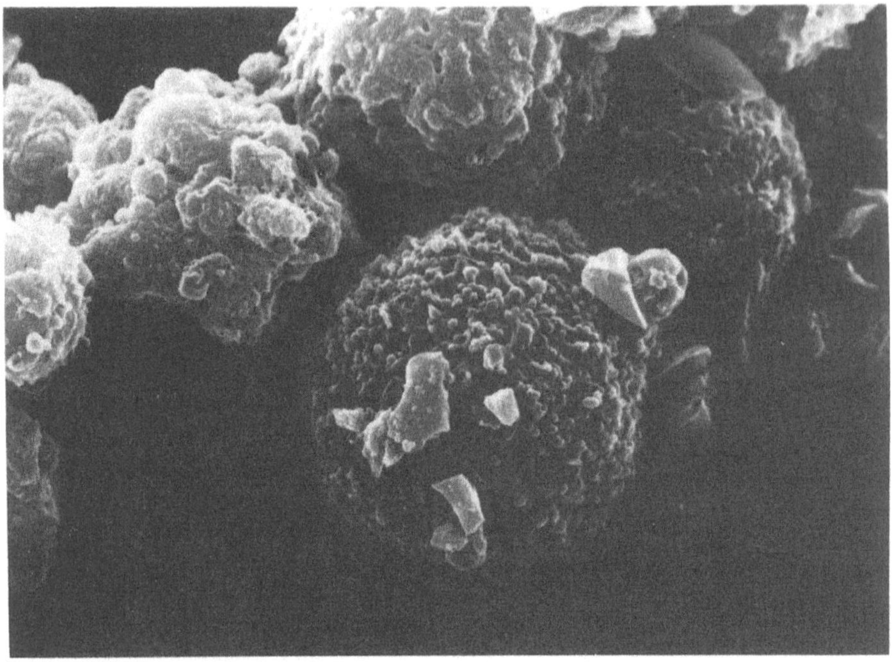

Fig. 2. Scanning electron micrograph of BAL cells, with quartz particles attached to the surface of an alveolar macrophage (original magnification × 3000)

with the Consort 30 Data Handling system (Becton Dickinson, Mountain View, USA). BAL cells were adjusted to a density of 1×10^6 cells per milliliter in phosphate-buffered solution (PBS); 5×10^7 fluorescent monodispersed polystyrene microspheres (1.91 μm in diameter) were added to 1 ml cell suspension. Cells and microspheres (ratio 1:50) were maintained in suspension using a shaker platform at 37 °C. After 60 min of incubation, the suspension was placed on ice for 5 min, washed twice, resuspended in ice-cold PBS, and measured immediately. Ten thousand events were analyzed for fluorescence, 90° light scatter, and volume at a flow rate of 120–150 events per second. Signals were displayed as volume/side scatter dot plots or fluorescence frequency distribution histograms. Using volume/scatter dot plots, alveolar marcrophages were characterized according to their volume and 90° scatter distributions. Fluorescence distributions of macrophage-phagocytized spheres were used to calculate the percentages of cells containing one to five spheres or more than five spheres (Fig. 3).

Chemiluminescence Assay

BAL cells were adjusted to 5×10^5 cells per milliliter in Ca^{2+}- and Mg^{2+}-free PBS; 200 μl cell suspension, 650 μl barbital (Veronal)-buffered salt solution and 100 μl (Lucige-

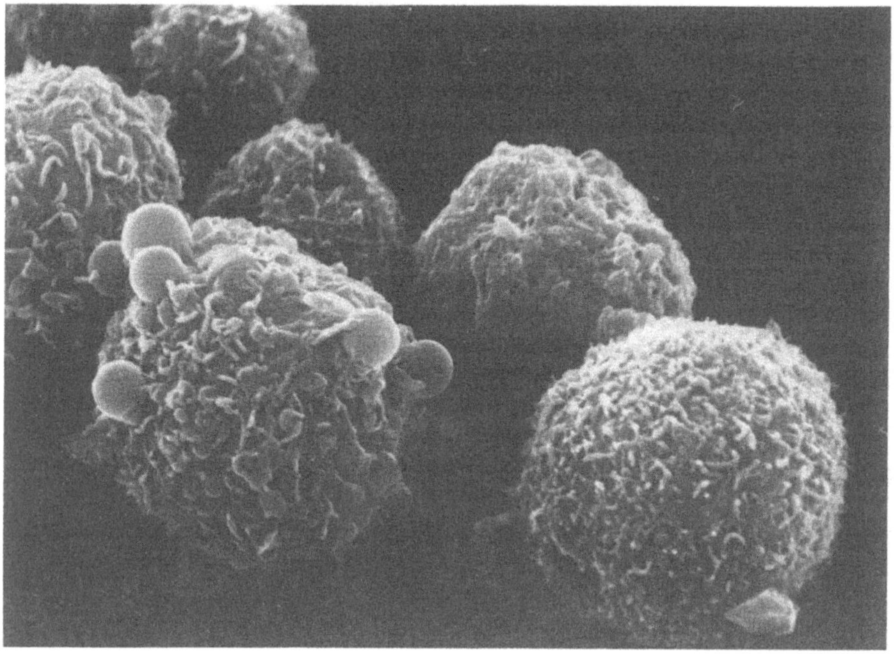

Fig. 3. Scanning electron micrograph of BAL cells with polystyrene microspheres (1.91 μm in diameter) attached on to and partly ingested by an alveolar macrophage (original magnification × 3000)

nin [10,10'-dimethyl-9,9'-biacridinium nitrate]), 1 μ*M*, Sigma, Munich, FRG) were placed in polystyrene vials. Following 10 min of incubation at 37 °C in the dark, the reaction was started, using either 20 μl phorbol myristate acetate (12.5 μ*M*, Sigma) or 50 μl opsonized zymosan suspension (12.5 mg/ml, Sigma). Photon emission was measured for 30 min in a six-channel Biolumat (LB 9505, Berthold, Wildbad, FRG).

Static Respiratory Compliance

To measure static pressure-volume curves of the lung, the animals were anesthetized as described for BAL and intubated with cuffed endotracheal tubes. Airway pressure was measured using a P23 ID Statham transducer. The animals were placed in a supine position and ventilated with an Engström ventilator at a tidal volume of 15 ml/kg. Prior to each measurement, the animals were paralyzed with 2 mg/kg suxamethonium chloride (Lysthenon, Hormon-Chemie, Munich, FRG), and the lungs were hyperinflated three times to a lung volume corresponding to a tracheal pressure of 30 cm H_2O. Following hyperinflation, the animals were allowed to exhale to functional residual capacity (FRC). Then the lung was inflated from FRC in stepwise volume increments of 20 ml up to a lung volume corresponding to a tracheal pressure of 30 cm H_2O using a Hamilton super syringe.

After each volume increment, breath was held for 5 s to allow airway pressure to stabilize. Pressure signals were recorded and plotted against volume increments. Respiratory compliance, obtained by linear regression analysis of the straight part of each pressure-volume curve, and inflated volume, taken as the mean increase in volume from 0 to 30 cm H_2O, were calculated for each animal.

Statistics

Results are expressed as means ± standard error of mean (SEM) for each parameter studied. Statistical significance was determined by the Kruskal-Wallis test, and individual group comparisons were made using the Mann-Whitney U-test. Differences with $p < 0.05$ were considered significant.

Results

The exposure conditions were tolerated well by all animals. No signs of indisposition were observed during compression, dust exposure, or decompression. The body weight of the animals did not change significantly during the observation period of (so far) 24 months.

Five months after the start of exposure, the proportional distribution of BAL cells was slightly changed as compared with baseline values. The percentage of alveolar macrophages was significantly ($p < 0.05$) decreased in the quartz-exposed group, whereas the percentage of lymphocytes increased (Fig. 4). However, the total number of BAL cells was augmented in the quartz-/compressed air-exposed group as early as 3 months after the start of exposure. After 5 months, this effect was apparent in both quartz groups, with higher levels in the combined quartz/compressed air group (Fig. 5). Chemiluminescence of BAL cells was significantly ($p < 0.05$) impaired as early as 1 month after the start of exposure in the quartz/compressed air group.

Following prolonged exposure of 22 months, no significant differences in the viability of BAL cells and the volume of recovered lavage fluid were observed between the four groups (Table 1). However, the total number of BAL cells and the percentage of neutrophils were markedly increased in both quartz-exposed groups. In addition, an increasing number of mast cells appeared in the BAL of both quartz-exposed groups. Phagocytosis of polystyrene beads was impaired in both dust groups, with significantly lower levels in the combined quartz-/compressed air-exposed group. A dramatic increase in LDH activity was determined in the BAL supernate of both dust-exposed groups. In addition, elevated levels of phosphatidylglycerol were found in the BAL of both quartz-exposed groups (Table 1). Respiratory static compliance was significantly ($p < 0.05$) lowered, from 21.8 ± 2.2 ml/mmHg in the control group to 13.6 ± 1.3 ml/mmHg in the quartz-exposed group and to 14.7 ± 2.2 ml/mmHg in the quartz-/compressed air-exposed group.

Both macroscopic and pathohistological evaluations of open lung biopsy samples revealed increased manifestation of silicotic granulomas, fibrosis, and quartz deposition in the quartz-exposed group as compared with the quartz-/compressed air-exposed group (M. Rosenbruch, personal communication, 1986).

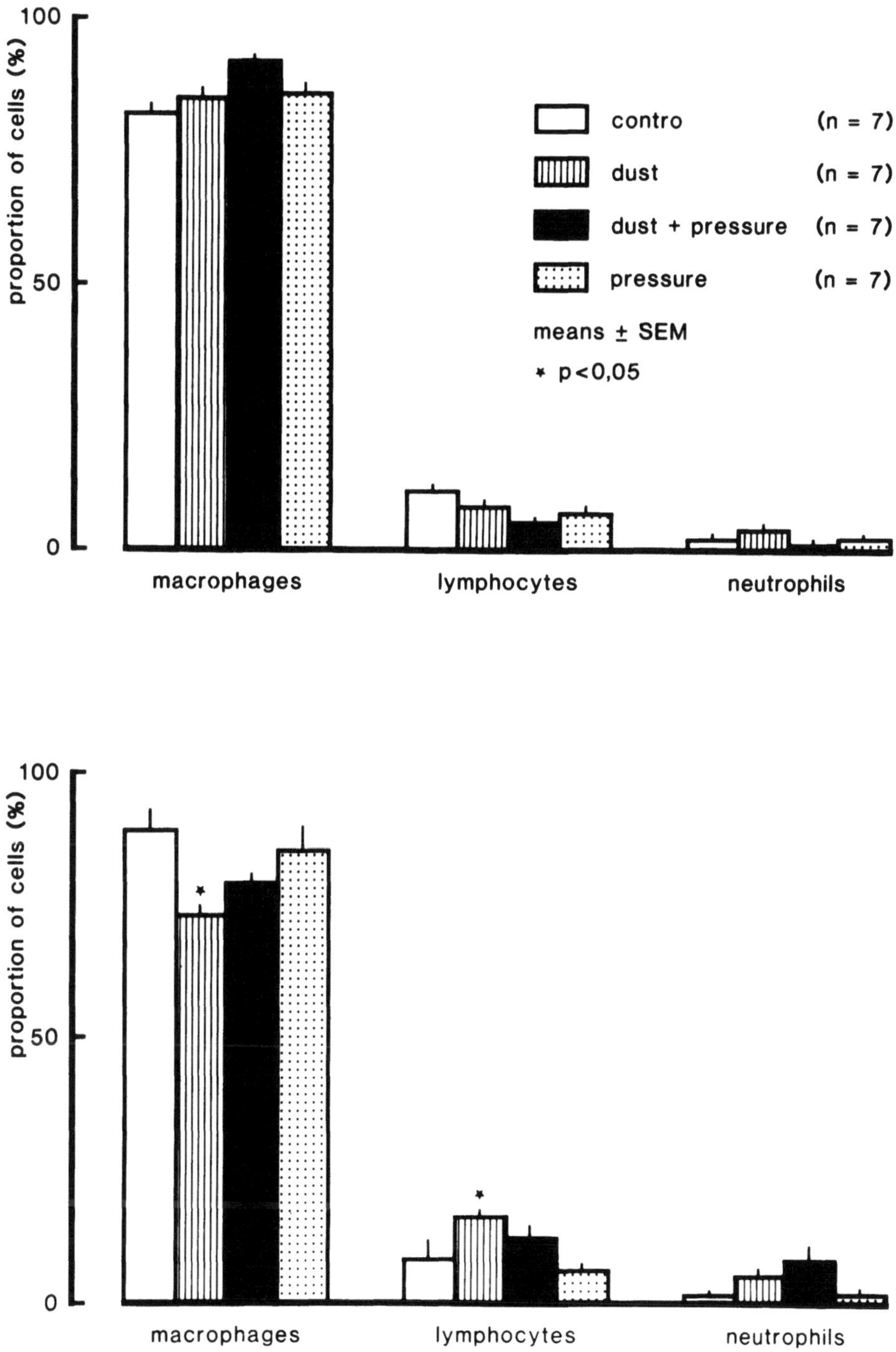

Fig. 4. Proportional analysis of BAL cell populations prior to (*top*) and 5 months after (*bottom*) start of exposure

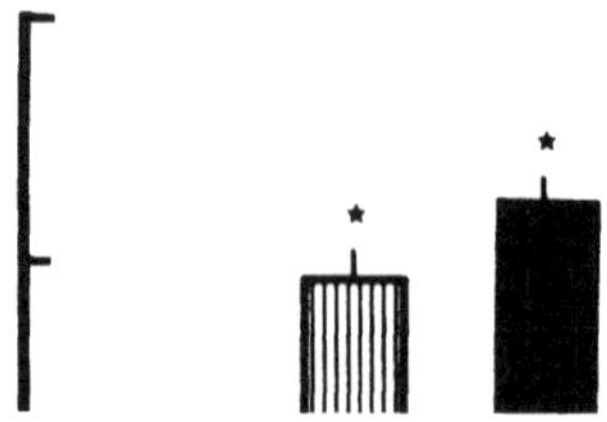

References

1. Distelmeier H (1981) Zur Anwendung von Spritzbetonbauweisen im Tunnelbau unter Druckluftbedingungen. In: Düsseldorfer Messegesellschaft (ed) Tunnel 81, vol 1, p 197
2. Ziskind M, Jones RN, Weill H (1976) Silicosis. Am Rev Resp Dis 113: 643–665
3. Stankus RP, Salvaggio JE (1985) The inorganic dust pneumoconioses. Clin Rev Allergy 3: 235–247
4. Davis GS (1986) Pathogenesis of silicosis: current concepts and hypotheses. Lung 164: 139–154
5. Reiser KM, Last JA (1986) Early cellular events in pulmonary fibrosis. Exp Lung Res 10: 331–355
6. Van Liew HD (1983) Mechanical and physical factors in lung function during work in dense environments. Undersea Biomed Res 10: 255–265
7. Krombach F, König G, Wander A, Lersch C, Hammer C (1985) Effect of repeated bronchoalveolar lavage on free lung cells and peripheral leukocytes. Transplant Proc 17: 2134–2136
8. Armbruster L, Breuer H, Gebhart J, Neulinger G (1984) Photometric determination of respirable dust concentration without elutriation of coarse particles. Particle Characterization 1: 99–101
9. Steinkamp JA, Wilson JS, Saunders GC, Stewart CC (1982) Phagocytosis: flow cytometric quantitation with fluorescent microspheres. Science 215: 64–66
10. Zimmerman BT, Canono BP, Campbell PA (1986) Silica decreases phagocytosis and bactericidal activity of both macrophages and neutrophils in vitro. Immunology 59: 521–525
11. Scheuchzengruber WJ, Eskew ML, Zarkower A (1985) Effects of prolonged inhalation of silica and olivine dust on immune functions in the mouse. Environ Res 38: 389–399

Table 1. Analysis of BAL constituents (mean ± SEM) following prolonged exposure to quartz and/or compressed air

	Group			
	Control n = 5	Quartz n = 7	Quartz and compressed air n = 5	Compressed air n = 5
Fluid recovery (%)	79.7 ± 1.1	81.4 ± 0.9	80.3 ± 0.9	82.0 ± 1.4
Viability (%)	74.7 ± 4.7	79.1 ± 1.8	79.3 ± 3.4	68.8 ± 4.6
Total cells ($\times 10^6$)	14.4 ± 1.9	70.9 ± 9.8[a]	72.0 ± 4.2[a]	5.6 ± 1.4
AM (%)	89.5 ± 1.3	69.1 ± 3.0[a]	69.8 ± 4.4[a]	88.0 ± 2.7
Lymphocytes (%)	5.8 ± 1.8	6.8 ± 1.0	9.0 ± 2.5	2.8 ± 0.4
Neutrophils (%)	0.3 ± 0.2	10.0 ± 2.3[a]	11.5 ± 3.1[a]	0.2 ± 0.2
Mast cells (%)	0.3 ± 0.2	11.6 ± 1.7[a]	9.5 ± 3.8[a]	3.6 ± 0.9
Phagocytic cells (%)	52.2 ± 7.6	35.0 ± 0.5[a]	21.5 ± 2.1[ab]	54.8 ± 8.5
LDH (units/liter)	1.3 ± 1.3	82.6 ± 23.0[a]	84.7 ± 9.1[a]	3.2 ± 1.1
Phosphatidylglycerol (μM)	3.0 ± 0.9	9.5 ± 1.2[a]	7.4 ± 2.2[a]	4.4 ± 1.3

AM, alveolar macrophages; LDH, lactate dehydrogenase
[a] $p < 0.05$ vs. control group
[b] $p < 0.05$ vs. quartz-exposed group

supernate. However, at the present stage of the study, a clear judgement cannot be made on the effects of compressed air on the development of experimental silicosis. Further investigations, which will in part be carried out in cooperation with other departments of our clinic or other institutes, have to be awaited. These investigations include the study of various soluble factors of both the BAL supernate and alveolar macrophage cultures, such as eicosanoids, interleukin (IL)-1, IL-2, and procollagen III peptide; the evaluation of X-ray examinations; scanning and transmission electron microscopy of BAL cells; detailed analysis of various parameters of lung function; and both the qualitative (histological) and the quantitative (morphometric) examination of lung tissue sections. In addition, in vitro studies on the effects of hyperbaric conditions on the interactions of free silica and alveolar macrophages should support the in vivo findings.

In conclusion, an experimental model was established for the development of silicosis in a compressed air environment, which allows the longitudinal study of cytological, functional, radiological, and pathohistological parameters during long-term exposure to silicogenic and hyperbaric conditions.

Acknowledgements. This study is part of the German BMFT grant No. 01 VD 492/7 and is being carried out in cooperation with the TBG (Tiefbau-Berufsgenossenschaft, Munich), Stuva (Studiengesellschaft für unterirdische Verkehrsanlagen e. V., Köln), the Medical Institute for Environmental Hygiene of the University of Düsseldorf (Director, Prof. Dr. H. W. Schlipköter), and the Institute for Occupational Diseases of the University of Munich (Director, Prof. Dr. G. Fruhmann). The authors thank Dr. G. Klima for scanning electron microscopy, Ms. G. Höbel for preparing the illustrations, and Ms. L. Rieder for typing the manuscript.

References

1. Distelmeier H (1981) Zur Anwendung von Spritzbetonbauweisen im Tunnelbau unter Druckluftbedingungen. In: Düsseldorfer Messegesellschaft (ed) Tunnel 81, vol 1, p 197
2. Ziskind M, Jones RN, Weill H (1976) Silicosis. Am Rev Resp Dis 113: 643–665
3. Stankus RP, Salvaggio JE (1985) The inorganic dust pneumoconioses. Clin Rev Allergy 3: 235–247
4. Davis GS (1986) Pathogenesis of silicosis: current concepts and hypotheses. Lung 164: 139–154
5. Reiser KM, Last JA (1986) Early cellular events in pulmonary fibrosis. Exp Lung Res 10: 331–355
6. Van Liew HD (1983) Mechanical and physical factors in lung function during work in dense environments. Undersea Biomed Res 10: 255–265
7. Krombach F, König G, Wander A, Lersch C, Hammer C (1985) Effect of repeated bronchoalveolar lavage on free lung cells and peripheral leukocytes. Transplant Proc 17: 2134–2136
8. Armbruster L, Breuer H, Gebhart J, Neulinger G (1984) Photometric determination of respirable dust concentration without elutriation of coarse particles. Particle Characterization 1: 99–101
9. Steinkamp JA, Wilson JS, Saunders GC, Stewart CC (1982) Phagocytosis: flow cytometric quantitation with fluorescent microspheres. Science 215: 64–66
10. Zimmerman BT, Canono BP, Campbell PA (1986) Silica decreases phagocytosis and bactericidal activity of both macrophages and neutrophils in vitro. Immunology 59: 521–525
11. Scheuchzengruber WJ, Eskew ML, Zarkower A (1985) Effects of prolonged inhalation of silica and olivine dust on immune functions in the mouse. Environ Res 38: 389–399

The Role of Surgery in Cancer Metastasis of the Lung: Results and Trends

L. SUNDER-PLASSMANN, H. DIENEMANN, and G. HEBERER

Until recently, the presence of lung metastases was generally believed to represent the final stage of a metastatic disease, in which the insignificant benefit from surgery would not justify its inherent risks [11]. Meanwhile, however, the benefit- risk ratio has changed dramatically, and furthermore, prognosis has been improved by chemotherapy. Today the final outcome of pulmonary surgery for lung metastases is dependent upon both total eradication of cancer tissue from the lung and the sensitivity of tumor cells to chemotherapy.

In the late 1950s, surgery of lung metastases was limited to either palliative resection in the presence of central necrosis and infection, bleeding, aspiration, and intractable pain or the elective resectional procedures in solitary or multiple lesions limited to one lung; a long disease-free interval from curative resection of the primary tumor was another precondition. In the University Surgical Clinic in Munich, only 36 patients met these criteria from 1955 to 1978, whereas since 1978, 186 patients have been operated on for the same reason, but on the basis of widened rules for indication (Table 1).

Prerequisites

Prerequisites for surgery of lung metastases today are: (a) the primary tumor must be resectable or controllable in a curative way; (b) extrapulmonary metastases must be

Table 1. Types of primary tumor in patients in whom resection was performed for metastatic lung cancer (University Surgical Clinic, Munich, Grosshadern). Compared with the few patients operated upon from 1955 to 1978 [8], 186 patients had resection from 1978 to November 1986 on the basis of widened rules for indications and as an adjunct to chemotherapy

Primary tumor	No. of patients	
	1955–1978	1978–11/1986
Hypernephroma	6	32
Testicular germ cell cancer	2	26
Colorectal carcinoma	3	23
Osteosarcoma	5	16
Breast cancer	2	12
Malignant melanoma	7	10
Others	11	67

Surgical Research:
Recent Concepts and Results
Baethmann/Messmer (Eds.)

excluded by computerized tomography (CT) scan or bone scan; (c) patients have to be at low operative risk, and surgical resection must be the most effective means to remove the lesions from the lung. Indications are given within or without a combined program of surgery and chemotherapy, surgery being sometimes only an adjuvant procedure between the chemotherapy cycles. In a chemotherapy program, the surgery indicated may be made up for histological exploration of (a) unrelated lesions that came up during or despite chemotherapy or (b) residual lesions showing partial remission in response to chemotherapy, which might consist of necrosis, mature tissue, or residual cancer. In primary tumors insensitive to chemotherapy [2], the aim and indication for radical surgery is – beyond histological evaluation – prolongation of survival and/or palliation in the presence of necrosis, infection, aspiration, bleeding, or pain.

Today, in contrast to the surgical routine some years ago, not only unilateral late solitary lesions but also bilateral multiple metastases appearing synchronously with the diagnosis of the primary tumor are operated on. Both indications have their special aspects [4, 5, 8–10].

The Solitary Lesion

A solitary lesion appearing years after eradication of the primary tumor may be the onset of a general manifestation of a hematogenous spread as well as a final sign of solitary invasion of tumor cells. The importance of the solitary lesion is relative because to date no diagnostic tool exists that would demonstrate all nodules present in the lung tissue: even scans in 4-mm layers usually do not detect a significnt number of lesions. Thus, surgical exploration usually brings out more nodules than are demonstrated in the CT scan [1, 3, 7]. Therefore, there is no real difference in the indication for a surgical intervention between the scan finding of a solitary lesion and that of multiple bilateral lesions. Also, with conventional whole lung tomography and CT scanning, in 1%–2% of all operations the surgeon will intraoperatively find a situation of miliary metastatic spread where tumor tissue eradication is no longer possible. Thus, the policy of "wait and see" for 8 weeks after detection of a nodule in the lung does not add information which could change the indication for surgery. Therefore, surgery is usually performed without delay. However, this does not interfere with the chemotherapy program for special primary tumors (e.g., osteosarcoma, testicular seminoma, or breast cancer), where the primary choice is chemotherapy. Chemotherapy should not be applied for a newly detected solitary nodule in these patients either, however, unless histological exploration of the nodule has proven its relation to the primary tumor.

Case 1

One year after radical mastectomy, a solitary nodule of 1-cm diameter was detected in the right lower lung lobe of a 67-year-old female. With no histological exploration, different chemotherapy modalities were applied without affecting the nodule. Its growth was carefully followed radiologically until it reached the size of an orange, at which time surgery could no longer be avoided. Resection of the lower lobe revealed on osteogenic sarcoma. It transpired that chemotherapy had been performed without careful evaluation of the histological report on the primary tumor removed in another hospital. Indeed, according to this report, the primary tumor was an unusual osteogenic sarcoma of the breast, insensitive to the chemotherapy regimen applied for 1 year.

Case 2

Six months after duodenohemipancreatectomy for adenocarcinoma of the pancreas, a solitary lung nodule was detected in the right upper lobe of a 64-year-old male, without further metastatic spread in other organs. Thoracotomy revealed a squamous cell carcinoma of the bronchus (pT 1, pN 0), and right upper lobectomy improved the patients chance of cure.

Multiple Synchronous Metastases

Sometimes, diagnosis of pulmonary metastatic spread precedes diagnosis of the extrapulmonary primary tumor. If the primary site can be resected and extrapulmonary metastases are excluded, resection is performed if no other effective treatment is available (hypernephroma [2], head and neck carcinoma, or soft tissue sarcoma). To date, there is no conclusive evidence that the number of metastases and the disease-free interval have any prognostic significance. Thus, resection is also performed in these patients without delay. In tumors sensitive to chemotherapy (e.g., testicular cancer), surgical resection is, of course, preceded by chemotherapy, and adjuvant surgery is performed to explore residual nodules. Especially in the case of testicular germ cell tumors under cisplatin-based chemotherapy, large pulmonary masses may disappear, leaving only residual nodules that have to be investigated. Necrotic tissue or mature teratoma is frequently found in these lesions, and adjuvant surgery helps to decide whether to continue or to stop chemotherapy in these cases.

Results

Operative Procedures

Contrary to radical tumor surgery in primary lung cancer, resection of lung metastases has to preserve as much lung tissue as possible. Wedge resection or enucleation is therefore performed in approximately 70% of all operations. Whenever possible, segmentectomy is preferred to lobectomy, and pneumonectomy is reserved for the exceptional case. The open Nd Yag laser system has already been applied in selected cases. In diffuse metastatic spread inoperable with conventional techniques, there seems to be a chance with laser coagulation of the lesions, without removing them. Our own experience in this field, however, is limited to two patients. A mortality from 1% to 4% is given in the literature for this type of surgery, with 1.2% in our own statistics for 186 patients [3–5, 7–10]. There is a tendency to perform sternotomy in all these patients, even when only unilateral lesions are suspected on the basis of the CT scan [3, 7, 10]. Routine mediastinectomy is also performed by some authors [10]. This, however, is followed by a higher mortality (4%) than occurs in the individual transpleural or transsternal procedure (approximately 1% [3, 5, 9]). So far, no conclusive data have shown any significant benefit from routine radical surgery (sternotomy plus mediastinectomy) as far as long-term survival or local recurrence of metastatic disease are concerned. In our own group of 56 patients presenting with bilateral metastases, only 32 have been operated on by sternotomy; in the rest, bilateral thoracotomy has been performed within a 10-day period, with a mortality of 0%.

Long-Term Survival

Overall 5-year survival rates of 25%–40% have repeatedly been reported [5, 7, 9, 10]. At first glance this may seem to demonstrate the overall efficacy of resection in those patients where an alternative therapy does not exist. In our own statistics, the cumulative 5-year survival rate according to Kaplan and Meier was 38%. However, because long-term survival is strictly dependent upon the histology of the primary tumor, overall figures can vary greatly according to the selection of patients with respect to primary tumors. Factors such as size and number of metastases, tumor doubling time, and disease-free interval can only be evaluated in terms of prognostic relevance when analyzed in a group *with identical primary tumors*. It is evident that a patient with a germ cell tumor highly sensitive to chemotherapy has a much better prognosis – even in the face of 20 synchronous, large bilateral metastases – than a patient with a malignant melanoma and only one small metastasis, with a disease-free interval of 1 year. To evaluate in detail the relative importance of secondary factors like number and size of metastases, the most important factor, i.e., the primary tumor, has to be taken into account, and long-term survival curves have to be calculated for identical primary tumors (Fig. 1). Testis teratoma with an 80% 5-year survival rate, has the best prognosis in our own statistics and in others [4, 5]. However, it still seems impossible to prove that surgery in these patients has any additional effect on long-term survival because no prospective data exist on chemotherapy without surgery in these patients. On the other hand, patients with malignant melanoma in our hands had a 2-year survival rate of less than 10%, and yet two patients in the group operated on before 1978 survived for more than 10 years. In the individual patient, it seems fair to expect prolongation of life from surgery in special circumstances, i.e., when surgery has removed the last source of tumor cells from the body; however, in the overall group, the life-saving effect of surgery for cancer metastatic to the lung has yet to be proven.

We have made a retrospective comparison of hypernephroma patients who all had radical primary tumor resection from the onset of lung metastases (Fig. 2). After 1 year, patients operated on for lung metastases ($n = 23$) seem to be significantly better off than the group of patients that refused surgery ($n = 36$); however, these data need to be supplemented. Surgery for lung metastases has proven to be efficacious in both the presence and absence of a chemotherapy program for the underlying primary

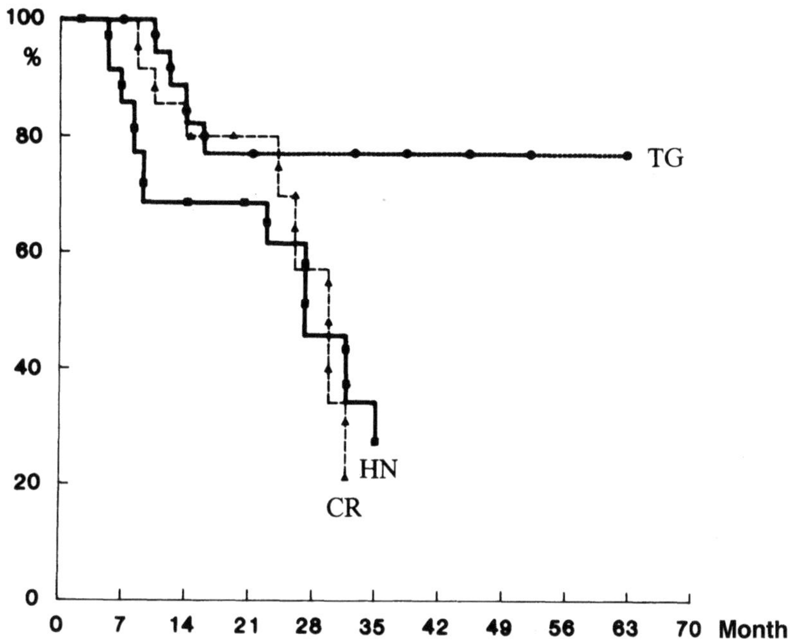

Fig. 1. Cumulative long-term survival rate (according to Kaplan-Meier) following resection of pulmonary metastases is dependent upon the primary tumor: for testicular glandular cancer (*TG*, n = 21), 5-year survival rate is 80%; for colorectal carcinoma (*CR*, n = 18), the 3-year survival rate is 20%; for hypernephroma (*HN*, n = 23), the 3-year survival rate is 26%. For *TG*, the mean survival is 64 months; for *CR*, 24 months; for *HN*, 28 months

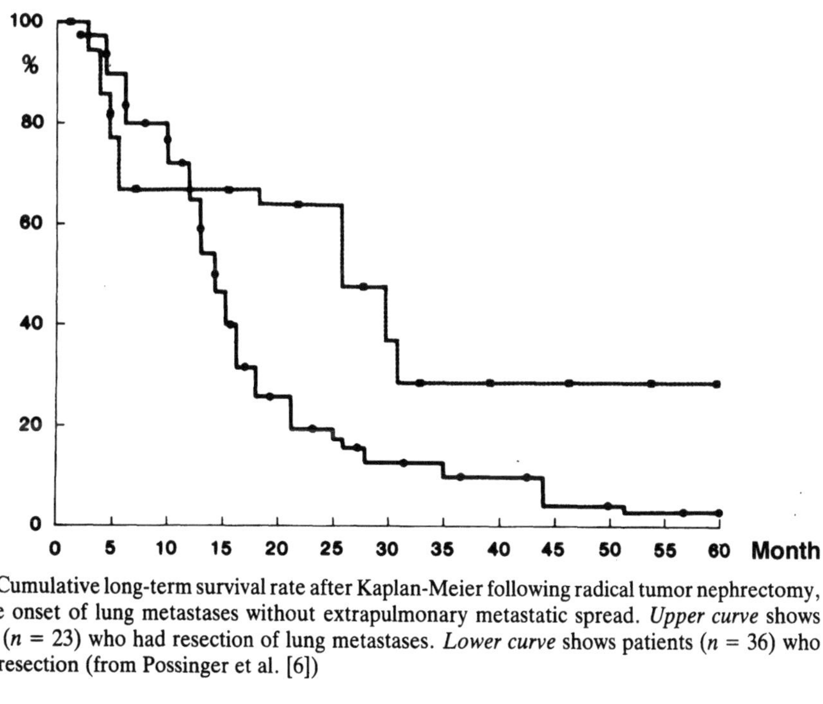

Fig. 2. Cumulative long-term survival rate after Kaplan-Meier following radical tumor nephrectomy, from the onset of lung metastases without extrapulmonary metastatic spread. *Upper curve* shows patients (n = 23) who had resection of lung metastases. *Lower curve* shows patients (n = 36) who refused resection (from Possinger et al. [6])

tumor. In the individual case, however, a prognosis of long-term survival is difficult to make since at the time of thoracotomy neither the surgeon nor the oncologist is able to say whether the lesions in the lung – be they solitary or multiple, large or small, unilateral or bilateral – are the initial signal of a general invasion and growth of tumor cells all over the body or the final manifestation of the last surviving tumor cells in a patient whose immune system has been able to stop further tumor cell mitoses.

References

1. Cooper JD, Nelems JM, Pearson FG (1978) Extended indications for median sternotomy in patients requiring pulmonary resections. Ann Thorac Surg 26: 413–418
2. De Kernian JB, Berry D (1980) The diagnosis and treatment of renal cell carcinoma. Cancer 45: 1947–1968
3. Johnston MR (1983) Median sternotomy for resection of pulmonary metastases. Thorac Cardiovasc Surg 85: 516–520
4. Mandelbaum J, Jaw PB, Einhorn LH, Williams StD, Rowland RG, Donohue JP (1983) The importance of one-stage median sternotomy and retroperitoneal node dissection in disseminated testicular cancer. Ann Thorac Surg 36: 524–527
5. Mc Cormac PM, Martini N (1979) The changing role of surgery for pulmonary metastases. Ann Thorac Surg 28: 139–143
6. Possinger K, Wagner H, Beck R, Staebler A, Schmid L, Vollmann B, Wilmanns W (1987) Prognosefaktoren beim Adenocarcinom der Niere. Rec Res Cancer Res (in press)
7. Regal AM, Hart T, Takita H (1982) Median sternotomy for resection of metastatic lung lesions. Abstracts XIV World Congress on Diseases of the chest, American College of Chest Physicians, Toronto, October 10–15, p 221
8. Stelter WJ, Sunder-Plassmann L, Heberer G (1983) Lungenmetastasen – Stellenwert der Resektion im onkologischen Therapiekonzept. Chirurg 54: 513–520
9. Sunder-Plassmann L, Ernst P, Heberer G (1986) Surgery of cancer metastatic to the lung: extended indications and results. Thorac Cardiovasc Surg 34: 82
10. Vogt-Moykopf J, Meyer G (1986) Surgical technique in operations on pulmonary metastasis. Thorac Cardiovasc Surg 34: 76
11. Vosschulte K (1962) Lunge. In: Hellner H, Nissen R, Vosschulte K (eds) Lehrbuch der Chirurgie. Thieme, Stuttgart, p 490

II. Novel Technologies in Surgery and Medicine

Extracorporeal Shock-Wave Lithotripsy of Gallstones*

M. DELIUS

Introduction

The history of extracorporeal shock-wave lithotripsy began in 1969. In the 1960s Häusler from the Technical University of Saarbrücken and Hoff from Dornier, an aircraft and technology company, had cooperated in investigating certain effects of high-speed phenomena. Häusler had shown a relation between the size of a body destroyed by shock waves and the duration of the shock-wave impulse. Hoff, on the other hand, had been working on the biological effects of shock waves. When considering practical applications of their knowledge, Häusler in 1969 conceived the idea of using shock waves for kidney-stone destruction, and in 1970 he was able to destroy kidney stones in a water-filled tube with a high-speed water drop [11]. As it was known from Hoff's previous work that shock waves can pass through body tissue, the concept of contact-free kidney-stone destruction was thereby born.

The concept of stone destruction itself was not new. The destruction of ureteric and vesical stones by electrohydraulic lithotripsy had been developed in the Soviet Union already in 1959 by Goldberg [10]. He had applied an idea of the physicist Jutkin from Leningrad who had destroyed plates made of china under water by electrical discharge. And vesical stones had been destroyed at the tip of a catheter which had to be in close contact to the stone surface. But the concept of Häusler and Dornier was different: the site of shock-wave generation was separated from the site of shock-wave action.

In 1973 Dornier approached the University of Munich for cooperation. In contrast to Häusler, who had the idea of a ringlike shock-wave generator, Hoff's group at Dornier had developed a different method of shock-wave generation, the electrode-ellipsoid system. Brendel from the Institute for Surgical Research considered the method useful only if shock waves were administered from outside the body without prior surgical intervention. Thus, the concept of extracorporeal shock-wave lithotripsy was realized for practical application.

Animal experiments for kidney-stone destruction were started with the Dornier shock-wave generator in 1975 at the University of Munich Institute for Surgical Research by Chaussy, a member of the institute at that time [3, 4]. These experiments were supported by the Bundesministerium für Forschung und Technologie. In 1980 the first kidney-stone destruction in humans was performed at this institute in cooper-

* Supported by Bundesministerium für Forschung und Technologie, Dornier GmbH, Germering, and Kurt-Körber-Stiftung, Hamburg.

Surgical Research:
Recent Concepts and Results
Baethmann/Messmer (Eds.)

ation with the Department of Urological Surgery [5] and in 1982 clinical routine began there.

Shock Waves for Gallstones

Destruction of gallstones was first considered in 1978 by Brendel [2]. The first question to be answered was, whether shock waves can destroy gallstones in vitro. Experiments performed at Dornier and at the institute confirmed this possibility. However, the degree of susceptibility of gallstones to destruction by shock waves varied widely.

To test gallstone destruction in vivo human gallstones were implanted surgically into canine gallbladders [1]. To improve visibility in the first experiments a T drain was implanted into the gallbladder with a subcutaneous reservoir for direct instillation or removal of contrast material. In the first dogs administered with 300–750 shock waves, stone disintegration was achieved in only 66%. After increasing the number of shock waves to 800–1200 this rate was improved to 90%. However, the size of the remaining stone fragments varied. In several animals these were fairly large; most animals had fragments in the gallbladder larger than 0.5 cm. These results were in contrast to those obtained in vitro.

This discrepancy between the in vitro and the in vivo results could be due either to insufficient shock-wave pressure in the gallbladder or to poor positioning of the stones localized by an X-ray system. The former possibility, however, was excluded by implantation of a pressure probe into the gallbladder, which confirmed pressures high enough to destroy stones. The latter, on the other hand, was a great problem. Stone disintegration could be followed by X-ray in the beginning, but the fragments then disappeared from the screen and could no longer be identified. Many shock waves were administered without observable target on the X-ray screen. There was no improvement of localization after removal of contrast material from the gallbladder via T drain or by administration of cholecystokinin. It was concluded that X-rays are not suitable for gallstone localization. Experiments on dogs showed ultrasound visualization also to be unsuitable. Ultrasound imaging was especially difficult, as the gallbladder slipped forward when the animals were placed in a prone position in the tub, thus covering the gallbladder by ribs. These problems were not encountered when small stones from human gallbladders were implanted into the common bile duct of dogs. Contrast material was administered via T drain; visualization was good and, thus, also the results.

The most serious side effect observed in dogs after gallstone destruction was pulmonary hemorrhage. This occurred at the diaphragmatic surface of the lower right lobe, which had presumably been in the high-pressure field of the shock wave. Although this did not cause clinical symptoms in the dogs, it was considered intolerable for application in humans. Therefore, the mechanisms leading to lung hemorrhage and the extent of hemorrhage expected in humans were studied. In separate experiments pressure probes were implanted into the pleural cavity between the lung and the diaphragm in dogs [9]. At various distances from the probe 1000 shock waves were administered for the study of hemorrhage at the site of probe implantation. The probes were positioned on two axes in relation to the shock-wave field: on the long

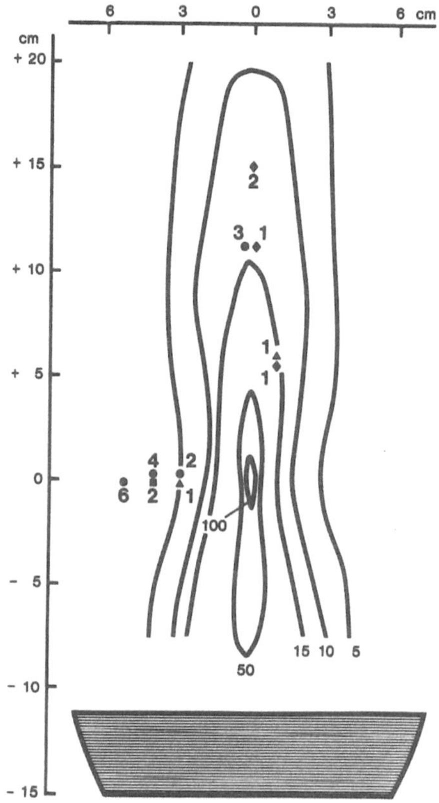

Fig. 1. Incidence of lung hemorrhage in relation to the shock wave pressure field. *Rhombi,* beagle with lung hemorrhage; *squares,* beagles withoug lung hemorrhage; *triangles,* boxer with lung hemorrhage; *circles,* boxer without lung hemorrhage. Pressure profiles were determined in water; pressure is given in Megapascal (MPa)

axis of the field and on a perpendicular axis through the second focus (Fig. 1). On the second axis lung hemorrhage did not occur at the site of pressure registration if the distance from the focus was 4 cm or more. At 3 cm hemorrhage was questionable. On the long axis of the field hemorrhage occurred even at 15 cm distance from the second focus. This distance correlated with the pressures registered, for pressure on the second axis was less than one-third of that observed on the long axis. It was concluded from this experiment that lung hemorrhage could probably be prevented in humans if the distance of the long axis of the shock-wave field to the lung was more than 3–4 cm. Other side effects after in vivo gallstone destruction were small hemorrhages in the liver and gallbladder wall; these, however, were not considered as a contraindication to use shock waves in humans.

As some gallstones were difficult to destroy by shock waves, a more powerful ellipsoid was constructed by Dornier, with the same performance at 15 kV as the earlier one at 20 kV. To test tissue damage by this ellipsoid in relation to that by the former one a separate experiment was performed. Three groups of dogs were exposed to 1500 shock waves, aimed at the same point of the gallbladder wall as earlier for study of tissue damage to liver and to gallbladder. Tissue damage caused by the new ellipsoid with 15 kV and that caused by the former ellipsoid were similar. In the high-pressure field of the shock wave the liver capsule was damaged and showed fibrinous deposits; in the liver parenchyma multiple small hemorrhages were seen. The gallbladder mucosa was focally destroyed, with thickening of the underlying wall. There was a slight increase of damage to the liver when using the new ellipsoid with 20 kV. It was concluded from this experiment that the use of 15 kV is advisable for the destruction of gallstones in humans.

The size of gallstone fragments destroyed by shock waves in vivo was varied and undefined. Autopsy had to be performed in the days following shock wave application. No data on fragment passage from the gallbladder could be obtained. In a separate experiment human kidney stone fragments of defined size were implanted into gallbladders of dogs [8]. Liver and pancreas enzymes were monitored in blood during the following 5 weeks as was the amount of fragments in the gallbladder. Approximately two-thirds of the fragments had left the gallbladder regardless of their size. Enzyme elevations in blood occurred significantly more often in dogs with a maximal fragment size of 4 mm than in those with 2 mm. Furthermore, papillary changes were detected in the former group. It was concluded from this experiment that stone fragments after gallstone destruction should be as small as possible, i. e., in the range of 2 mm.

In January 1985 the first patient was treated at the Institute for Surgical Research in cooperation with the Department of Internal Medicine II of the University of Munich. By July 1987 approximately 200 patients had been treated for gallbladder stones with extracorporeal shock waves. This number is still too small to draw final conclusions. Gallstone desruction by shock waves will be used extensively by the end of 1987, when Dornier will have installed gallstone lithotripters in more than ten clinical departments. Our goal is to make gallstone destruction comparable for the patient to a visit at the dentist: fast and, if necessary, repeated treatments on an outpatient basis.

Mechanisms of Shock Wave Action

Destruction of kidney stones by extracorporeal shock waves is the treatment of choice nowadays in the majority of cases, while destruction of gallbladder stones by shock waves is an alternative to conventional treatment for a subset of patients [13]. In contrast to the large practical experience with shock waves under clinical conditions, little is known about their mechanisms of action.

Two fundamentally different mechanisms are proposed: a direct action on the concrement and an indirect action through the surrounding medium. In the case of the former the stone is destroyed by pressure or tensile forces exerted in the stone after the wave has entered and which exceed cohesive forces. Reflection of the wave at the posterior stone surface may be particularly important here. In the case of indirect action, on the other hand, the shock wave may induce changes in the surrounding medium leading to stone destruction.

The second possibility was tested in an experiment with gallstones from the same gallbladder. The stones were placed into two different media with similar impedance. Since reflection of the shock wave at the stone surface depends on the impedance of the surrounding medium, the shock wave entering the stone is similar in both media. It was found that gallstones could be destroyed in one medium only. This clearly suggests that gallstones are destroyed by mechanisms imparted by the medium.The mechanism of stone destruction can hardly be explained in any way other than by cavitation, i.e., formation of gas bubbles in a fluid (cf. [7]). This mechanism can even damage hard metals. Cavitation is known to be produced by the lithotripter in water, as shown by the pitting of aluminium foils [6]. Cavitation is also observed by ultrasound.

In the liver, shock waves cause cavitation in vivo as observed by ultrasound. It can be seen in vessels, probably in veins. After several hundred shock waves a reflex from stationary air is observed in the high-pressure field of the wave. As tissue damage was observed in the same area, it is highly probable that this was caused by cavitation. Tissue damage in canine kidneys by shock waves was examined electron-microscopically [12]. Directly after shock-wave application, the capillaries and venular walls were torn, with extravasation of blood cells. There was no damage to tubular cells, or tubular structures. This suggests that cavitation occurs primarily intravascularly and/or interstitially but not in the cells.

Outlook

Further work on shock waves at the Institute for Surgical Research is concentrating on two major issues: on whether shock waves can be used for tumor therapy and on their biological effects. The effects of shock waves on tumor cells in vitro and on tumor growth in vivo are being examined. Since effects of shock waves on tumors are limited, studies for combination modalities are also under way.

References

1. Brendel W, Enders G (1983) Shock waves for gallstones: animal studies. Lancet I: 1054
2. Brendel W, Chaussy C, Schmiedt E, Eisenberger F (1979) Berührungsfreie Zertrümmerung von Nierensteinen – eine neue Therapie? In: Alexander von Humboldt-Stiftung (ed) Wissenschaftliche Zusammenarbeit und Austausch zwischen Deutschland und Japan. Bonn, pp 197–204
3. Chaussy C (1982) Extracorporeal shock wave lithotripsy, 2nd edn. Karger, Basel
4. Chaussy C, Eisenberger F, Wanner K (1977) Die Implantation humaner Nierensteine – ein einfaches experimentelles Steinmodell. Urologe A 16: 35–38
5. Chaussy C, Brendel W, Schmiedt E (1980) Extracorporeally induced destruction of kidney stones by shock waves. Lancet I: 1265–68
6. Coleman A, Saunders J, Crum L, Dyson M (1987) Acoustic cavitation generated by an extracorporeal shock wave lithotripter. Ultrasound Med Biol 13: 69–76
7. Crum L (1982) Acoustic cavitation In: Proceedings of the 1982 IEEE ultrasonics symposium. IEEE, New York, pp 1–11
8. Delius M, Enders G, Brendel W (1987a) Passage of stone fragments from canine gallbladders. Surg Obstet Gynecol (in press)
9. Delius M, Enders G, Heine G, Stark J, Remberger K, Brendel W (1987b) Biological effects of shock waves: lung hemorrhage by shock waves in dogs – pressure dependence. Ultrasound Med Biol 13: 61–67
10. Goldberg V (1979) Eine neue Methode der Harnsteinzertrümmerung – elektrohydraulische Lithotripsie. Urologe B 19: 23–27
11. Häusler E, Kiefer W (1971) Anregung von Stoßwellen in Flüssigkeiten durch Hochgeschwindigkeitswassertropfen. Verhandlg Dtsch Physikal Ges (VI) 6: 786
12. Liebich HG, Delius M, Enders G, Xuan Z, Brendel W (to be published) Biological effects of shock waves: ultrastructural changes in canine kidneys – dose dependence and time course
13. Sauerbruch T, Delius M, Paumgartner G, Holl J, Wess O, Weber W, Hepp W, Brendel W (1986) Fragmentation of gallstones by extracorporeal shock waves. New Engl J Med 314: 818–822

Breakdown of Tumor Microcirculation Induced by Shock-Waves or Photodynamic Therapy*

A. E. GOETZ, R. KÖNIGSBERGER, J. FEYH, P. F. CONZEN, and W. LUMPER

Introduction

Differences between blood vessels of normal tissue and those of tumors have long been known to exist [18], however, few efforts have been made to exploit this knowledge for therapy of malignancies. Recently the enhancement of tumor damage by induction of ischemia has been proposed as a promising treatment for tumors [4]. This currently involves the application of moderate heat [20], the use of embolic substances, e.g., autologous thrombin and cyanoacrylates [24] or clamping the supplying vessels of the tumors [5]. It has been suggested that these methods lead to an occlusion of tumor blood supply, blocking nutrition of the tumor and thus leading to ischemia in the tumor and to tumor cell death.

The present paper focuses on photodynamic therapy (PDT) and shock-wave treatment of tumors to ascertain whether these treatments act by means of a similar mechanism. The effectiveness of PDT with hematoporphyrin derivative (HpD) has already been demonstrated in more than 2000 patients [16]. In contrast, treatment of tumors by shock waves is still in its initial experimental phase, and even experimentally no tumor cure has yet been demonstrated.

HpD-PDT has been reported to affect the microcirculation in nonmalignant tissue [3]. Experiments have shown that L1210 cells taken from mice that received HpD did not respond to light irradiation in vitro whereas tumors in vivo did respond. This finding supports the conception of tumor microcirculation as the main target of PDT [17]. The reduction of blood flow in bladder tumors and in rat mammary carcinomas points in the same direction [19, 21]. However, the exact mechanisms leading to this phenomenon and to tumor killing in vivo remain controversial. As for shock-wave application, we recently demonstrated in an in vivo microcirculatory preparation that shock waves induce transient arteriolar vasoconstriction. Furthermore, we observed petechial hemorrhages, extravasation of macromolecules, and intravascular thrombosis affecting predominantly the small venules [2].

Corresponding to these findings electron micrographs have revealed damage to the vascular endothelium of venules and postcapillaries (F. Hammersen, unpublished results). With the exception of arteriolar vasoconstriction such findings have been dependent upon the number of shock waves applied to intact tissue.

* Supported by the Kurt-Körber-Stiftung and by the Bundesministerium für Forschung und Technologie.

Surgical Research:
Recent Concepts and Results
Baethmann/Messmer (Eds.)

These findings on shock-wave application led us to investigate in detail the effects of shock waves on tumor tissue. The present investigation was performed to evaluate the microcirculatory effects in tumor tissue and surrounding tumor-free areas of PDT-HpD and of shock-wave treatment. In addition, we have studied the effects of shock waves on tumor growth and on the survival rate of tumor-bearing animals.

Material and Methods

Transparent aluminium access chambers were implanted into the dorsal skinfold of male Syrian golden hamsters as described previously [8, 11]. In addition, permanently indwelling catheters were implanted into the right carotid artery and into the right jugular vein. Following at least 48-h recovery from microsurgery and anesthesia, preparations fulfilling the criteria of intact microcirculation were utilized for implanting 40000–60000 tumor cells of the amelanotic hamster melanoma A-Mel-3 into the center of the chamber preparation. For evaluation of tumor growth microphotographs of the chamber preparation were taken using a Wild MPS 55/51 photoautomat. After 3–4 days, functioning tumor microcirculation was established; at 6–7 days after tumor- cell implantation the mean diameter of tumors was about 6 mm. These tumors were used for the acute experiments. Details regarding the various physiological parameters studied, such as capillary density, segmental volume flow and tissue oxygenation of tumors, are described elsewhere [1, 9, 10].

HpD-PDT Experiments

Fifteen male Syrian golden hamsters were studied. HpD (Photofrin II) was administered intravenously in a dosage of 5 mg/kg body weight. Photofrin II (Photofrin Medical, Inc., Cheektowaga, N. Y.) is a fraction of HpD, 90% of which consists of material responsible for in vivo photosensitization. This HpD consists mainly of dihematoporphyrin ether (DHE).

After 4 h FITC-dextran (150000 dalton) and FITC-labeled erythrocytes were administered intravenously. Both markers served for evaluating vascular diameters and blood-cell velocity, respectively. Between 5 and 9 h after HpD application single-vessel irradiation was performed. This period was chosen since previous experiments using time-resolved laser-fluorescent microscopy had demonstrated a tumor-selective accumulation of HpD at this time [12]. A 75-W Xenon high-pressure arc was utilized as excitation source. Irradiation intensity was in the order of 350 mW/cm^2, and excitation wavelength ranged between 450 and 490 nm. Microcirculatory effects were studied using a barrier filter at 515 nm. This spectral filtering was necessary to visualize the fluorescently labeled red cells and FITC-dextran 150. While irradiating circular areas with a diameter of 50–70 μm the microcirculatory effects were transferred via a low light level television camera to a TV monitor and stored on videotape. The videoscreens were later analyzed off-line at magnifications of 1200 X. In separate experiments total chamber irradiation was performed using illumination by quartz lamp at an irradiation intensity of 300 mW/cm^2. The microcirculatory effects were monitored using the above-mentioned photomacroscope.

Shock Wave Treatment

Twenty-seven male Syrian golden hamsters with an amelanotic hamster melanoma were studied. The tumor-bearing animals were anesthetized by pentobarbital 6–7 days after tumor-cell implantation for studying shock-wave induced alterations in tumor microcirculation within the amelanotic hamster melanoma A-Mel-3 and the surrounding adjacent tumor-free tissue. The plastic cover slide was carefully removed and replaced by a transparent Teflon membrane. To protect the animals from drowning in the warm-water bath (37 °C) during shock-wave exposure, the hamsters were placed in water-tight plastic tubes. The chamber preparation with its central window area projected over this tube via a longitudinal slit into the water bath. The transparent tube was continuously superfused with a mixture of oxygen and air (fraction of oxygen, 0.4).

Prior to, during and 8 min after shock-wave exposure fluorescent or colored videophotomacroscopy was performed. Prior to and after videorecording the chamber preparations were photographed using the above-mentioned photoautomat. To evaluate the presence of perfusion within the tumor area, sodium fluorescein (376 mol. wt.) and FITC-dextran 150 were administered intravenously. For shock-wave treatment chamber preparations were positioned horizontally with the intact epidermis in the direction of the electrode. The window area was exactly centered in the second focus by the intersection of two laser beams. The shock waves were generated by a Dornier lithotripter made for experimental use. In this system shock waves are generated by an underwater spark discharge. The discharging electrode is positioned in the focus of a rotationally symmetric semiellipsoid. The shock wave is propagated spherically, reflected by the walls of the ellipsoid, and concentrated in the second focus. In this area pressures of about 80 MPa are reached. The pressure field has a diameter of about 1.5 cm. The areas were exposed to 100 shock waves at a voltage of about 15 kV. Three groups were formed: a control group (n = 7), a group receiving 100 shock waves (n = 10) and a group to which an additional 100 shock waves were applied 24 h later (n = 10).

For evaluating tissue perfusion a digital-image analyzing system of Hamamatsu Photonics Inc. was utilized [13]. Prior to application of the fluorochromes the video image was digitized and stored in a 16-bit videoframe memory of the image processor. Following intravenous administration of the fluorochromes the video-image was transferred to a second video frame memory. Subsequently the fluorochrome image was subtracted from the baseline image. The subtracted image demonstrated accumulation of the fluorochromes after intravenous application. Accumulation of the dyes was checked repeatedly over a period of 30 min. Thus even if the vessels were obscured by hemorrhage, perfusion of the tissue could be monitored by visualizing the diffusion of the dye into the hemorrhage.

Results

HpD-PDT

Complete *arteriolar vasoconstriction* in the adjacent tumor-free tissue was observed within 30–90 s (diameter, 43–64 μm; n = 8). Stasis within precapillaries and capillaries originating from the constricted arterioles was noted. Microvessel diameters in venules (diameter, 8–54 μm, n = 15) and in tumor vessels (diameter, 8–26 μm; n = 49) remained unchanged. In venules of the surrounding tumor-free tissue and in tumor vessels the appearance of amorphous conglomerates was observed. The intravenous application of acridine orange, an in vivo marker of platelets [22], demonstrated that these amorphous intravascular structures consisted mainly of platelet aggregates. Thus HpD-PDT induced an *intravascular thrombosis* in tumor vessels and in venules of the adjacent tissue. The time until stasis induced by the intravascular platelet aggregation ranged between 5 and 35 min and between 1 and 11 min in venules and in tumor vessels, respectively. These results are summarized in Fig. 1. The irradiation time necessary for inducing stasis was not dependent on any of

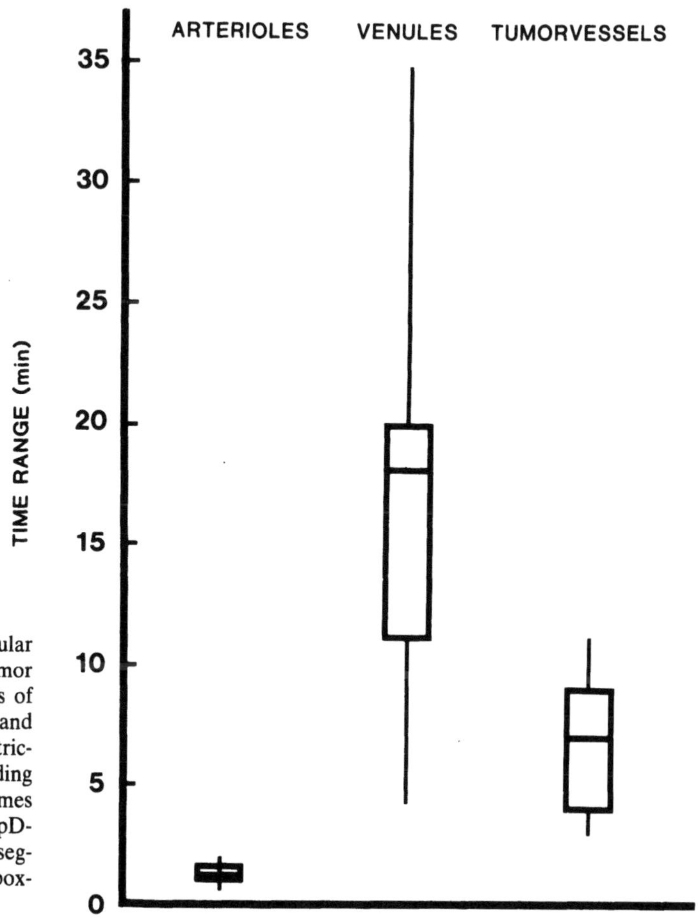

Fig. 1. HpD-PDT induces intravascular thrombosis in the tumor vessels and in venules of the adjacent tissue and arteriolar vasoconstriction in the surrounding tumor-free areas. Times until stasis after HpD-PDT of the vascular segments are given in box-plots

the microcirculatory parameters measured, i.e., no correlation with blood cell velocity, microvessel diameter, or volume flow could be demonstrated. Besides of these phenomena integral irradiation of the total chambers showed petechial hemorrhages selectively within the tumor areas (Fig. 2).

Shock Wave Treatment

In the control group no significant changes of the microcirculatory parameters, blood cell velocity, vessel diameter, or segmental volume flow were found when keeping the animals in the warm-water bath for a period necessary for shock-wave treatment.

When applying 1 × 100 shock waves to the tumor-bearing chamber preparations a constant finding in the surrounding tumor-free tissue was constriction of all arteriolar microvascular segments, i.e., of arcading, transverse and terminal arterioles and of precapillaries. As evaluated by videomicroscopy arteriolar vasoconstriction began here within seconds, reached its maximum after about 20–30 s and tended to release after 4–10 min. In addition, microhemorrhages were detected at the site of small venular microvascular segments. In these areas leakage of macromolecules and the appearance of amorphous conglomerates were observed. As in the experiments using HpD-PDT, acridine orange was injected, and we were able to identify the amorphous intravascular structures as platelet aggregates. Within the tumor complete hemorrhage after application of 100 shock waves was noted. Quantifying hemorrhage by planimetry indicated a statistically significant difference to the surrounding tumor-free tissue. Only 50% of the adjacent tissue area was hemorrhagic (Fig. 3).

The fluorescent dyes FITC-dextran 150 and sodium fluorescein were not found in the tumor 30 min after shock-wave treatment. After 12 h reperfusion began at the edge of the tumor area. At 24 h after shock-wave treatment all tumors were reperfused. However, we were unable to differentiate whether reperfusion occurred in previously occluded vascular channels or in newly formed blood vessels. Due to the complete hemorrhage of the tumor, no exact quantitative analysis of the microcirculatory blood flow within the tumor area after reperfusion was possible. We were only able to assess whether perfusion was present or not.

These effects on tumor blood flow led us to treat a third group of animals with an additional 100 shock waves 24 h after the first shock-wave exposure. The additional 100 shock waves induced an increase of hemorrhagic areas in the surrounding tumor-free tissue. Perfusion in the surrounding tumor-free tissue after the second administration of 100 shock waves was noted about 10 min after shock-wave application. Within the tumor, breakdown of microcirculation lasted for more than 24 h, indicating persisting ischemia (Fig. 4).

Tumor growth curves in the control group and in animals treated with shock waves are shown in Fig. 5. Fifteen days after tumor-cell implantation the chamber preparation in the control group was completely covered by the amelanotic hamster melanoma. Tumor growth in the animals treated with 100 shock waves was significantly delayed 3 days after shock-wave treatment, but did not differ significantly from the controls 5 days later. In group 3, the hemorrhagic area 48 h after the second 100 shock-wave application was significantly smaller than the tumor mass in the control group. It is possible that the hemorrhagic area consisted only of necrotic material,

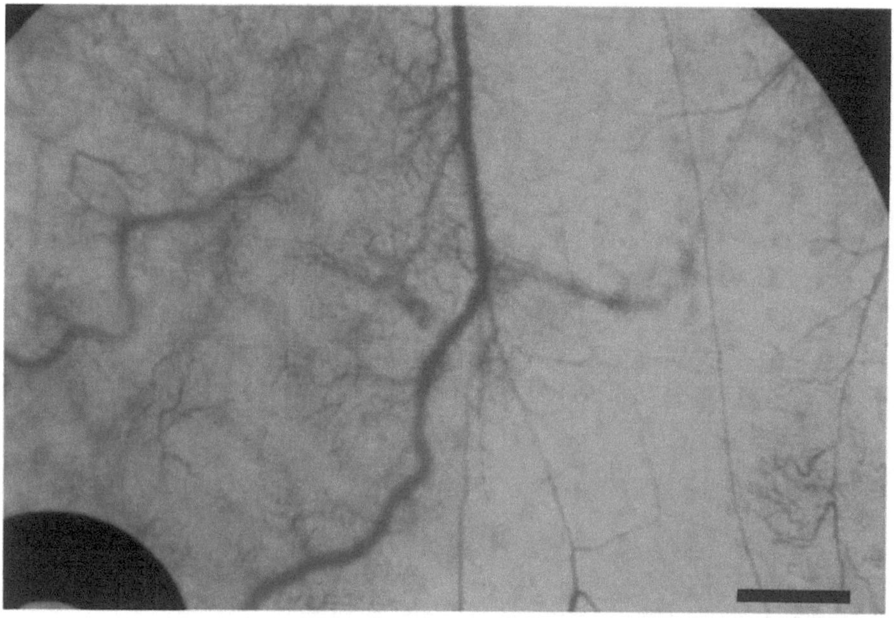

a

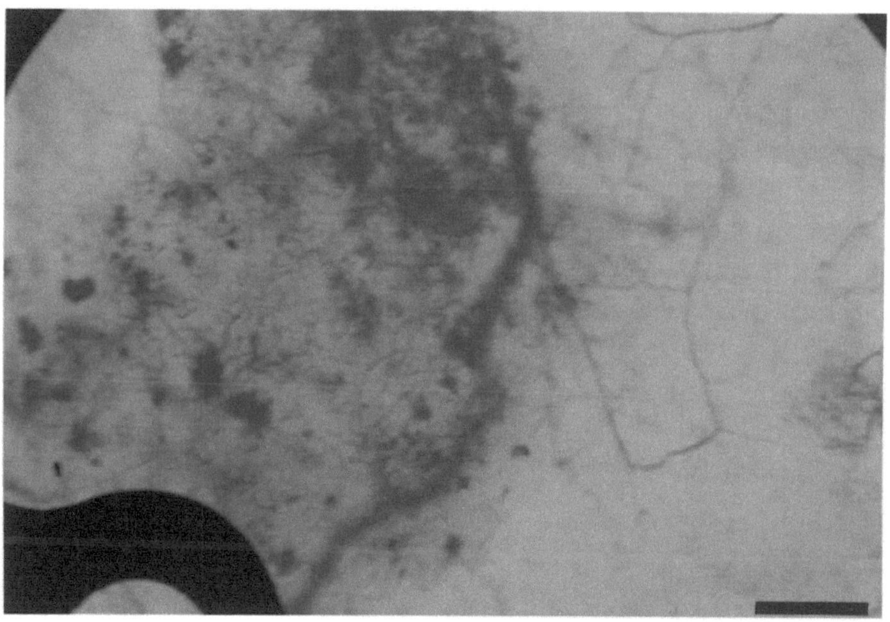

b

Fig. 2a,b. Photomacroscopic images of a skin-fold chamber preparation with an amelanotic hamster melanoma in the left part of the image prior to **a)** and after **b)** HpD-PDT of the total chamber. In the tumor area petechial hemorrhages are recognized and in the surrounding tumor-free tissue arteriolar vasoconstriction is visible. The disappearance of venular segments is due to an intravascular thrombosis in the venules. *Bars* indicate 1 mm

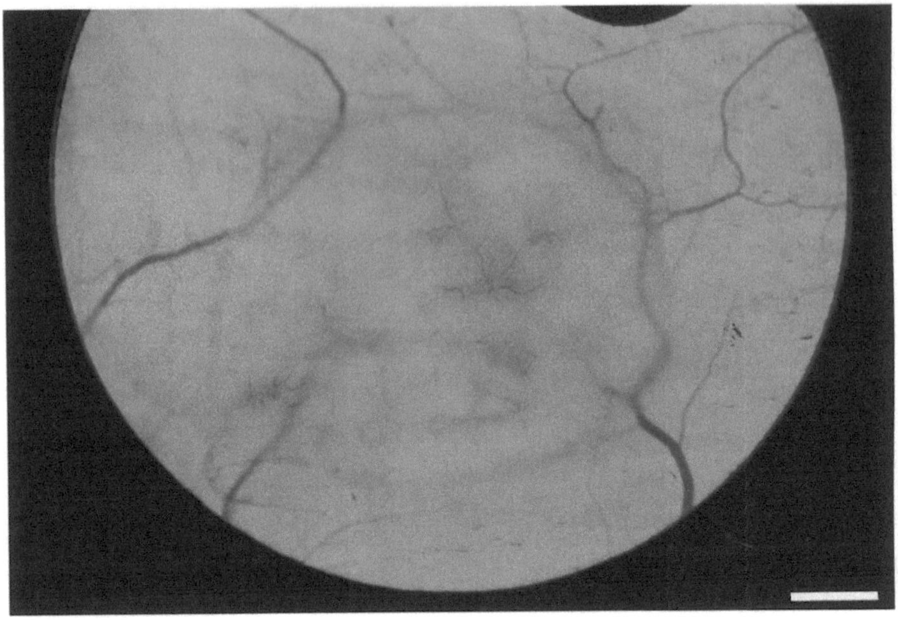

a

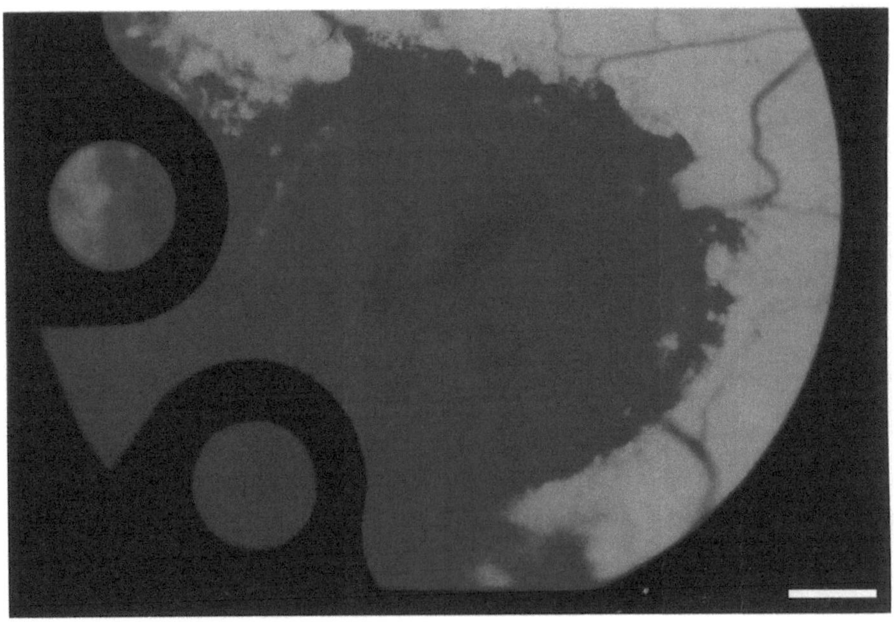

b

Fig. 3a, b. Photomacroscopic images of a skin-fold chamber preparation with a hamster amelanotic melanoma in the center prior to **a)** and after **b)** application of 100 shock waves. Total hemorrhage of the tumor area is visible as opposed to a partial hemorrhage in the surrounding tumor-free tissue. *Bars* indicate 1 mm

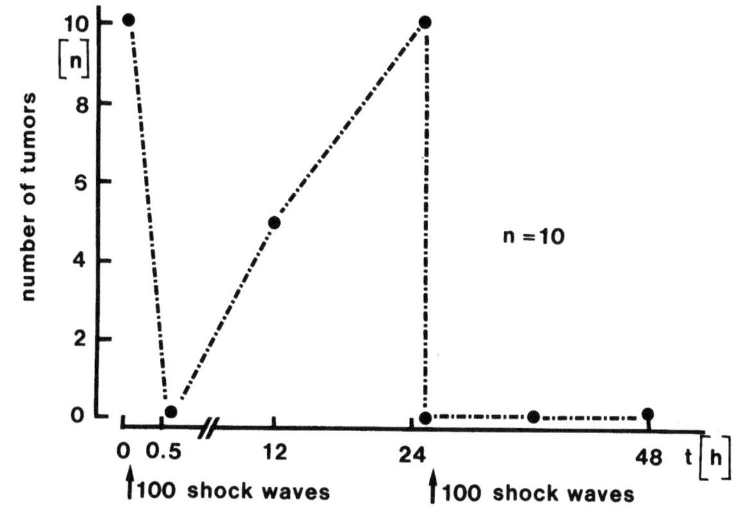

Fig. 4. Number of perfused tumors as evaluated by videofluorescent microscopy at 30 min, 12 h and 24 h after initial application of 100 shock waves and at 30 min, 12 h and 24 h after application of additional 100 shock waves

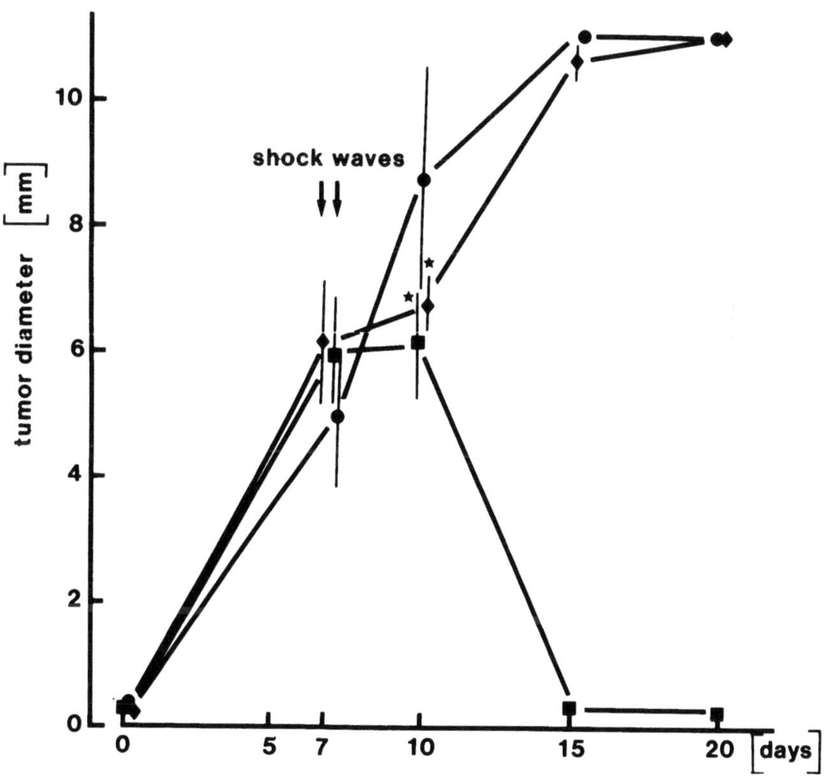

Fig. 5. Tumor growth curves in control and in shock-wave treated animals. *Circles,* control ($n = 7$); *rhombi,* 1 × 100 shock waves ($n = 10$); *squares,* 2 × 100 shock waves ($n = 10$). Mean values and standard deviations (*vertical lines*) are given; *asterisks* indicate $p < 0.05$ versus control

since no perfusion was present in this area at that time. Five days later an apparent reduction of the tumor mass was observed. The newly formed blood vessels at the edges of hemorrhagic areas did not show the typical chaotic angioarchitecture of the amelanotic hamster melanoma. As indicated by comparison of photomacroscopic images the original vasculature could be demonstrated in part.

Figure 6 demonstrates the survival rate of control animals and that of animals treated with shock waves. Maximum survival in the control group was 32 days and in the group treated with 1 × 100 shock waves 63 days. In group 3, with application of 2 × 100 shock waves within 24 h, 70% of the animals are currently alive after more than 130 days. Two animals in this group were lost due to hemorrhagic shock after removal of the catheter by the animals themselves, and a third died from rectum prolapse. In the control group one animal died 9 days after tumor-cell implantation due to hemorrhagic shock after biting off the indwelling arterial catheter. In group 2, one animal died 9 days after tumor-cell implantation due to rectum prolapse. All other animals died from metastasis and tumor cachexia.

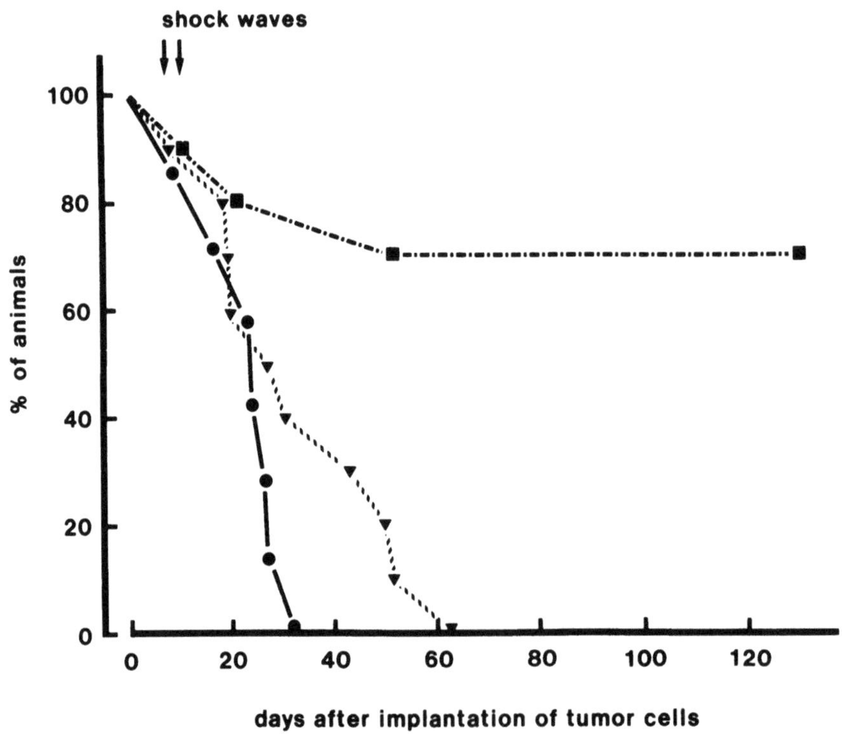

Fig. 6. Survival rate of tumor-bearing animals in the control and the shock-wave treated groups. Death of animals in all groups within the first 15 days after tumor cell implantation was induced either by hemorrhagic shock after biting the permanently indwelling catheters or by rectum prolapse. In the group of animals treated with 2 × 100 shock waves two animals died from hemorrhagic shock and a third from rectum prolapse. *Circles,* control ($n = 7$); *triangles,* 1 × 100 shock waves ($n = 10$); *squares,* 2 × 100 shock waves ($n = 10$)

Discussion

The present investigations demonstrate that damage to the vascular supply of tumors can be induced by HpD-PDT as well as by shock-wave treatment. In addition we found that reperfusion began immediately after shock-wave treatment in the normal tissue surrounding tumor areas, whereas ischemia in the tumor persisted. PDT seems to induce similar effects. This is supported by recent findings of Star et al. (1986) who tested the viability of tumor cells by transplanting the exposed tumor tissue immediately after treatment into the flank of the same animal. Even when HpD-PDT with a four-fold lethal dose for the tumor was applied, all transplanted tumors regrew. The conclusion therefore appears valid that tumor killing by PDT is secondary to destruction of the tumor microcirculation.

Our investigation provides some insights into the mechanisms of PDT-induced ischemia in tumors. In contrast to other experiments we have shown that the breakdown of tumor microcirculation is due mainly to intravascular thrombosis and, in contradistinction to others, we observed no vasoconstriction or vascular collapse of tumor vessels [16, 21]. In addition, we suggest that the immediate vasoconstriction of the arterioles supplying the tumor tissue contributes to the long-lasting tumor-selective breakdown of microcirculation. It may be of interest that tumor ischemia by similar mechanisms was observed in this study after shock-wave treatment; this has also been reported following treatment using the same type of chamber and tumor with hyperthermia [7].

Thus the three different methods seem to act via common mechanisms leading to ischemia of the tumor. The most intriguing question therefore to be answered in future studies is what mechanisms are responsible for inducing circulatory arrest of tumor microcirculation. In the context of these enormous intravascular changes it seems to be important to reconsider the specific characteristics of the vascular system of tumors. Our findings in the case of this particular tumor accord with those shown by other investigators studying different experimental tumors regarding certain basic characteristics of tumor microcirculation [6, 9, 10, 14, 15, 23]. Large differences in vessel diameter within a short microvascular segment are observed and tumor vessels are dilated, tortuous and exhibit redundant curvatures. Wide sinusoides may be found as well as a critical reduction of capillary density insufficient for an adequate supply of the tissue. In addition, blood flow is extremely nonhomogeneous: high- and low-perfusion areas and shunt perfusion may be found simultaneously. One of the most important characteristics is "insufficient secondary neoangiogenesis." Mesenchymal cells may participate in the lining of the vascular wall; wide endothelial gaps can be seen, allowing extravasation of red blood cells and of macromolecules. Endothelial edema is sometimes present as well. These findings are in part responsible for the appearance of intravascular thrombi. This is accompanied by an enhanced microhematocrit in tumor microvessels 100% above the level of normal tissue (Goetz, unpublished results). In addition each factor (hypoxia, anoxia, and acidosis), contributes to an enhanced rigidity of red blood cells and thereby to an increased vascular resistance of tumor microcirculation.

It seems plausible that therapeutic induction of a breakdown in tumor microcirculation may be accomplished more easily in this state of circulatory dysfunction than in normal tissue. All methods reported thus far, e.g., hyperthermia, PDT and shock waves, induce arteriolar vasoconstriction in the surrounding tumor-free tissue and formation of intravascular thrombosis of tumor vessels, as well as selective hemorrhage in tumor areas. These factors contribute to a further increase of vascular resistance to tumor microcirculation, leading finally to complete ischemia. A vicious circle is thus activated leading to no-reflow in the tumor and, eventually, self-destruction particularly of the tumor center. For a successful treatment of tumors it is necessary however, that not a single tumor cell survives. Therefore, damage to the vasculature surrounding the tumor tissue is also desired.

In summary, in addition to besides showing mechanisms of action of PDT and shock waves we have been able to demonstrate that shock-wave treatment itself may lead to regression of the tumor. Our conclusions are, however, restricted to the skin-fold chamber preparation. Studies are therefore needed in an intact tumor model to test whether tumor treatment may be performed by using shock waves. It must nevertheless be noted that an enhanced vulnerability of tumor vasculature as opposed to surrounding tumor-free tissue has been demonstrated. Identical findings were obtained by photodynamic therapy with HpD. The effects induced by HpD-PDT and shock-wave treatment are novel, promising modalities for inducing ischemia in tumor tissue. They provide further support for the use of tumor microcirculation as the main target for tumor therapy.

References

1. Asaishi K, Endrich B, Goetz A, Messmer K (1981) Quantitative analysis of microvascular structure and function in the amelanotic melanoma A-Mel-3. Canc Res 41: 1898–1905
2. Brendel W, Delius M, Goetz A (1987) Effect of shock waves on the microvasculature. Progr Appl Microcirc 12: 41–50
3. Castellani A, Pace GP, Concioli M (1963) Photodynamic effect of haematoporphyrin on blood microcirulation. J Pathol Bacteriol 86: 99–102
4. Denekamp J, (1984) Vasculature as a target for tumor therapy. Progr Appl Microcirc 4: 28–38
5. Denekamp J, Hill S, Hobson B (1983) Vascular occlusion and tumor cell death. Eur J Cancer Clin Oncol 19: 271–275
6. Eddy HA (1980) Alterations in the tumor microvasculature during hyperthermia. Radiology 137: 512–521
7. Endrich B (1984) Mikrozirkulation maligner Tumore. PhD Thesis, University of Heidelberg
8. Endrich B, Asaishi K, Goetz A, Messmer K (1980) Technical report. A new chamber technique for microvascular studies in unanesthetized hamsters. Res Exp Med 177: 125–134
9. Endrich B, Goetz A, Messmer K (1982a) Distribution of microflow and oxygen tension in hamster melanoma. Int J Microcirc Clin Exp 1: 81–99
10. Endrich B, Hammersen F, Goetz A, Messmer K (1982b) Microcirculatory blood flow, capillary morphology and local oxygen pressure of the hamster amelanotic melanoma A-Mel-3. J Natl Cancer Inst 68: 475–485
11. Goetz A, Endrich B, Laprell C, Meßmer K (1981) An experimental model for prolonged studies of the microcirculation. Bibl Anat 20: 65–68
12. Goetz A, Feyh J, Schneckenburger H, Conzen P, Jocham D, Unsoeld E (1985) Quantitative in vivo measurement of Photofrin II in tumor- and tumor-free tissue. In: Jori G, Perria C (eds) Photodynamic therapy of tumors and other disease. Libreria Progretto Editore, Padova, pp 405–408
13. Goetz A, Feyh J, Ortner H, Conzen P, Brendel W (1987) Digital on-line subtraction on videomicroscopic images for detection of hematoporphyrin-derivative fluorescence. Int J Microcirc Clin Exp 6: 71
14. Hammersen F, Osterkamp-Baust U, Endrich B (1983) Ein Beitrag zum Feinbau terminaler Strombahnen und ihrer Entstehung in bösartigen Tumoren. Mikrozirk Forsch Klin 2: 15–51

15. Hammersen F, Endrich B, Messmer K (1985) The fine structure of tumor blood vessels. Int J Microcirc Clin Exp 4: 31–43
16. Kessel D (1984) Porphyrin localization: a new modality for detection and therapy of tumors. Biochem Pharmacol 33: 1389–1393
17. Musser DA, Datta-Gupta N (1984) Inability to elicit rapid cytocidal effects on L1210 cells derived from porphyrin-injected mice following in vitro photoirradiation. J Natl Cancer Inst 2: 427–434
18. Ribbert H (1904) Über das Gefäß-System und die Heilbarkeit der Geschwülste. Dtsch Med Wochenschr 30: 801–803
19. Selman SH, Kreimer-Birnbaum M, Klaunig JF, Goldblatt PJ, Keck RW, Britton SI (1984) Blood flow in transplantable bladder tumors treated with hematoporphyrin derivative and light. 44: 1924–1927
20. Song C (1982) Physiological factors in hyperthermia. In: Dethlefson LA, Dewey WC (eds) Cancer therapy by hyperthermia, drugs and radiation. NCI Monogr 61: 169–176
21. Star WM, Marijnissen PA, van den Berg-Blok AE, Versteeg JAC, Franken KAP, Reinhold HS (1986) Destruction of rat mammary tumor and normal tissue microcirculation by hematophorphyrin derivative photoradiation observed in-vivo in sandwich observation chambers. Cancer Res 46: 2532–2540
22. Tangelder GJ, Slaaf DW, Reneman RS (1982) Fluorescent labeling of blood platelets in vivo. Thrombosis Res 28: 803–820
23. Warren BA (1979) Tumor angiogenesis. In: Petersen HI (ed) Tumor blood circulation. CRC Press, Boca Raton, pp 49–75
24. Young A (1981) Therapeutic embolisation. Br Med J 283: 1144–1145

New Treatment Concepts for Insulin-Dependent Diabetes Mellitus

B. U. von Specht, A. Dibelius, and H. Königsberger

Today's routine therapy of insulin-dependent diabetes mellitus (IDDM) is a good example of how treatment of symptoms may help the patient stay alive without curing him. The discovery of insulin by Banting and Best in 1922 and its introduction in clinical therapy lowered early diabetes lethality dramatically. Despite many attempts however, a prevention of late diabetic complications and of their contribution to common morbidity and lethality has not yet been achieved [1]. A major point of any therapy of diabetes remains whether the late-diabetic syndrome can be cured or prevented. Total endocrine-replacement therapy seems a promising attempt toward reaching this goal [2, 3]. Nevertheless, before its becoming a routine therapy many problems must be solved. Therefore, grafting either of the whole pancreas or of isolated islets of Langerhans and the related problems remain an important matter for experimental research.

Up to now experimental and clinical segmental pancreas allografts combined with postoperative administration of immunosuppressive agents such as cyclosporin A (CsA) have shown considerably longer survival times than have comparable islet allografts [4, 5]. The surgical technique of the former, however, is more complex, and management of the unnecessary exocrine part of the organ has not been solved satisfactorily. Duct-occlusive techniques may cause islet atrophy due to organ fibrosis, while open-duct procedures, although functioning in some animal models, may lead to incurable ascites.

Pancreatic islet transplantation is a promising approach, but there are problems to overcome here as well. First, as described by many authors, the relatively low yield of islets isolated from a single pancreas limits the application of one-donor – one-recipient transplantation in clinical application [6]. Second, it is striking that, while CsA provides significant prolongation of allograft survival in clinical and experimental segmental pancreas, transplantation seems to be less effective for islet grafts, especially for those transplanted across a major histoincompatibility barrier [7, 15]. A further problem of both pancreas and islet transplantation is a possible influence of the autoimmune process which leads to complete B cell destruction and, thus, to diabetes. This autoaggression may also destroy the graft after transplantation. Pancreatic transplantation in identical twins with IDDM [8] and experimental transplantation in the BB/Wistar rat [9] in an animal model of autoimmunologically induced diabetes have provided evidence that the persisting autoimmune process plays an important role in the destruction of transplanted B cells.

Surgical Research:
Recent Concepts and Results
Baethmann/Messmer (Eds.)

In order to solve these problems we have investigated in a strongly histoincompatible rat model whether it is possible to prolong islet graft survival by CsA to an extent comparable to that of pancreas grafts if the islet preparation is highly purified. A further aim of this study was the development of an one-donor – one-recipient model. With regard to both histocompatibility and autoimmunological factors the uncertain role of appropriate timing as well as the question as to the most effective immunosuppressive treatment have been studied by islet transplantation in a BB/W rat colony which was newly established in Munich. Islets were, therefore, transplanted both at early stages of diabetes with active autoimmunity and at late stages, in order to investigate differences in graft survival and the effectiveness of pre- and/or postoperative CsA.

A one-donor – one-recipient model can be established by increasing the yield of islets isolated from a single donor pancreas. For this purpose collagenase digestion for the isolation of islets was modified [10]. A major modification involved in vivo perfusion of the donor pancreas with neutral red for the labeling of islets and omission of a Ficoll gradient for cell isolation. Details are described elsewhere [11]. Neutral red permits specific identification of islets and excludes impurities of the transplant preparation by small lymph nodes and acinar tissue which are assumed to induce rejection of islet allografts [12–14]. Ficoll itself may affect the integrity of the islets and insulin secretion. It was possible to isolate 800–1000 islets from one pancreas, making possible a one-donor – one-recipient transplantation. In vitro glucose stimulation and perfusion tests showed the impaired function of isolated islets. The number of islets grafted was sufficient to decrease diabetic blood glucose levels in the recipients immediately following intraportal transplantation. The recipients were made diabetic by previous intravenous injection of streptozotocin. Isogeneic transplanted animals remained normoglycemic for an observation period of up to 240 days. Allogeneic islet grafts transplanted across a major histocompatibility complex (MHC) barrier without immunosuppression were rejected between 3 and 9 days after transplantation. In recipients treated with CsA long-term prolongation of graft survival was observed. Glucose levels remained normal for 28–150 days with three animals having a normoglycemic survival beyond this period (Fig. 1). Functional tests and histological sections proved functioning grafts.

In contrast to previous reports prolongation of allogeneic islet graft survival by CsA was found. In order to compare the validity of these results whole pancreata were grafted microsurgically in the current model using the same immunosuppressive treatment. CsA prolonged mean graft survival from 4.7 to 37.0 days, which is comparable to findings of other authors [15]. Our results on islet transplantation showed for the first time that long-term allogeneic islet-graft survival can be achieved by CsA and the employment of an isolation method which provides a higher yield of purified islets that are more effectively depleted of contaminating cells (Tables 1, 2). Both factors may have contributed to the substantial prolongation of islet-allograft survival [16].

After a successful colony of BB/W rats was established, our further interest focused on the role of autoimmunological mechanisms of the disease on islet allo- and isografts. Using the same technique of islet transplantation as in the above experiments, three different immunosuppressive regimens were investigated: (a) isogeneic and allogeneic islet transplantation without immunosuppression, (b) postoperative

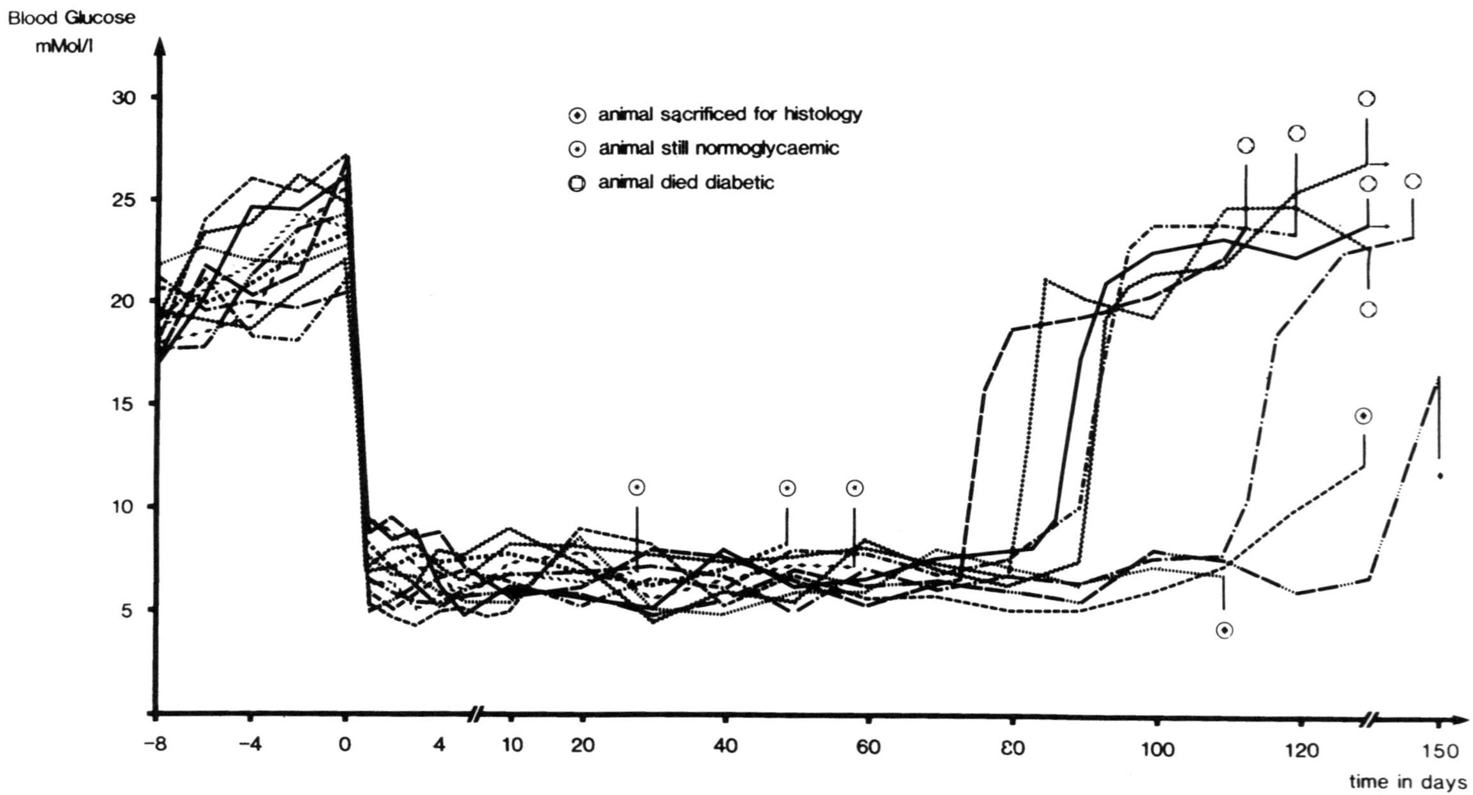

Fig. 1. Blood glucose levels after allogeneic (strong MHC barrier DA-Lewis) intraportal islet transplantation with CsA (30 mg/kg b. w. i. m. at day 0, 1, and 2 posttransplantation) ($n = 12$). Recipients were made diabetic by an i.v. injection of 65 mg/kg b.w. streptozotocin. Grafts were considered rejected when glucose levels rose again above 16.5 mmol/l, as determined by the glucose dehydrogenase method using an autoanalyzer

Table 1. Islet graft survival time in three groups: (1) isogeneic transplantation (DA-DA) (2) allogeneic without immunosuppression (DA-) (3) allogeneic with CsA 30 mg/kg b. w. i. m. at day 0, 1, and 2 after transplantation (DA-Lew). About 1000 islets using a neutral red isolation technique were transplanted to diabetic recipients intraportally. Recipients were made diabetic by injection of 65 mg/kg b. w. streptozotocin i. v.

Donor-recipient strain	n	Graft survival (days)	Mean survival (days)
Isogeneic DA → DA	6	> 53[a], < 63[a], > 68[a], 124, 200[b], 240[b]	124.6 ± 78.9
Allogeneic DA → Lewis	8	3, 4, 5, 5, 5, 5, 8, 9	5.5 ± 2.0
Allogeneic DA → Lewis + 3 × CsA 30 mg/kg b. w. on days: 0, 1, 2	12	> 28[a], > 49[a], > 59[a], 73, 82, 88, 94, 110[b], 111, 117, 129[b], 150[b]	90.8 ± 35.1

[a] Animal still normoglycemic
[b] Animal sacrificed for histology

Table 2. Survival of heterotopic pancreas grafts

	n	Graft survival (days)	Mean graft survival (days)
Isogeneic Lewis → Lewis	8	38[a] > 60 > 60 > 60 44[a] 25[b] > 60 > 60	> 50.9 ± 13.6
Allogeneic DA → Lewis	6	4 7 5 3 4 5	4.7 ± 1.4
Allogeneic DA → Lewis ± 3 × CsA 30 mg/kg b. w. on days: 0, 1, 2	9	30 42 26 15[a] 44 52 41 14[b] 69	37.0 ± 17.8

Pancreata were grafted using microsurgical techniques. The duct was drained into the peritoneal cavity. Grafts were considered technically successful if the recipient survived the first days after transplantation
[a] Animal died normoglycemic
[b] Graft removed

CsA administration, and (c) pre- and postoperative immunosuppression with CsA. Animals were divided into short- and long-term diabetic recipients. In the controls islets of nondiabetic BB/W rats were transplanted to isogeneic recipients made diabetic by streptozotocin. Thus, the degree of histocompatibility in the colony could be tested and the influence of an autoimmunological process ruled out. BB/W rats are not strictly inbred, but the transplantation experiments and mixed lymphocyte cultures revealed a status of the colony close to isogenicity. Nevertheless, transplantation between BB/W rats can be considered pseudoisogeneic.

Spontaneous diabetes of the BB/W rat was cured by transplantation of about 1000 islets. Glucose-tolerance tests and histological examinations revealed normal graft

Table 3. Islet graft survival time in diabetic BB/W recipients without immunosuppression

		n	Graft survival (days)	Median of graft survivals (days)
"Pseudo"-isogeneic: n. diab. BB/W → diab. BB/W	a) short-term diabetic	10	5, 6, 7, 7, 8, 10, 12, 12, 15, 18	9
	b) long-term diabetic	10	15, 19, 20, 25, 28, 32, 32, 34, 37, 38	30
Allogeneic: Lewis → diab. BB/W	a) short-term diabetic	8	2, 3, 3, 4, 4, 4, 5, 7	4
	b) long-term diabetic	9	3, 3, 4, 5, 6, 8, 8, 8, 9	6

Short-term diabetic: stable diabetic situation up to 20 days
Long-term diabetic: stable diabetic situation longer than 12 weeks. Recipients' routine insulin therapy stopped at day of transplantation

function. Therefore, the one-donor – one-recipient concept that was already successful in the model of streptozotocin-induced diabetes is also viable in the BB/W model. All transplantation groups (allogeneic and isogeneic, with and without immunosuppression) had a significantly shorter graft survival in short-term as compared to long-term diabetic recipients. The allograft group without immunosuppression (Table 3), however, showed the smallest difference (at a low level of statistical significance). In the pseudoisogeneic group islets of those animals with recent onset of diabetes were destroyed significantly faster than in the long-term diabetic animals. Postoperative CsA treatment led to a considerable prolongation of graft survival in all groups except in the pseudoisogeneic transplanted short-term diabetic recipients, in which only a slight prolongation could be observed, indicating a high degree of autoaggression (Table 4). Additional pretreatment of recipients with CsA prolonged islet-graft

Table 4. Islet graft survival time in diabetic BB/W recipients with postoperative immunosuppression (CsA 25 mg/kg b.w. i.m. at day 0, 1, 3, 7 posttransplantation)

		n	Graft survival (days)	Median of graft survivals (days)
"Pseudo"-isogeneic: n. diab. BB W → diab. BB W	a) short-term diabetic	8	17, 19, 21, 21, 22, 25, 26, 26	21.5
	b) long-term diabetic	10	35, 45, 61, 62, 71, 72, 77, 85, 92, 101	71,5
Allogeneic Lewis → diab. BB/W	a) short-term diabetic	9	48, 51, 54, 55, 61, 63, 64, 68, 72	61
	b) long-term diabetic	9	68, 71, 78, 81, 82, 85, 88, 93, 94	82

Short-term diabetic: stable diabetic situation up to 20 days
Long-term diabetic: stable diabetic situation longer than 12 weeks

Table 5. Islet graft survival time in diabetic BB/W recipients with pre- and postoperative immunosuppression. (CsA 10 mg/kg b. w. i. m. at day 9, 6, 3 before transplantation and CsA 25 mg/kg b. w. at day 0, 1, 3, 7 posttransplantation)

		n	Graft survival (days)	Median of graft survivals (days)
"Pseudo"-isogeneic:				
n. diab. BB W → diab. BB/W	a) short-term diabetic	10	48, 56, 69, 70, 73 74, 78, 79, 82, 89	73,5
	b) long-term diabetic	9	69, 88, 91, 98, 98, 101, 109, 117, 124	98
Allogeneic:				
Lewis → diab. BB/W	a) short-term diabetic	10	63, 68, 72, 78, 79 81, 83, 86, 88, 93	80
	b) long-term diabetic	9	88, 89, 94, 94, 99, 101, 103, 109, 128	99

Short-term diabetic: stable diabetic situation up to 20 days
Long-term diabetic: stable diabetic situation longer than 12 weeks

survival in all groups as compared to postoperative treatment alone (Table 5). Especially graft survival in the pseudoisogeneic short-term diabetic group was considerably improved. The results obtained in the pseudoisogeneic group confirm the hypothesis of islet-cell destruction by the basic diabetic process in the BB/W rat. Accordingly, it is assumed that the highly active autoimmunological process early in diabetes was responsible for the faster destruction of transplanted islets in the short-term diabetic recipients. In the allografted groups without immunosuppression (Fig. 3a) almost no difference in survival was found between early- and late-stage diabetic recipients. This can be explained by the dominating role of histoincompatibility for rejection. Suppression of allograft rejection by a postoperative CsA treatment, however, presumably rendered the autoimmunological response in the recipient more important for islet graft survival. Additional immunosuppressive pretreatment was administered to influence this situation and to make the recipient susceptible for the graft.

Presuming that the pathogenesis of IDDM in humans is similar to that of the BB/W rat, the results on islet or pancreas transplantation may underline the significance of an appropriate timing for transplantation and that of the actual immunological state of the recipient. If it is considered necessary to perform transplantation in early diabetes to stabilize the metabolic situation and to prevent diabetic complications, preoperative immunosuppression with CsA may be beneficial in improving control of the disease process as a basis for better graft survival.

Two major efforts may dominate future therapy of IDDM: on the one hand, prevention of diabetes by immunosuppressive treatment of patients at risk of developing diabetes, and, on the other, pancreas or islet transplantation. The problem with the former is evident, i. e., side-effects of immunosuppression at a time when it is not certain whether diabetes becomes manifest at all. Immunosuppression after clinical onset of diabetes could be too late, because almost 90% of the B-cell mass is already destroyed by then. Before islet transplantation becomes a clinical routine several problems must be solved, and obtaining a sufficient yield of islets from a single human pancreas is one of the greatest challenges at the moment.

References

1. West KM (1982) Hyperglycaemia as a cause of longterm complications. In: Keen H, Jarrett RJ (eds) Complications of diabetes. Arnold, Londons, pp 13–17
2. Federlin K, Bretzel RG (1984) The effect of islet transplantation on complications in experimental diabetes of the rat. World J Surg 8: 169–178
3. Landgraf R, Landgraf-Leurs MMC, Burg D, Kampik A, Castro LA, Abendroth A, Illner WO, Land W (1986) Long-term follow-up of segmental pancreas transplantation in type 1 diabetes. Transpl. Proc. 18: 1118–1124
4. Gray DWR, Morris PJ (1984) Cyclosporine and pancreas transplantation. World J Surg 8: 230–235
5. Sutherland DWR (1981) Pancreas and islet transplantation. Diabetologia 20: 161–185
6. Kamp CB, Knight MB, Sharp DW, Lacy PE, Ballinger WF (1973) Transplantation of isolated islets into the portal vein of diabetic rats. Nature 244: 447
7. Rynasiewicz J, Sutherland DER, Kawahara K, Gorecki P, Najarian JS (1980) Cyclosporin A prolongation of segmental pancreas and islet allograft function in rats. Transpl Proc 12: 270–274
8. Sutherland DER (1984) Twin to twin transplantation: reversal and reenactment of pathogenesis of type I diabetes. Trans Assoc Am Physicians 97: 80–87
9. Naji A, Silvers WK, Barker CF (1981) Islet transplantation in spontaneously diabetic rats. Transpl Proc 13/1: 826–828
10. Lacy PE, Kostianovsky M (1967) Method for the isolation of intact islets of Langerhans from the rat pancreas. Diabetes 16: 35–39
11. Dibelius A, Königsberger H, Walter P, Permanetter W, Brendel W, v. Specht BU (1986) Prolonged reversal of diabetes in the rat by transplantation of allogeneic islets from a single donor and cyclosporine treatment. Transplantation 41/4: 426–431
12. Lafferty KJ, Prowse, SJ (1984) Theory and practice of immunoregulation by tissue treatment prior to transplantation. World J Surg 8: 187–197
13. Lacy PE (1984) Experimental immunoalteration. World J Surg 8: 198–203
14. Bowen KM, Andrus L, Lafferty KJ (1980) Successful allotransplantation of mouse pancreatic islets to nonimmunosuppressed recipients. Diabetes 29 (Suppl.): 98–104
15. Rynasiewicz, JJ, Sutherland DER, Ferguson RM, Souifflet JP, Morrow CHE, Goetz FC, Najarian JS (1982) Cyclosporin A for immunosuppression: observation in rat heart, pancreas and islet allografts models and in human renal and pancreas transplantation. Diabetes 31 (Suppl) 4: 92–108
16. Dibelius A, Königsberger H, Permanetter W, Walter P, Brendel W, v. Specht BU (1986) Prolonged pancreatic islet allograft survival by cyclosporine compared to whole pancreas allograft survival. Transpl Proc 18/5: 1167–1168
17. Königsberger H, Dibelius A, Permanetter W, Walter P, Brendel W, v. Specht BU (1987) Influence of postdiabetic onset time and immunosuppressive treatment on islet grafts in the spontaneous diabetic BB/W rat. Transplantation (in press)

Computer Applications in Surgical Research*

R. Schosser, H. Forst, W. Gross, C. Weiss, H. Zeintl, and K. Messmer

Introduction

Among surgeons the application of computer science and technology is still considered to be of minor importance because operating skills and experience do not profit from data processing. In other medical fields, such as radiology and anesthesiology, the advantages of employing computers were recognized much earlier and have led to the development of new diagnostic and therapeutic procedures, e. g., sonography, NMR tomography, monitoring in the ICU, and computer controlled closed-loop infusion [11]. In surgical research computers are becoming increasingly popular, but the range of applications is still limited. Personal computers today have a performance comparable to that of mainframe computers 15 years ago, but these are used primarily for simple applications such as word processing.

In the following we describe applications of computers in surgical research and give a few typical examples as to how they have been realized in our department.

Applications

In a given unit of experimental surgery the spectrum of research is usually confined to a limited number of scientific fields, e. g., immunology, circulation, and biochemistry. Some applications described below may therefore be of varying relevance for particular institutions while others may be useful to all surgical research units, irrespective of their major fields of interest.

Data Acquisition

With regard to data acquisition two fundamental types of experiments must be distinguished: the in vitro and the in vivo. Further subdivision is possible as to whether the data produced are evanescent or permanent. A histological section is permanent and can be evaluated at any time; the related experiments are in vitro and not time-critical with respect to data acquisition. In contrast the change in blood pressure upon application of epinephrine is evanescent. The characteristics of a pressure curve can be evaluated only if a continuous registration *during* the action of the drug has been taken; such data are in vivo and time-critical.

* Supported by Forschungsschwerpunkt 16.2 Baden-Württemberg

Surgical Research:
Recent Concepts and Results
Baethmann/Messmer (Eds.)

Data obtained from experiments may be classified as qualitative or quantitative. The assessment of the quality of granulation in a healing wound cannot be measured by physical methods. Qualitative data must be classified and categorized in order to obtain figures. Blood pressure, on the other hand is a quantitative measurement and is obtained directly in terms of numbers.

The amount of data produced depends upon their type and upon whether they are time-critical or not. A qualitative categorial observation produces a single figure per measurement. A blood pressure registration obtained from measurements at intervals of 5 s over a 20-min period yields a total of 240 such figures.

Data acquisition can be carried out on-line or off-line. In the on-line mode the computer is connected directly to the measuring equipment (sensor, amplifier) via an analogue or digital interface. Observed values are transferred into the computer memory immediately after the measurement has taken place. In the off-line mode, the data are either entered manually into a computer terminal or read from floppy disk or magnetic tape which, in turn, was written previously by a measuring device or another computer connected to the measuring equipment.

Computers are used most efficiently for real-time applications with a plethora of data. There are, however, methods which although not time-critical produce large amounts of data, e.g., gamma spectrometry for blood flow measurements by means of radioactive microspheres [21, 22]. Although evanesence of data is no problem here, these methods are relatively time-critical because they are practical only if the measurements can be finished within a reasonable period of time. As compared to other methods in experimental surgery the analyses of images produces the largest mass of data (262144 numbers per image of 512 × 512 pixels resolution and 256 gray levels) and therefore generally requires the aid of a computer.

An illustration of a real-time application with large amounts of data is provided by our system for assessing local and global contractility and the dynamic geometry of heart ventricles. Local contractility is measured by means of miniaturized-piezoceramic transducers implanted into the myocardium. The ultrasonic transit-time method yields a continuous signal, representing the distance between transducers. Global myocardial contractility is determined from the derivatives of intraventricular pressures. Dynamic ventricular geometry is also assessed by sonomicrometry: transducers are implanted into the septum and the opposite ventricular free walls, measuring the septolateral diameters of both ventricles. An additional pair of transducers is attached to the left ventricular myocardium perpendicular to the septolateral axis, yielding the anterior-posterior diameter of the left ventricle [7].

Our data acquisition system consists of a hemodynamic monitoring unit for ECG and four pressures (Fig. 1). The analogue signals are digitized each at a rate of 500 Hz using an analogue digital converter and then transferred to the computer. The ultrasonic dimension gauge processes signals of four transducers simultaneously. Equipped with its own microprocessor, the sonomicrometry unit outputs digital data which can be transferred directly into the computer using a serial line. The computer is a PDP11/23 (Digital Equipment Corporation, Maynard, MA, USA). The program provides functions such as subtraction and summation of signals and calculation of their derivatives. Scatter plots are available for any pair of parameters, allowing the study of pressure-dimension loops (Fig. 2). Graphic routines draw readings or scatter plots of the signals in different colors on a 512 × 512 graphic display or on a plotter.

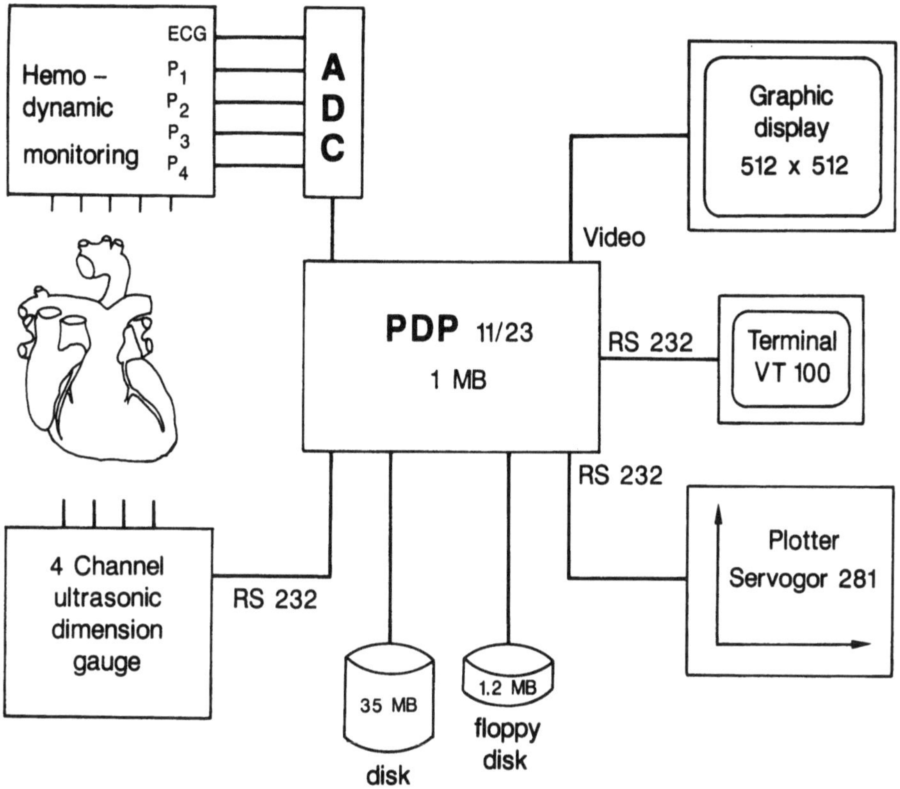

Fig. 1. Computer system for the assessment of local and global myocardial contractility and dynamic geometry of the heart ventricles. *ADC,* analog digital converter; $p_1 - p_4$, pressure curves; *RS 232,* asynchronous serial line

Gamma spectrometry is an example of a relatively time-critical application. This is used to calculate the relative amounts of radionuclides in a tissue sample containing microspheres with different radioactive labels. Each radionuclide has a characteristic energy spectrum, which must be recovered from the complex spectrum of the mixture using special mathematical procedures. Data acquisition from gamma spectrometry as performed in our laboratory is shown in Fig. 3. We use a sample changer unit Model 5260 (Packard Instruments Inc., Downers Grove, IL, USA) with a 3"-NaJ(Tl) detector and a capacity of 300 sample tubes of 1-inch diameter. The electrical pulses obtained from the detector are conditioned (amplified and rectangularized) and entered into a multichannel pulse-height analyzer, MCA Series 40 (Canberra Industries Inc., Meriden, CT, USA). The MCA is a special microcomputer dedicated to real time data acquisition and the generation of energy spectra (Fig. 4). It is connected to a second computer PDP11/24 via a high-speed serial link. After each measurement the MCA sends the spectrum of 1024 channels to the PDP. While the MCA is already measuring the spectrum of the following sample, the current spectrum is analyzed with the program MIC-III, which is a completely new and substan-

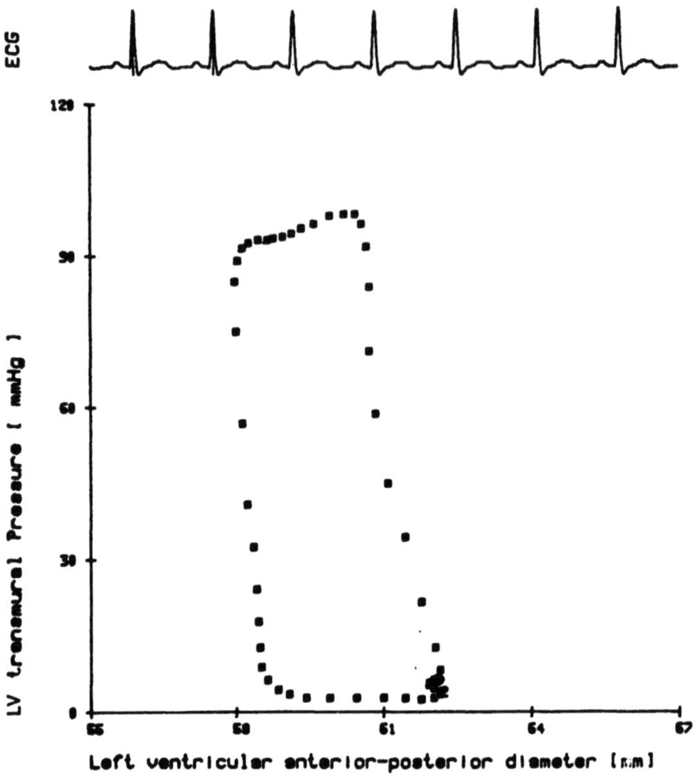

Fig. 2. Plot obtained from the system shown in Fig. 1. *Right side,* the following curves are shown *(from top to bottom):* ECG, left ventricular pressure *(LVP)*, first derivative of LVP *(dp/dt)*, mean intrathoracic pressure (p_{th}), septolateral diameter of the left ventricle (DLV_{sl}), anterior-posterior diameter of the left ventricle (DLV_{ap}). *Left side, at top* the ECG; *below,* a pressure-dimension loop of the left ventricular transmural pressure versus the anterior-posterior diameter

tially improved version of MIC-II [22] with a modified linear regression algorithm for spectrum deconvolution. The amount of data produced by the MCA and analyzed with the PDP for a typical experiment (300–400 samples) is 300000–400000 numbers. An electronic scale is also connected to the PDP, and the weights of tissue samples are transferred automatically upon pushing a button on the scale.

Process Control

Data are occasionally acquired not only to quantify characteristics of a subject but also to control certain parameters within the experiment. Such an application, referred to as "process control", is based on a closed-loop system consisting of a sensor as input device, the computer, and an output device. A typical example is deliberate hypoten-

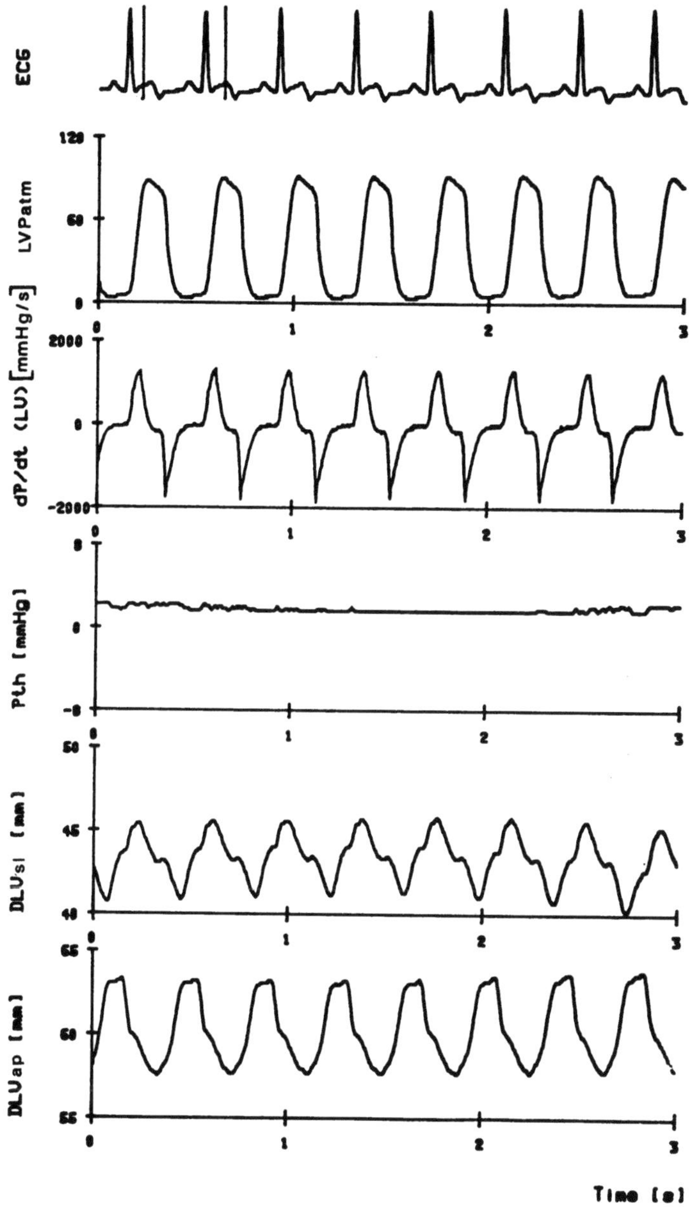

Fig. 2. (Continued)

sion by infusion of a short-acting hypotensive drug, e.g., sodium nitroprusside [3, 14, 18]. Blood pressure is monitored at intervals of a few seconds and compared with the desired level. If actual pressure is higher or lower than the preset value, the infusion rate is increased or decreased so as to maintain constant pressure.

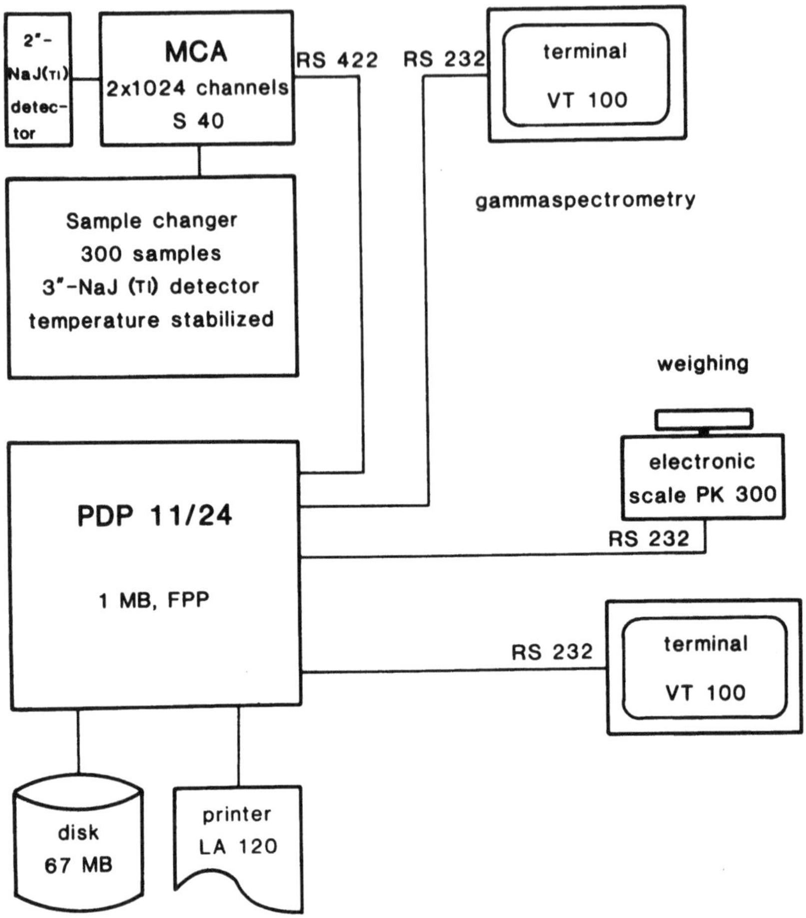

Fig. 3. Computer system for gamma spectrometry. The multichannel pulse-height analyzer (MCA) controls the sample changer and an additional external detector, used for samples with high activity. The MCA is connected to the computer via a high-speed serial line (RS 422), while the other components are connected with medium-speed serial lines (RS 232)

Another application of process control in experimental surgery is the maintainance of a low arterial blood pressure level during hemorrhagic hypotension as a shock model using a combined withdrawal/infusion pump. In our microcirculation laboratory we control the position of a microscope stage in two dimensions (x, y axes) to a precision of 1 μm by means of stepping motors connected to the computer (Fig. 5). This device is used to relocate regions of interest within the translucent hamster skinfold chamber or the hairless mouse ear for the sequential assessment of microhemodynamic parameters such as vessel diameter, red blood cell velocity, and functional capillary density [15, 27].

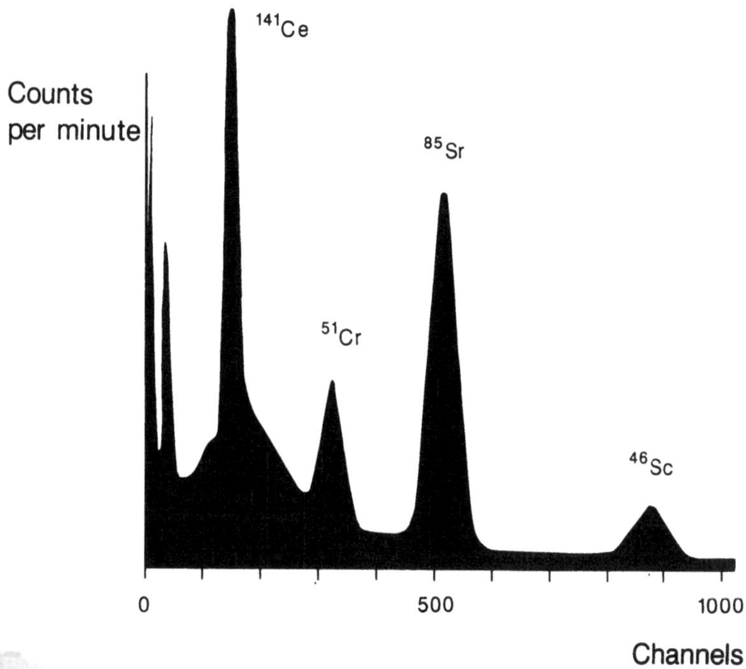

Fig. 4. Complex gamma spectrum containing four nuclides: ^{141}Ce, ^{51}Cr, ^{85}Sr, ^{46}Sc. Gamma spectrometry resolves the contributions of each nuclide

Image Processing

Data in medical research and experimental surgery are often extracted from images. For diagnostic purposes a qualitative description is frequently sufficient, e.g., the presence or absence of a fracture in X-ray images. In research, however, where differences and changes of parameters must be confirmed by means of statistical techniques, qualitative (subjective) information must be transformed into quantitative (objective) data in terms of numbers, using digital image processing. In addition, individuals can grasp the general content of an image very quickly, but their perception may fail to distinguish fine contrasts. The computer can compensate for this deficiency in the human visual system by means of contrast enhancement and pseudocolor presentation.

Digital image processing is used in microcirculation research for evaluation of images obtained from intravital microscopy (Fig. 5) [15, 27, 28, 29]. Video signals produced from television cameras or recorders are digitized and processed in a special image processor unit, connected to and controlled by, in our case, the PDP11/24. With this system stereological evaluations are performed, e.g. determination of functional capillary density and calculations of surface area within a microscopic image. Now under development is the direct assessment of functional capillary density by sequential subtractions of a series of images obtained in equidistant time intervals. With this method non-movingstructures of an image can be eliminated while moving structures are enhanced, resulting in a tracing of the perfused microvessels.

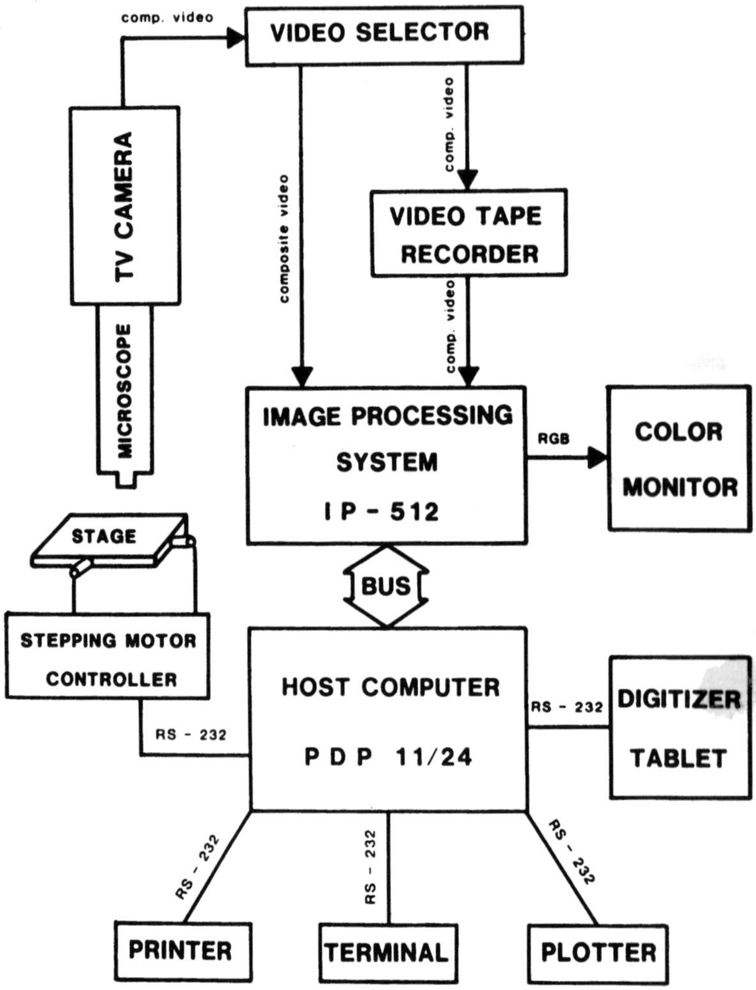

Fig. 5. Computer-assisted microcirculation analysis system (CAMAS). The image processing system is connected to the host computer via a high-speed system bus, the other components are linked with medium-speed serial lines (RS 232). The stepping motors of the microscope stage are controlled by the computer (process control)

Data Evaluation

Raw data obtained from experiments in the form of numbers are usually meaningless per se. It is impossible to draw a conclusion from a list of several hundreds or thousands of numbers representing blood flows or pressures or any other biological parameter. Only appropriate methods of evaluation, using statistical and/or graphical techniques, can reveal changes, patterns, and trends in a set of data and correlations between parameters. The process of data evaluation can be divided into the following steps:

- Data management and reduction
- Exploratory data analysis
- Inferential statistics
- Data presentation

Data Management and Reduction

That data are stored in a computer does not in itself mean that they are ready for evaluation. A prerequisite for successful analysis is a well-planned and organized structure both of data and of data files. Data are commonly evaluated by means of statistical software packages, such as BMDP or SAS [4, 5, 19, 20] or others [10, 26]. These packages provide not only statistical techniques but also data management facilities. For effective data management it is necessary to know the file and record operations supported by the software so that the data can be arranged accordingly. As to the structure of a file, statistical software generally distinguishes between records (rows) and variables (columns). The value of a variable on a given record is called an "observation." Fundamental operations for data management and reduction include the following:

- Joining records from several files side-by-side
- Merging records from several files sequentially
- Transposing observations into variables (and vice versa)
- Summarizing observations on a variable over several records

These operations allow data to be reshaped and combined as necessary. Whenever possible data should be stored in separate files, each containing the data of a particular phenomenon. An example could be an experiment in which 10 hemodynamic, 10 blood chemistry, and 15 blood flow parameters are measured. Here, values on one set of parameters (e.g., hemodynamics) may be measured more often than those on another (e.g., blood flow values). Combining these data into one merged data set could result in chaos.

Because it is easy to store large amounts of data with the computer, many scientists succumb to the temptation to do this. Once the storage space is filled with millions of numbers, however, it becomes difficult to find a point to begin data reduction. For this reason, if a mass of data is expected, a strategy for reduction should be worked out *before* data collection begins. The radioactive microsphere method [21, 22] produces large amounts of data, simply because the sample volume for measuring radioactivity is limited, and larger organs must therefore be divided into many samples. Statistical analysis, however, focuses on the organ, not on individual samples. Therefore, the organ blood flow must be summarized from the sample data. In a recent study we investigated the effect of a new drug on peripheral occlusive disease in a dog model using the microsphere method. The entire musculature of both hind legs was measured (except the flexor muscles of the thigh), yielding 334 muscle samples per animal. With four injections of microspheres we obtained a total of 10068 figures. These data were reduced by a factor of 1:105 to 96 figures, representing the flow in thigh and calf of either leg; this was done by means of only two operations (summarizing and transposing). The processing time needed for this data reduction was 2:32 min with BMDP and 2:06 min with SAS on a MicroVAX II computer (Digital Equipment Corporation, Maynard, MA, USA).

Exploratory Data Analysis

On the univariate level of exploratory data analysis data may be summarized using descriptive statistics such as measures of location (mean, median) and measures of dispersion (standard deviation, quantiles). Distribution of data can be visualized by means of histograms. Bivariate scatter plots show the interdependence of two variables. In many studies carried out in experimental surgery, however, several parameters are measured simultaneously within the same subject and the data obtained are therefore *multivariate.* The interrelationships among the variables are usually unknown. Studying the relations of any combination of two variables at a time by means of two-dimensional techniques shows only a facet of the complex totality because each plot is only a small detail.

Considerable efforts have been spent during the past two or three decades to develop graphic techniques to visualize multivariate data, e.g., bi-plots, glyphs, Andrews plots [1], and Kleiner-Hartigan trees [13]. Although some techniques are based on seemingly common concepts (flowers, trees), their interpretation is fairly abstract. A new approach to this problem was reported by Chernoff, who proposed "faces" to represent points graphically in k-dimensional space [2]. Each variable, standardized for the interval $[0 \leq x \leq 1]$, is assigned to one or more of 18 features such as size, location, rotation, curvature and density of hair, eyes, eyebrows, nose, mouth and face line. The result is a typical "physiognomy" for each subject as determined by its data.

The caricatural Chernoff faces were refined by Flury and Riedwyl, who added the feature of asymmetry, which allows the representation of 36 variables in one face [8, 9]. This method is now available for personal computers [24] and for the software package SAS. Figure 6 shows two extreme faces (all parameter values 0 or 1, respectively) and the average face (all parameter values 0.5). With this technique each subject is represented by an individual face. Looking at a series of faces it is strikingly easy to detect patterns and clusters of subjects, which would never have been found

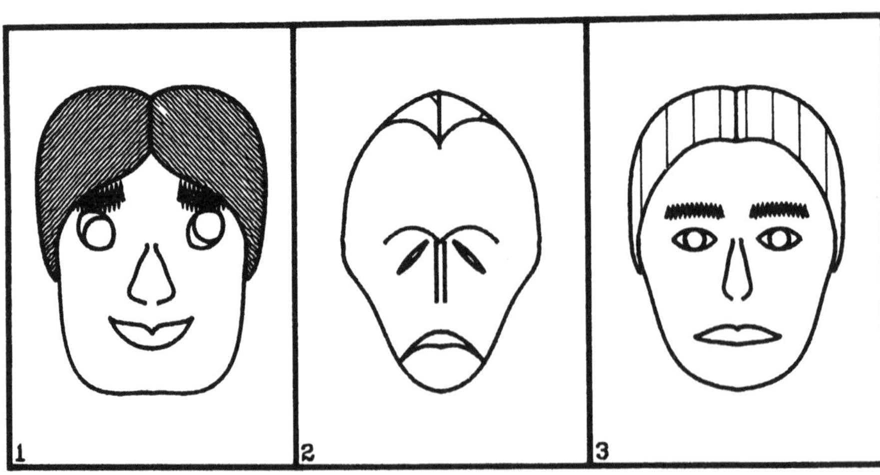

Fig. 6. Flury-Riedwyl faces. The *left* two faces are extremes, with all parameters set to 1 or 0, respectively. The *right* face is a "normal" face (all parameters set to 0.5). The faces have been drawn on the plotter Servogor 281

when looking only at numbers or bivariate plots. Changes within the same subject may be visualized by means of asymmetrical faces, for example half of the face representing the state before and the other half the state after treatment.

As compared to other graphical techniques, the advantage of Chernoff faces is the sensitivity of our perception to asymmetry, to small changes in facial expression, and to associations to the array of faces stored in our memory. The technique is an excellent tool to explore multivariate data and can be used to aid in cluster and discriminant analysis as well as to detect trends in time-series analyses.

Inferential Statistics

During the past two decades an increasing number of articles and studies has dealt with the statistical quality of medical publications (review in [25]). Most authors have concluded that statistics are used inappropriately in 50% or more of the articles published. A common finding is that such simple techniques as the *t*-test, χ^2-test and Wilcoxon signed-rank test are inappropriately applied to complex experimental designs and multivariate data sets. This holds in particular for experimental research in which the data are usually analyzed by the medical scientist himself without the assistance of a professional statistician. A typical example is the evaluation of animal studies on regional blood flow measured with the radioactive microsphere technique. The experimental design of these studies frequently involves two or more groups of animals and several consecutive measurements within each group. The use of the *t*-test and nonparametric tests for pairwise comparisons of groups and/or measurements is inappropriate here; rather, multifactorial analysis of variance for repeated measures or multiple regression techniques should be used for this type of experiment. Admittedly, these methods cannot be carried out on pocket calculators but require access to the considerable computer resources available only since the technical revolution of microcomputers began. Nowadays, however, all common statistical software packages are available on personal and microcomputers [26], and medical scientists can readily use them. A three-way analysis of variance for repeated measures, which was used to evaluate the study on peripheral occlusive disease mentioned above, was carried out on a MicroVAX II computer in approximately 30 s with each of the packages BMDP and SAS. Improving the quality of statistical analyses is one of the most important functions of computers in experimental surgery, and the lack of computing resources should no longer serve as an excuse for incorrect or inappropriate statistical analyses.

Data Presentation

The amount of information which humans can process in a given period of time is dependent on the way in which the data are presented. Data in graphic form are grasped much faster than mere figures and lengthy explanations of numerical results. Chernoff faces, for example, are not restricted to exploratory data analysis but may also be used to illustrate the results of multivariate statistical tests. A variety of graphic presentations are routinely available in statistical packages or may be tailored to specific needs using graphic software on a personal computer or the graphic tools of statistic software (e.g., SAS).

Communication

Communication is a fundamental pillar of science. Results of research have been distributed in manuscript form ever since the origin of science, but the exponential increase of written material today makes it impossible to keep abreast of all research by reading all journals that might have some relevance in a particular field of interest. For quick access to and economic selection of relevant literature it is necessary to use data bases such as Medline, which are maintained at large computing centers dedicated to information services. Among the 3000 public data bases available around the world, some are of particular interest for experimental surgery, e.g., the Laboratory Animal Data Bank (LADB) available from the Pergamon International Information Corporation's (PIIC) service Infoline [6].

Progressive specialization accompanies the rising number of scientists involved in complex research projects, and communication between the members of different project groups becomes increasingly important. Conventional communication techniques such as post and telephone are slow and expensive, particularly for international cooperative projects with scientists separated by long distances and several time zones. For several years computer networks have spread around the world, improving international communication and cooperation. Most popular in academic fields are the European Academic Research Network (EARN) and BITNET in the USA. Both networks, as well as a number of others, are interconnected via gateways and support nearly 1900 academic computing service centers. Any user of these computing centers can send messages, manuscripts, data, and programs to other users via a common electronic mailbox system. With each center having 500–1000 accounted users, a total of 950000–1900000 scientists are connected to one another around the clock by terminals. Similar networks are available for in-house and campus communication with personal computers, but these are rarely found in medical schools and institutions in Europe.

At the Department of Experimental Surgery, University of Heidelberg, we have established a heterogeneous network, which at present is one of the largest local area networks (LAN) for medical research in Germany [12, 16, 17, 23]. The basic concept here involved utilizing the capabilities and resources of personal computers (PC) to attain a maximum efficiency. We consider the PC a universal workstation in a distributed processing environment, which satisfies all needs in medical research. The universal workstation comprises the functions of:

- An autonomous PC for data entry and simple analyses, for word processing, graphical and other independent applications
- A host computer terminal to run interactive sessions in dialogue with the mainframe, start batch jobs, and transfer data to and from the host
- A communication terminal to transfer and receive electronic mail from other users

For the universal workstation concept, the LAN must:

- Connect the workstations with one another and provide software for file transfer and mailbox functions
- Connect to the local computer service centers via gateways and supply software for terminal emulation and file transfer

- Connect to remote computer service centers via the public wide area data network (X.25; in Germany, DATEX-P) with software for file transfer
- Support resource sharing in terms of publicly accessible disks for data and program storage, public printers for letter quality printing and high resolution graphics (e. g., laser printer) etc.
- Support public services such as Telex, Teletex, etc.

Our local area network NET/ONE (Ungermann-Bass Inc., Santa Clara, CA, USA) has been instituted during the past 2 years; its present configuration is shown in Fig. 7. The network conforms to IEEE standard 802.3 (Ethernet) for ISO levels 0–2 and to the industry standard protocol XNS for higher ISO levels. The transmission type is baseband and the rate is 10 Mbit/s which is equivalent to approximately 500 printed pages per second. The network consists of two 500 m segments of coaxial cable, connecting 11 main buildings of the campus "Theoretikum." A maximum of 64 PCs per building my be linked to the network, using eight multiplexers in parallel. The university (IBM) and hospital (Siemens) computing centers are connected via fiber-optic cable 500 m in length and a short coaxial segment (50 m). Additional hosts linked to the network are the PDP11/24 and the MicroVAX II of the Department of Experimental Surgery. EARN is accessed via the university computing center; the X.25 packet switched public data network is directly connected to the LAN by means of a packet assembler/disassembler (PAD). A maximum of 31 simultaneous computer sessions are possible at the moment (IBM 16, Siemens 8, PDP 1, MicroVAX 2, and remote X.25 hosts 4). Twenty-two research groups from 12 theoretical and clinical disciplines involved in cardiovascular research participate in the project and 17 PCs are presently connected to the network; we expect a further increase in the number of users.

Discussion

The applications described above do not represent a complete overview. We are well aware that numerous important applications of computers in experimental surgery have been omitted here, e. g., knowledge-based ("expert") systems to support diagnostic and therapeutic decision making. Our aim, however, has been to show the diversity of computer applications, their usefulness, and their impact on research itself by means of certain typical examples.

Regardless of how many computer resources are available, their utilization is dependent upon the acceptance of the scientists and the technical staff who must work with them. When we initiated training courses for the network users, the majority had only little if any conception as to the capabilities of the network; in fact, some were rather skeptical. During these courses users were invited to participate in a literature retrieval from Medline in their respective fields. Five minutes later they held some 10 or 20 references in their hands, for which they would have spent hours with Index Medicus in the library. They could observe how messages and manuscripts are transferred from Heidelberg to the USA in a few minutes. These were arguments which not even skeptics could resist.

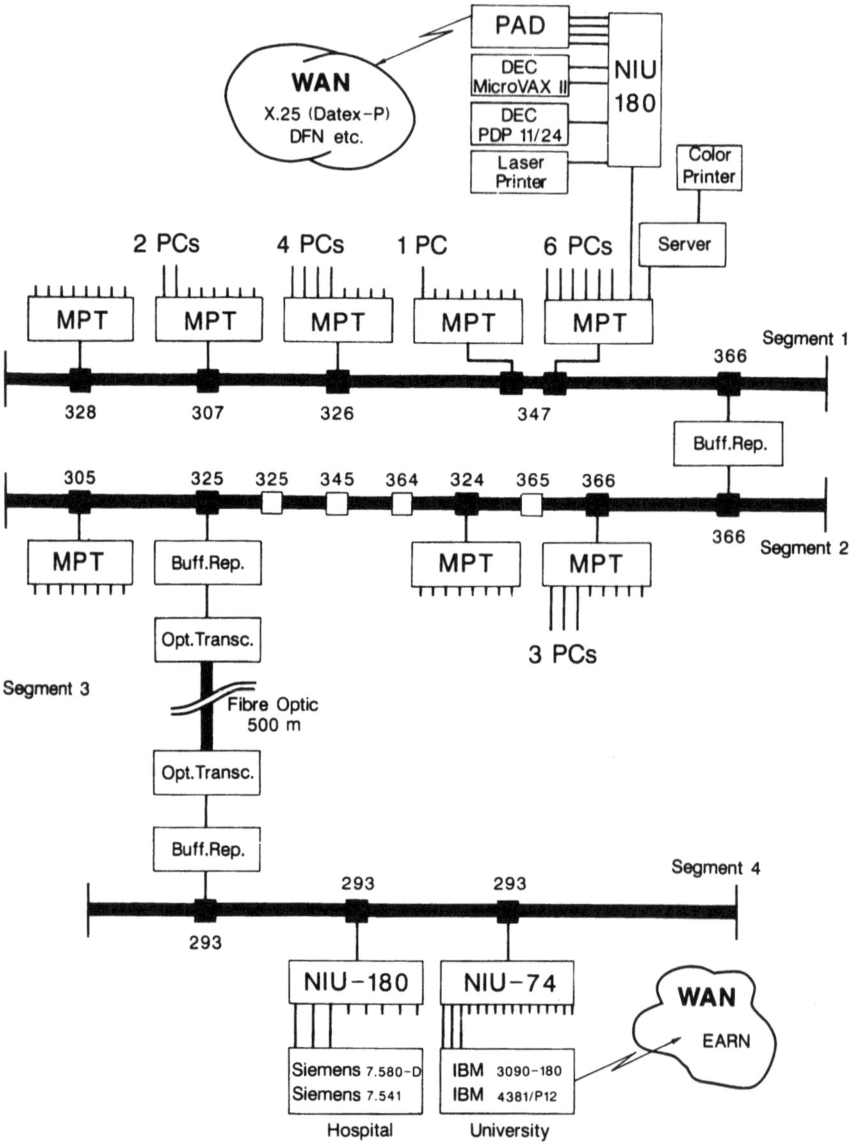

Fig. 7. Configuration of heterogeneous local area network at the University of Heidelberg. The length of the network is approximately 1550 m (two coaxial segments of 500 m, one fiber-optic segment of 500 m, and one coaxial segment of 50 m). *Numbers* below or above the boxes on the cable denote building numbers. The cable is installed in the basement, short connections lead to the multiplexers which are located on the intermediate floor of each building. *MPT,* multiport transceiver (= multiplexer); *Buff. Rep.,* buffered repeater to connect two segments; *Opt. Transc.,* optical transceiver, converts electrical to optical signals and vice versa; *NIU,* network interface unit, connects devices with different protocols to the network (180 = asynchronous serial lines, 74 = IBM 3270 controller; *PAD,* packet assembler-disassembler (converts X.25 protocol); *WAN* wide area network (Datex-P of the German Postal and Telecommunications Authorities); *DFN,* Deutsches Forschungsnetz (German Research Network), which connects the computer service centers of all universities in Germany

Other critical aspects are the resources in terms of money, time, and manpower which must be spent in establishing and maintaining an effective computer environment in a research department. The most common error is to expect a maximum of output from a minimum of input. With the exception of ready-to-use standard or customized application software, no benefit is gained merely from the physical presence of a computer. The development of a new application program requires months or years, depending on the number of computer scientists involved and on their experience. The image processing system for microcirculatory research, for example, consumed some 2 man-years and the LAN system some 3. However, once the program is in routine use, tremendous savings of time and manpower accrue to medical scientists. From our experience we estimate the costs for maintaining an effective computer environment at 20%–25% of both scientific staff and budget. In our department, three out of nine academic colleagues are involved in the development and maintainance of programs; two of these are mathematicians, and one is an electronics engineer.

Conclusions

An effective computer environment is indispensable for a modern department of experimental surgery. The department should have its own group of computer scientists who are responsible for the hardware, operating system, and application software, and who develop special application software in close cooperation with the medical scientists. According to modern concepts of distributed processing, a department should have its own computers which are embedded in both campus and wide area networks in order to utilize all capabilities offered by modern technology. Computer scientists who work in a department of experimental surgery should spend a substantial part of their efforts in motivating and educating their medical collegues; this function is as important as computers and programs themselves. A prerequisite for effectiveness, however, is allocating sufficient funds to the computer environment. This is repaid through an increased productivity on the part of the medical and technical staff, through improved reliability of the data, and through an improved statistical quality of the results.

References

1. Andrews DF (1972) Plots of high dimensional data. Biometrics 28: 125–136
2. Chernoff H (1973) The use of faces to represent points in k-dimensional space graphically. J Am Stat Ass 68: 361-368
3. de Asla RA, Benis AM, Jurado RA, Litwak RS (1985) Management of postcardiotomy hypertension by microcomputer-controlled administration of sodium nitroprusside. J Thorac Cardiovasc Surg 89: 115–120
4. Dixon WJ (ed) (1985) BMDP statistical software manual. University of California Press, Berkley
5. Engelman L, Hill MA, Dula M (1986) BMDP data manager manual. BMDP Statistical Software, Los Angeles
6. FASEB News (1983) Cooperative agreement with Pergamon International Information Corporation. Fed Proc 42: 2517

7. Forst H, Racenberg J, Peter K, Messmer K (1987) Right ventricular performance during mechanical ventilation with positive endexpiratory pressure. In: Kox W, Bihari D (eds) Septic shock and the adult respiratory distress syndrome. Springer, Berlin Heidelberg New York (in press)
8. Flury B, Riedwyl H (1981) Graphical representation of multivariate data by means of asymmetrical faces. J Am Stat Ass 76:757–765
9. Flury B, Riedwyl H (1983) Some applications of asymmetrical faces. Technical Report No. 11, Institut für Mathematische Statistik und Versicherungslehre, Universität Bern
10. Francis I (1983) A survey of statistical software. Comput Statist Data Analysis 1: 17–27
11. Hartung HJ, Osswald PM, Bender HJ (eds) (1985) Anwendungsgebiete der Computertechnologie in Anaesthesie und Intensivmedizin. Springer, Berlin Heidelberg New York Tokyo (Anaesthesiology and Intensive Care Medicine, vol 168)
12. Holzförster HJ, Schosser R, Zeintl H, Messmer K (1986) Konzept und Realisierung eines Lokalen Netzwerkes im Bereich der Medizin an der Universität Heidelberg. Springer, Berlin Heidelberg New York, p 512 (Med. Informatik und Statistik, vol 64)
13. Kleiner B, Hartigan JA (1981) Representing points in many dimensions as trees and castles. J Am Stat Ass 76: 260–276
14. Meline LJ, Westenskow DR, Pace NL, Bodily MN (1985) Computer-controlled regulation of sodium nitroprusside infusion. Anesth Analg 64: 38–42
15. Messmer K, Funk W, Endrich B, Zeintl H (1984) The perspectives of new methods in microcirculation research. In: Messmer K, Hammersen F, Zweifach BW (eds) Perspectives in methodology for studies of the microcirculation. Karger, Basel, pp 77–90 (Progr Appl Microcirc, vol 6)
16. Pfister M (1986) Test und Bewertung verschiedener LAN-Produkte zur Auswahl eines PC-LAN mit Verbindung zu Großrechnern für den FSP 16.2 der Universität Heidelberg. Thesis, University of Heidelberg/Professional School Heilbronn, Heilbronn
17. Pfister M, Holzförster HJ, Schosser R (1986) Testplan für die Bewertung und Auswahl von Lokalen Netzen im Bereich der Medizin. Springer, Berlin Heidelberg New York, p 516 (Med. Informatik und Statistik, vol 64)
18. Potter DR, Moyle JTB, Lester RJ, Ware RJ (1984) Closed loop control of vasoactive drug infusion – a preliminary report. Anaesthesia 39: 670–677
19. SAS Institute Inc. (1985) SAS user's guide: basics, Version 5 Edition. SAS Institute Inc., Cary
20. SAS Institute Inc. (1985) SAS user's guide: statistics, Version 5 Edition. SAS Institute Inc., Cary
21. Schosser R (1980) Durchblutungsmessungen mit radioaktiv markierten Microspheres. Methodik und rechnergestützte Auswertung. Thesis, University of Munich, Munich
22. Schosser R, Arfors KE, Messmer K (1979) MIC-II – A program for the determination of cardiac output, arterio-venous shunt and regional blood flow using the radioative microsphere method. Comput Program Biomed 9: 19–38
23. Schosser R, Weiß C, Holzförster HJ, Messmer K (1986) Anwendungsmöglichkeiten und Benutzeranforderungen an ein lokales Netzwerk in der Medizinischen Forschung. Springer, Berlin Heidelberg New York, pp 439–42 (Med. Informatik und Statistik, vol 64)
24. Schüpbach M (1984) ASYMFACE – Asymmetrical faces on IBM PC. Technical Report No. 16, Institut für Mathematische Statistik und Versicherungslehre, Universität Bern
25. Williamson JW, Goldschmidt PG, Colton T (1986) The quality of medical literature: an analysis of validation assessments. In: Bailar III, JC, Mosteller F (eds) Medical uses of statistics. NEJM Books, Boston, pp 370–391
26. Woodward WA, Elliott AC (1983) A survey of statistical packages on microcomputers. Comput Statist Data Analysis 1: 191–200
27. Zeintl H (1985) Computergestützte Kapillarerkennung und Kapillardichtebestimmung in der Intravitalmikroskopie. Thesis, University of Heidelberg, Heidelberg
28. Zeintl H, Tompkins WR, Messmer K, Intaglietta M (1986) Static and dynamic microcirculatory video image analysis applied to clinical investigations. In: Mahler F, Messmer K, Hammersen F (eds) Techniques in clinical capillary microscopy. Karger, Basel, pp 1–10 (Prog Appl Microcirc, vol 11)
29. Zeintl H, Endrich B, Funk W, Messmer K (1984) Kapillarlängenmessung – Ein Vergleich zwischen einer "exakten" und einer stereologischen, d.h. statistischen Methode. In: Kropatsch W (ed) Mustererkennung 1984 (Informatik-Fachberichte 87). Springer, Berlin Heidelberg New York Tokyo, pp 70–6

III. Intestinal Immunology

Immune System of the Gut*

G. ENDERS

The organism is exposed to an abundance of antigenic material on its intestinal mucosal surface. The antigenic load consists of bacteria, viruses, and food components, which may become harmful, as in the case of gastroenteritis and food allergy. Protection against this challenge in the gut is provided by an array of defense mechanisms, one of which is the mucosal immune system of lymphoid cells distributed along the intestine. These cells are widely and diffusely distributed or assembled in follicles such as Peyer's patches (PP) of the small intestine. In addition to these specific immune cells the intestine enjoys nonspecific protection through mucosal motility, the formation of mucus, gastric acid, and intestinal enzymes which can change the antigenicity of ingested material.

Specific Immune Defense System of the Gut

Regulation of the Specific IgA System

IgA is the specific immunoglobulin in secretions [1]; in the intestine it is produced by plasma cells in the lamina propria. After secretion from these cells dimeric IgA binds to cell surface receptors on epithelial cells. This complex is internalized and subsequently secreted into the gut lumen [2]. Functions of IgA include, among others, inhibiting adherence of bacteria, forming complexes with antigens for digestion and neutralizing antigens. Explaining regulation of the development of IgA-forming plasma cells is a matter of controversy. Kawanishi et al. [3] favor a T-cell-dependent differentiation of PP precursor cells, which migrate along the thoracic duct, the mesenteric lymph nodes and finally "home" in the lamina propria. Cebra and coworkers [4], on the other hand, suggest an antigen-driven local differentiation of IgA plasma cells without T-cell influence in the intestine.

To test these two hypotheses, we developed an animal model in which all PP in the intestine of rats were surgically removed. No regeneration of PP could be seen after several months [5]. This model therefore seems useful for investigating the role of PP for the frequency and distribution of IgA plasma cells. After 8–12 weeks the gut was immunohistologically investigated by peroxidase-labelled IgA-specific antibodies. In

* This work was supported in part by Deutsche Forschungsgemeinschaft grants EN 147/1–1 and EN 147/2–1

Surgical Research:
Recent Concepts and Results
Baethmann/Messmer (Eds.)

Table 1. IgA-secreting cells (mean) and cells with cytoplasmic IgA (cIgA; median) in the lamina propria of the small intestine, thoracic duct and mesenteric lymph nodes in controls and PP-deprived rats

	IgA-secreting cells		cIgA cells	
	Control	PP-deprived	Control	PP-deprived
Lamina propria	360 ± 20	40 ± 10*	34.9 (29–73)	12.25* (6–36)
Thoracic duct	n. d.	n. d.	1936 (1240–3184)	487* (0–1667)
Mesenteric lymph nodes	170 ± 30	45 ± 10*	3027 (826–10856)	1441* (29–2982)

cIgA cells of lamina propria as percent of all lamina propria cells; all other figures are numbers of cells $\times 10^6$. * $p < 0.05$

addition, cells were enzymatically isolated and tested for immunoglobulin secretion in agar. As shown in Table 1, both IgA-secreting cells (as determined by reverse hemolytic plaque assay) and cells with IgA in plasma (immunohistology) were diminished in PP-deprived animals, in comparison with control animals. In addition to plasma cells in the intestine, cells with Cytoplasmic IgA were found in the thoracic duct, mesenteric lymph nodes (MLN) and spleen. The thoracic duct and MLN showed a decrease of cells with cytoplasmic IgA, suggesting that removal of PP reduces IgA precursor cells, which normally recirculate through the thoracic duct to the small intestine.

It was further studied as to whether reduction in the overall number of IgA plasma cells in the intestine is accompanied by a reduction of antigen-specific cells in the lamina propria; PP-deprived and control rats were orally challenged with lipopolysaccharide (LPS) as antigen. After 2 weeks lymphoid cells from mesenteric lymph nodes, spleen, and lamina propria of the small intestine were analyzed for antibodies against LPS by a hemolytic plaque assay. As shown in Fig. 1, rats without PP had less anti-LPS-secreting cells in the lamina propria than control rats but considerably higher antigen responsive cells in the MLN and the spleen. A similar response was found when using antigens as different as sheep red blood cells and cholera toxin [6]. We conclude from these findings that disturbances in the first line of defense against oral antigens lead to a higher number of antigen-reactive cells in the other lymphoid organs.

Antigen Recognition in the Gut

A prerequisite for an immunologic reaction is recognition of the antigen by specialised cells, such as monocytes, macrophages, and dendritic cells in the lymph nodes and spleen. These cells are also found in the gut in the PP and the lamina propria. As these cells are separated by the intestinal epithelium from the antigen, specialized

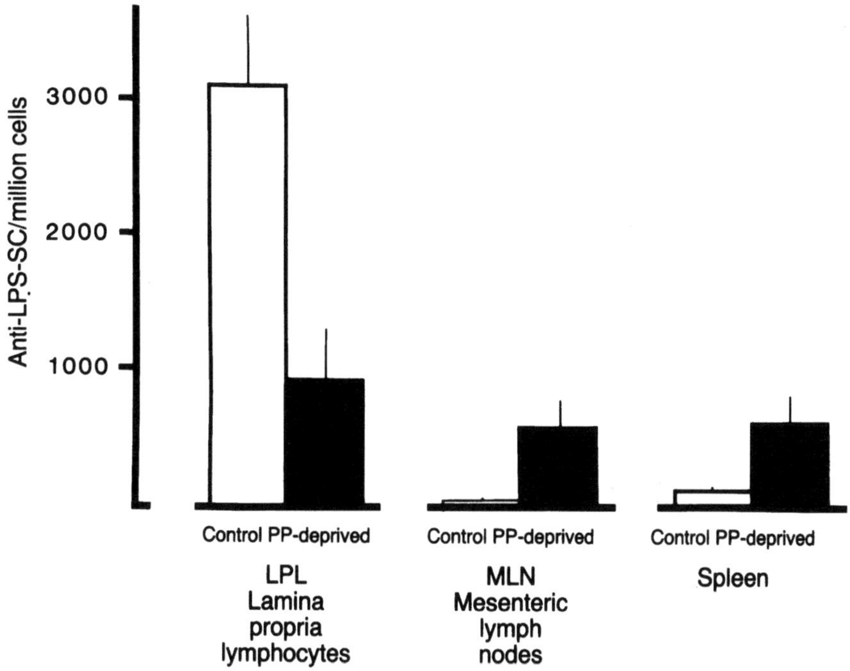

Fig. 1. Anti-LPS-secreting cells (mean ±) in the small intestine, mesenteric lymph nodes (MLN) and spleen of control and Peyer's patches deprived rats as tested by hemolytic plaque assay in vitro

epithelial cells which make contact with the antigen must transmit the information for immune recognition. Specialized cells of the intestine were described in 1974 by Owen and coworkers [7] and were designated as M cells due to their microfolds. M cells which cover PP are easily detected by electron microscopy. It has been demonstrated that intact proteins as well as pathogens are transported across these cells. Histology has revealed M cells to be in close contact with monocytes and dendritic cells, indicative of their cooperation in the immune response. The role of PP in antigen recognition could be shown by antigen challenge (cholera toxin) in isolated intestinal loops with or without PP [8] and in rats with surgical removal of PP [9].In both experiments a local immune response could not be detected. In the former, recirculating antigen-specific cells were not found in the thoracic duct, whereas in the latter a reduction of antigen-specific cells of only the IgA isotype was found. Therefore, antigen recognition must be possible in the absence of M cells and PP. However, loss of PP's regulatory influence causes alterations in the antibody response. Finally, the cells lack the "homing" propensity for the gut.

The hypothesis that PP are generally the location for recognition of orally administered antigens could be shown directly in another experiment using labelled, antigen-specific T cells from an in vitro T-cell line. After feeding the specific antigen, it was possible to show an accumulation of T cells in PP. Neither application of a nonspecific antigen nor control feeding attracted T cells into PP in control experiments. Recogni-

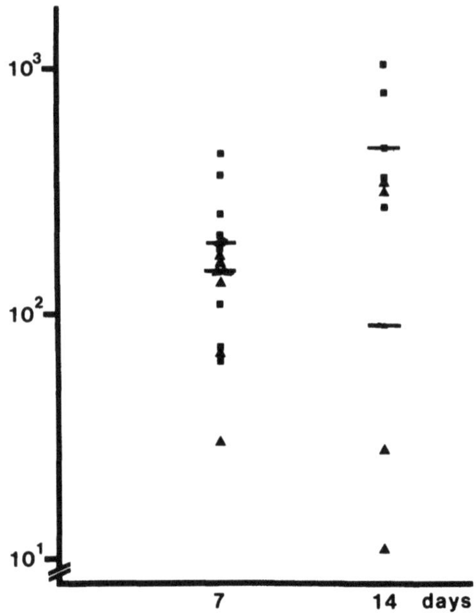

Fig. 2. IgA nitro-iodo-pleurel (NIP) (Anti-Nip (4-hydroxy-3 iodo-5 nitrophenyl) specific antibodies in serum of rats given i.v. AG-specific T cells. *Triangles,* controls; *squares,* animals fed with artificial AG (NIP); antibody concentrations given as reciprocal of final dilution

tion of the antigen in these patches resulted in a high systemic IgA response (Fig. 2). Thus, a regulatory influence of PP on recognition of a T-cell-dependent antigen is clearly demonstrated.

Non-specific Mucosal Defense System

The non-specific defense system consists of destruction of antigens by gastric acid or by proteolytic enzymes and inhibition of antigen contact with the luminal surface by mucus and motility. Abdominal surgery impairs the non-specific defense system. Dysfunction of the system may affect antigenicity and the contact time of ingested antigens.

The non-specific defense system of the gut is not well understood at present. In an attempt to elucidate interactions here, we studied the influence of gastric-acid loss on the response towards orally administered antigens in vagotomized rats. Preliminary results demonstrate dramatic alterations of immunoglobulin concentrations in bile, intestinal fluid, and serum after proximal gastric vagotomy. As shown in Table 2, the changes affect primarily IgA concentrations in serum, bile and intestinal fluid as well as total immunoglobulin concentrations in bile and small intestinal fluid. These changes do not result from an altered blood circulation but from the increased intestinal antigenic load. This could be shown by measuring concentrations of immunoglobulin and intestinal bacterial load over 6 weeks. IgA concentrations in bile and intestinal fluid increased continously, reaching a plateau after 4 weeks. Examination of intestinal bacterial load showed colonization of the upper small intestine by numerous bacteria in vagotomised animals. The immunoglobulins of the bile were in

Table 2. Total immunoglobulin and IgA concentrations of control rats and vagotomised rats in serum, bile and intestinal fluid (mg/ml, mean ± SE)

	Total Ig		IgA	
	Control	Vagotomised	Control	Vagotomised
Serum	40.7 ± 1.8	36.3 ± 2.0	0.25 ± 0.04	1.5 ± 0.4*
Bile	0.8 ± 0.1	3.1 ± 0.15*	0.1 ± 0.02	0.5 ± 0.1*
Intestinal fluid	0.07 ± 0.02	0.77 ± 0.08*	< 0.01	0.02 ± 0.003

*$p < 0.05$

most cases directed towards these bacteria (as assessed by indirect immunofluorescence). Specificity of the immunoglobulins of the biliary and intestinal fluid against gut antigens could also be shown in an experiment with vagotomized animals to which a defined antigen (LPS 055 B5) was orally administered (Fig. 3). The animals produced high concentrations of specific antibodies against the orally administered antigen in bile and serum, whereas control animals showed only traces (Fig. 3). We conclude therefore that after vagotomy the antigen was structurally unchanged, had a longer contact with intestinal epithelium and was immunogenic. While many studies have examined the regulation of the specific immune response to orally given antigens, only a few experiments have been conducted on the non-specific defense system. An antigen-specific nature of the non-specific defense mechanism has been shown for mucus production [10] and for motility [11], demonstrating even immunological memory. It has been shown [12] that antigens can be recognized even

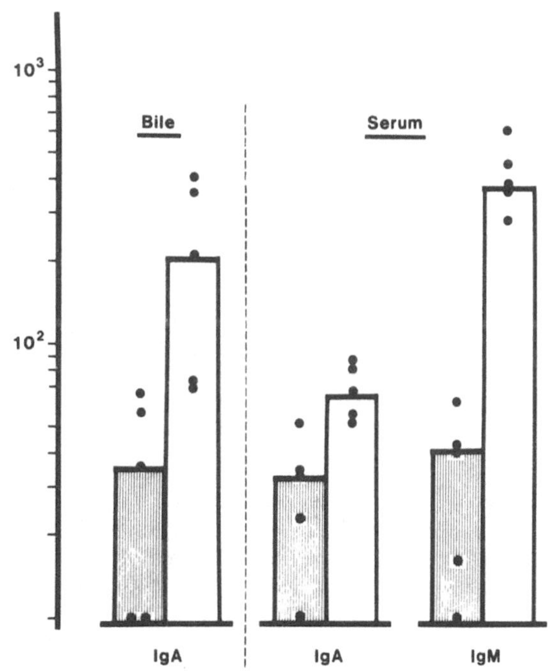

Fig. 3. LPS-specific antibody concentration in serum and bile of proximal gastric vagotomized rats (*unshaded bars)* and of control rats (*shaded bars)* (titer). IgG was not detectable in serum or bile, nor IgM in bile. *Columns* represent mean values

in the stomach; this recognition is associated with an increase in gastrin production. Whether these mechanisms are related to the immune defense system is not yet clear, however.

Conclusion

The antigenic conditions prevalent in the intestinal mucosal environment require potent immune mechanisms which must respond to luminal antigen. Lymphoid tissue organized in PP seems to have a strong regulatory influence on the specific immune response (IgA, intraepithelial T cells). The response is associated with its function as a source of IgA precursor cells and regulatory T cells, as well as its role in antigen presentation. In addition to these mechanisms an array of non-specific factors contribute to the defense system, e.g., in eliminating antigenicity (gastric acid, proteolytic enzymes) and in inhibiting direct contact of antigens with the intestinal luminal surface (mucus, motility). The mechanisms controlling the non-specific defense system of the gut are not well understood. Insight into these processes may be not only of scientific interest but also helpful in treating patients undergoing abdominal surgery.

Acknowledgements. The author wishes to thank A. Hauffe, J. Krumbach, A. Pfleiderer and B. Sinkula for excellent technical work and C. Chaudhry for typing the manuscript.

References

1. Tomasi TB, Plaut AG (1985) Humoral aspects of mucosal immunity. In: Gallin JJ, Fauci AS (eds) Advances in host defense mechanisms, vol 4. Raven, New York, pp 31–63
2. Brandtzaeg P (1980) Transport models for secretory IgA and IgM. Clin Exp Immunol 44: 221–232
3. Kawanishi K, Salzmann L, Strober W (1983) Mechanisms regulating IgA class specific immunoglobulin production in murine gut associated lymphoid tissue: II. Terminal differentiation of post switch sIgA bearing Peyer's patch B-cells. J Exp Med 158: 649–669
4. Cebra JJ, Cebra ER, Clough ER, Fuhrmann JA, Komisar JL, Schweitzer PA, Shahin RD (1983) IgA commitment: models for B-cell differentiation and possible roles for T-cells in regulating B-cells development. Ann NY Acad Sci 409: 25–38
5. Enders G, Gottwald T, Brendel W (1986) Induction of oral tolerance in rats without Peyer's patches. Immunology 58: 311–314
6. Enders G, Delius M, Ballhaus S, Brendel W (1987) Role of PP in the intestinal immune response to CT in enterically immunized rats. Infect Immun 55: 1997–1999
7. Owen RL, Johns AL (1974) Epithelial cell specialization within human PP: an ultrastructural study of intestinal lymphoid follicles. Gastroenterology 66: 189–203
8. Husband AJ, Gowans JL (1978) The origin and antigen dependent distribution of IgA containing cells in the intestine. J Exp Med 148: 1146–1160
9. Enders GA, Brendel W (1987) The influence of Peyer's patches on the organ specific distribution of IgA plasma cells. Immunology (in press)
10. Lake AM, Bloch KJ, Neutra MR, Walker WA (1979) Intestinal goblet cell mucus release: II. In vivo stimulation by Ag in the immunized rat. J Immunol 122: 834–837
11. Palmer JH, Castro GA (1986) Anamnestic stimulus-specific myoelectric responses associated with intestinal immunity in the rat. Am J Physiol 250: G266–273
12. Krämling HJ, Enders G, Teichmann RK, Demmel T, Merkle R, Brendel W (1987) Antigen induced gastrin release: an immunologic mechanism of gastric antral mucosa. Adv Exp Med Biol (in press)

Absorption of Macromolecules and Particles from the Gut

J. SEIFERT, and W. SASS

Introduction

The energy supply of living organisms is provided by the functioning of the gastrointestinal tract. Since food is not presented in an absorbable condition, the tract is equipped with digestive systems, such as acid production in the stomach, the various enzymes of the pancreas and salivary glands, the bile of the liver and the hormones of the gut. The autonomous nervous system, i.e. the vagus and the sympathic nerves, begin and control the absorption processes.

Apart from the knowledge that macromolecules as well as particles are degraded to absorbable smaller elements by these digestive mechanisms [1], it is known that newborn babies can absorb macromolecules such as gammaglobulin from the gut in an undegraded form [2]. By this means newborn children are protected against infections via the absorption of substances from the milk of the mother. This is necessary at a time when resistance to infection is not operating. In adults the ability to absorb macromolecules in undigested form with their original, biological activity is commonly thought to be lost. Experimental data from adult animals and humans, however, demonstrate that the adult organism is also capable of absorbing intact macromolecules from the gut.

Absorption of Radioactively Labeled Horse Gammaglobulin

Labeling proteins with isotopes such as ^{125}I or ^{131}I offers a simple method for tracing the route of absorption. With radioactivity which normally is bound tightly to the protein [4], it can be observed whether proteins are absorbed. Furthermore, it is possible to evaluate the macro- and micromolecular conditions in which proteins are present after absorption. For the following investigations 50 mg gammaglobulin from horses were radioactively labelled. By chromatography via Sephadex G 25 gel, labelled protein was separated from unbound label [5]. Rats, dogs, and humans were fed with 50 mg radioactively labelled horse gammaglobulin. As shown in Table 1, radioactivity appeared in blood of humans and animals during an observation time of 6 h. The increase of radioactivity in blood indicates that gammaglobulin was absorbed but does not answer the question as to whether the protein was in a macromolecular or in a degraded condition. Therefore, immunological tests were performed to identify macromolecules with specific antibodies. With anti-horse gammaglobulin from rab-

Surgical Research:
Recent Concepts and Results
Baethmann/Messmer (Eds.)

Table 1. Radioactivity in blood of humans, dogs, and rats* after enteral application of radioactively labelled horse gammaglobulin (% of applied dosage in 1 ml)

	Observation time						
	Before	1 h	2 h	3 h	4 h	5 h	6 h
Humans (n = 3)	0.0	0.0025 ±0.0005	0.0020 ±0.0003	0.0027 ±0.0005	0.0024 ±0.0004	0.0020 ±0.0001	0.0018 ±0.0001
Dogs (n = 4)	0.0	0.0092 ±0.0025	0.0088 ±0.0020	0.0078 ±0.0020	0.0050 ±0.0022	0.0072 ±0.0021	0.0061 ±0.0018
Rats (n = 4)	0.0	–	–	0.25 ±0.10	–	–	0.32 ±0.05

*Values for rats determined only after 3 h and 6 h

bits, horse gammaglobulin can be precipitated. In the agar gel diffusion technique according to Ouchterlony [6], serum from humans and animals fed with horse gammaglobulin was tested against anti-horse gammaglobulin. Precipitating lines indicated that horse gammaglobulin was present in the serum of humans and animals after an absorption time of 6 h. With this test system it is possible to demonstrate that macromolecules are absorbed from the gut, since degraded protein fragments do not react with the antiserum.

Quantitative Demonstration of Absorbed Proteins

To ascertain how much of the absorbed horse protein was in macromolecular or degraded form, radiochromatography was performed with serum of fed animals and humans. With this method it is possible to separate labeled proteins according to their molecular weight. Chromatography showed that 99% of radioactivity was bound to the protein after labeling and before the protein was administered. After oral application and absorption, we found 20% in dogs, between 4% and 10% in rats and 15% in humans in the macromolecular, undegraded form in serum (Table 2). This investigation shows that adult animals and humans are able to absorb macromolecules in a macromolecular state from the gut. The amount of high molecular weight proteins absorbed form the gut is, however, different from species to species.

Table 2. Immunological demonstration of protein absorption through the intestinal wall using agar gel diffusion technique; quantitative separation of absorbed proteins in serum by radiochromatography in high and low molecular weight proteins; biological activity after absorption tested by lymphocytotoxic titer

	Precipitate	High-molecular	Low-molecular	Lymphocytotoxic titer
Before	–	–	–	1:4
After	+++	10%	90%	1:64

Biological Activity of Macromolecular Proteins after Absorption

To determine whether macromolecules were transferred from the lumen of the gut to the blood without loosing biological activity, a protein was used with characteristics which can be tested before and after absorption. The horse gammaglobulin used reacts against human lymphocytes and destroys lymphocytes in the presence of complement. This ability can be tested in vitro by the lymphocytotoxic titer. Before enteral application the horse gammaglobulin had a lymphocytotoxic titer of 1:1024. After absorption no significant increase of titer was found in the blood of the animals. This was probably due to dilution of the absorbed macromolecular proteins by the blood. Therefore, an increase of antibody titer was studied in a system with a lower flow rate and which takes part in the absorption process. This is the thoracic duct, which has a flow rate of 1 ml/min in rats. By cannulating the thoracic duct, lymph can be collected almost quantitatively. To study the biological properties of the absorbed protein, rats were fed with 5 ml (250 mg) of an antilymphocytic gammaglobulin from horses with a lymphocytotoxic titer of 1:1024. The lymphocytotoxic titer in the lymph of the rats was 1:4 before application of the antilymphocytic gammaglobulin. Six hours after application the titer was significantly increased to 1:32. Under these conditions, it was possible to demonstrate the biological activity of the absorbed protein.

The next questions were whether macromolecules are all absorbed in the same way, and which factors influence their absorption. It is conceivable that absorption of macromolecules is a passive process which depends upon molecular weight, i.e., the bigger the molecule, the lower the absorption rate. A further question was whether "self" and "nonself" properties of macromolecules and a pre-existing immunological memory play a role in absorption for these substances. Investigations were performed on proteins of different molecular weight and biological properties. Furthermore, the immune response against these proteins was manipulated.

Comparison of Absorption of Macromolecules of Various Molecular Weights

The smallest molecule tested in these experiments on rats was insulin, with a molecular weight of 5700 dalton. The next larger molecule, which was investigated in the same experiments, was a proteolytic enzyme of plant origin (bromelain) with a mean molecular weight of 33000 dalton. The second largest molecule tested was haemoglobin with a molecular weight of 64000 dalton. The largest molecule was a gammaglobulin. All animals received equivalent amounts of the test proteins. Time of absorption was 6 h in all experiments. After this period the amount of test protein remaining in the gut was determined. Absorption was calculated from the remaining amount and the applied dose. Test proteins were studied by radiochromatography with various Sephadex gels. Table 3 shows that there was no relationship between absorption rate and molecular size. Horse gammaglobulin, the largest molecule studied, was absorbed at a higher rate than the smaller bromelain and bromelain was better absorbed than insulin. Hence, the theory that smaller molecules are better absorbed than larger ones must be rejected, ruling out passive diffusion as a mechanism of absorption.

Table 3. Absorption rate and percentage of macromolecules in serum after absorption

	Absorption rate (% applied dose)	Macromolecules (% in serum)	Macromolecules (mg/animal)
Insulin	72	10	7.2
Bromelain	40	40	16.0
Haemoglobin	69	1.2	0.7
Horse gammaglobulin	54	10	5.4

Influence of the Immune Response on the Absorption of Antigenic Proteins

To investigate whether the systemic immune response influence absorption of proteins, rabbits were immunised against human gammaglobulin until precipitating antibodies could be detected in serum. Absorption studies with human gammaglobulin were then performed with the immunized animals. In a second investigation human serum albumin was tested for absorption. The results were compared with control experiments with untreated, nonimmunized animals. Whereas nonimmunized animals absorbed 88% of the gammaglobulin load within 4 h, immunized animals absorbed only 57%. If, however, the immunized animals were fed with a protein against which they were not sensitive, e.g., human serum albumin, the absorption rate was normal (approximately 80%). Thus, the systemic immune response influences markedly and specifically absorption of antigenic proteins.

Absorption of Particles

In a next step, it was tested whether particles are taken up from the gut, reaching blood and lymph. For this purpose rats received intraduodenally natural particles, i.e., *Lycopodium* spores (mean diameter, 35 μm) and *Urtica* pollen (mean diameter, 16 μm). The animals were then subjected to drainage of the thoracic duct. Resorption of the particles was studied under light microscopy in the collected lymph. Distinction from blood cells is possible on the basis of their characteristic shape and size. Figure 1 shows the number of particles observed in the thoracic duct lymph. In general, only a small fraction of particles was absorbed. An early maximum at 20 and 60 min was followed by a later increase after 80 and 140 min. This indicates that the absorption of particles is a discontinuous process.

Further studies were made as to the mechanism of particle absorption. Scanning electron microscopy revealed particles to be localized on the M cells of the Peyer's patches. The microfolds of M cells evidently caught the particles (Fig. 2a), and the M cell thereafter descended (Fig. 2b). Particles were later observed in deeper parts of the Peyer's patches attached to or phagocytized into macrophages (Fig. 3). As far as a general purpose of macromolecular or even particle absorption is concerned, it is conceivable that the phenomenon is associated with immunological processes involved in the distinction of "self" and "nonself". Thus, cellular as well as humoral immunological processes may be stimulated if antigens are administered orally.

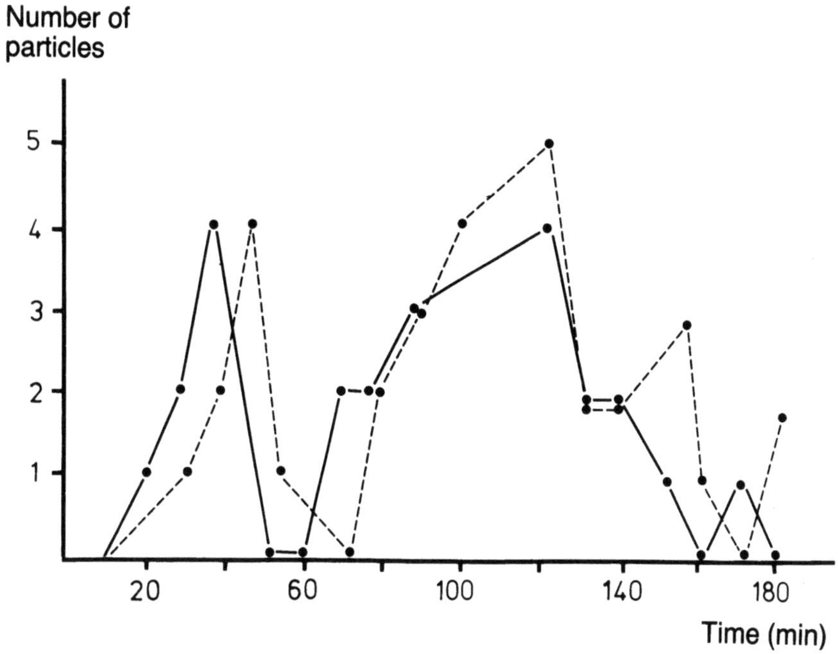

Fig. 1. Number of particles in lymph of thoracic duct after enteral application. *Solid line,* 16 μm *Urtica* pollen ($n = 6$); *broken line,* 35 μm *Lycopodium* 5 pores ($n = 4$)

Response of Lymphocytes in Peyer's Patches and in Thoracic Duct after Administration of an Immunogenic Protein

Rabbits were immunized against human gammaglobulin (HGG). Immunized animals were fed either with HGG or, in control experiments, with human serum albumin (HSA). The number of lymphocytes in the thoracic duct was counted over 4 h. Thereafter, Peyer's patches were dissected and histologically investigated. The number of lymphocytes in the thoracic duct of HGG-fed animals was twice as high as that in control animals fed only with HSA (Fig. 4). Even 1 h after feeding, the differences were highly significant. It is inferred from this that more lymphocytes were mobilized after feeding an immunogen to sensitized animals.

Histological investigations of Peyer's patches confirm this observation. In the dome region of a lymph follicle, but also at the base, masses of lymphocytes were observed in animals which were sensitized and fed with HGG (Fig. 5). The draining lymph vessels at the base of the lymph follicles were filled with lymphocytes too (Fig. 6). These findings also suggest that lymphocytes are mobilized if an antigenic protein is presented orally. The function of the mobilization of lymphocytes is as yet unclear.

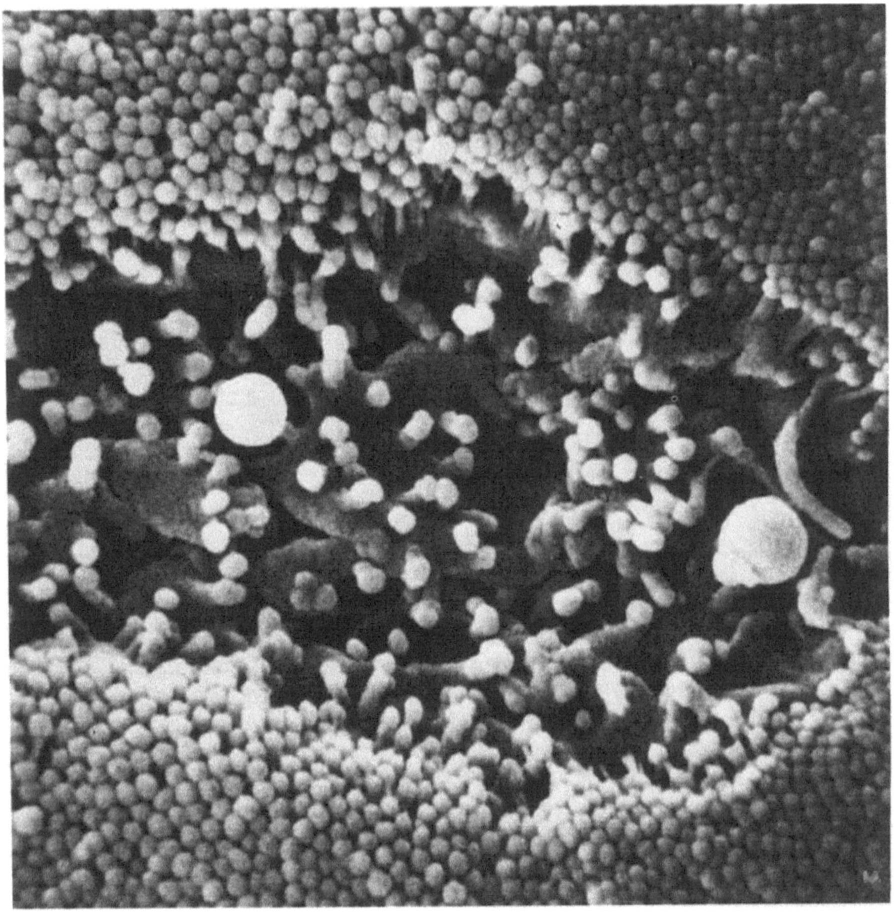

Fig. 2a, b. a) Two particles on the surface of an M cell, demonstrated by scanning electron microscopy. **b)** An M cell catches a particle by its microfolds. The M cell seems to be deeper than the other mucosa cells

Humoral Response in the Gastrointestinal Tract after Enteral Administration of an Immunogenic Protein

Not only cellular but also humoral immune reactions may be expected if antigenic proteins are enterally administered to immunized animals. The type of response was elucidated by the following investigations. Rabbits were immunized against HGG until precipitating antibodies appeared in the serum. The amount of antibodies found was 450 μg/ml [7]. The animals were then fed with HGG. During an absorption period of 6 h the amount of circulating antibodies was frequently tested. As shown in Fig. 7, the amount of circulating antibodies decreased significantly to 170 μg/ml.

To investigate the mechanism of elimination of antibodies after oral challenge, rabbit anti-HGG was radioactively labeled and intravenously injected into untreated

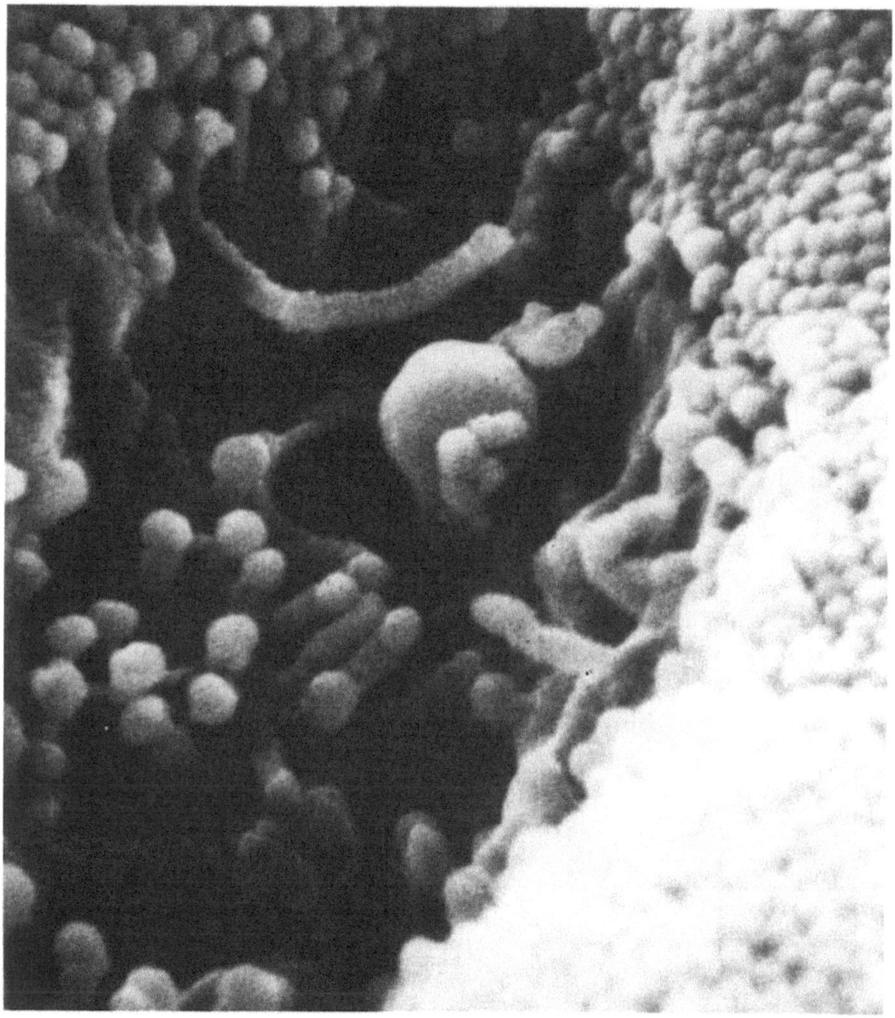

Fig. 2b

animals. Thereafter, animals were fed with HGG. Control animals intravenously received radioactively labeled normal rabbit serum and were also fed with HGG. After 4 h of absorption the animals were killed, and the radioactivity measured in the wall of the gut. Table 4 demonstrates that animals receiving radioactive antibodies had significantly more radioactivity in the intestinal wall than control animals. It can thus be concluded that circulating antibodies were fixed in the wall of the gut after the antigen was enterally administered, raising the possibility that an antigen-antibody reaction had taken place.

Such a reaction may be indirectly detectable, e. g., by consumption of complement, release of histamine, and an increase of blood flow in the affected tissue. These parameters were therefore studied in animals which were sensitized against HGG and

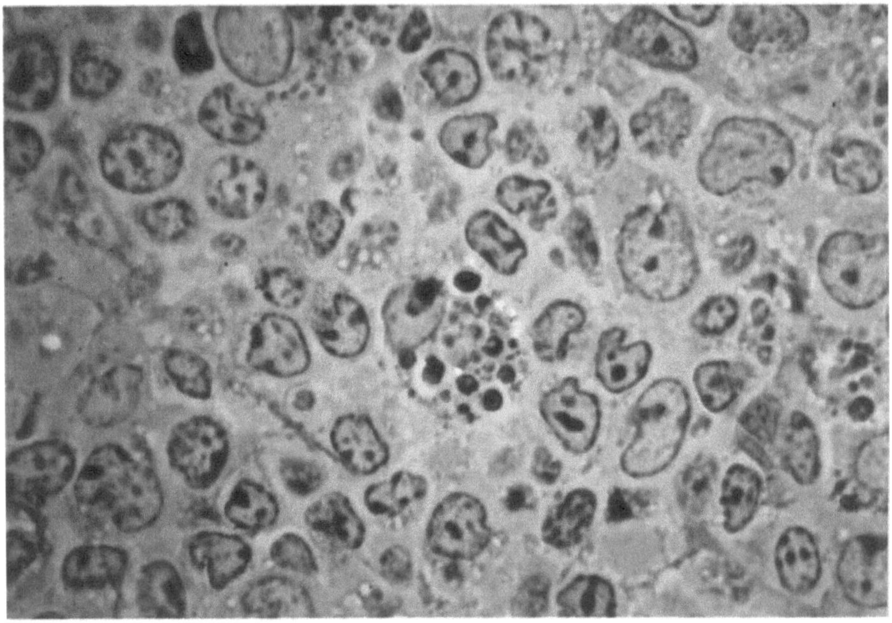

Fig. 3. Macrophage of a follicle of Peyer's patches with absorbed or ingested particles (*white dots in the center)*

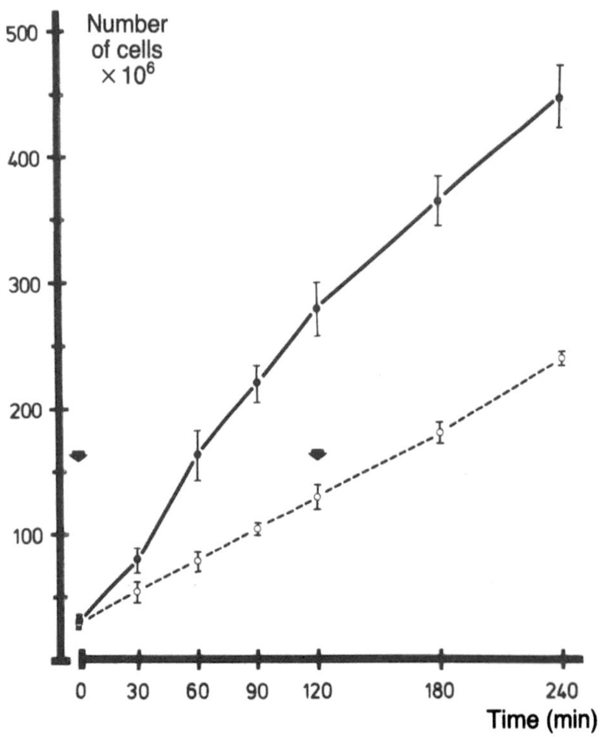

Fig. 4. Number of lymphocytes in thoracic duct of immunized rabbits after antigen feeding *(arrows)* with HGG (*solid line)* and of controls after feeding with human serum albumin (*broken line*)

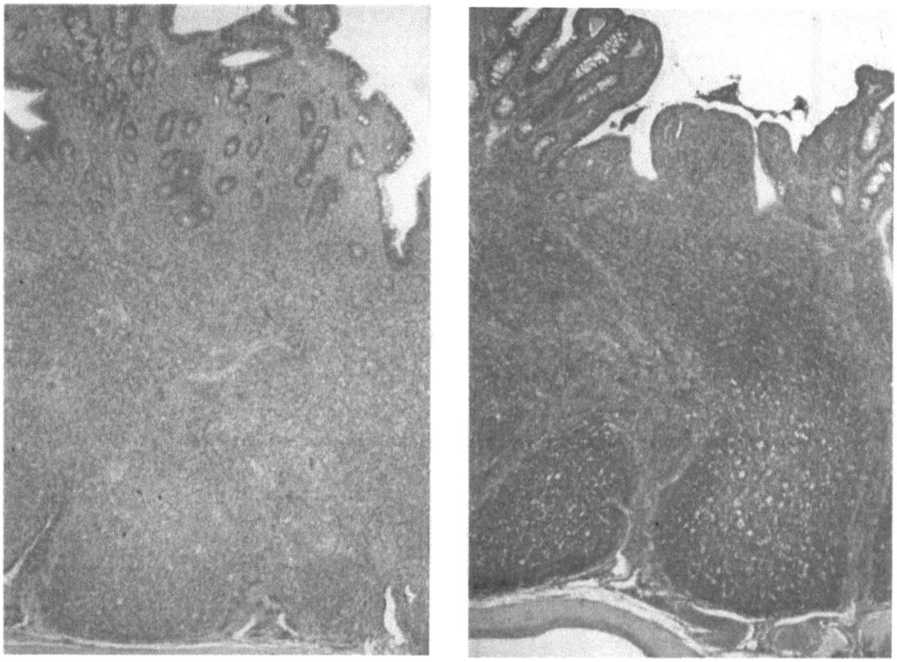

a b

Fig. 5a, b. Lymph follicle of Peyer's patches in rabbits after administration of HGG. **a)** Control rabbits, oral application of HGG; **b)** immunized rabbits, antigen feeding of HGG

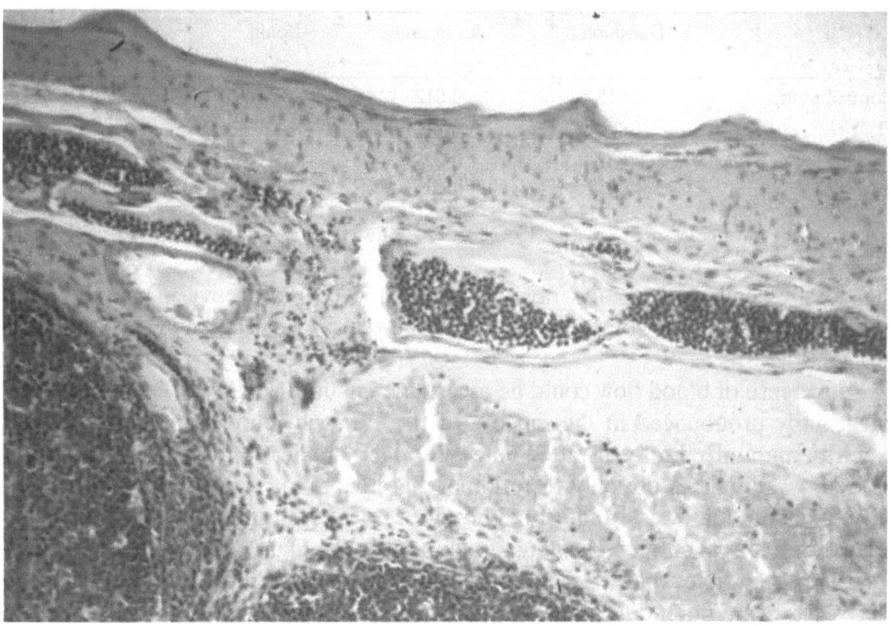

Fig. 6. Lymph vessels at base of lymph follicle filled with lymphocytes in animals immunized against HGG and fed with the immunogen (HGG)

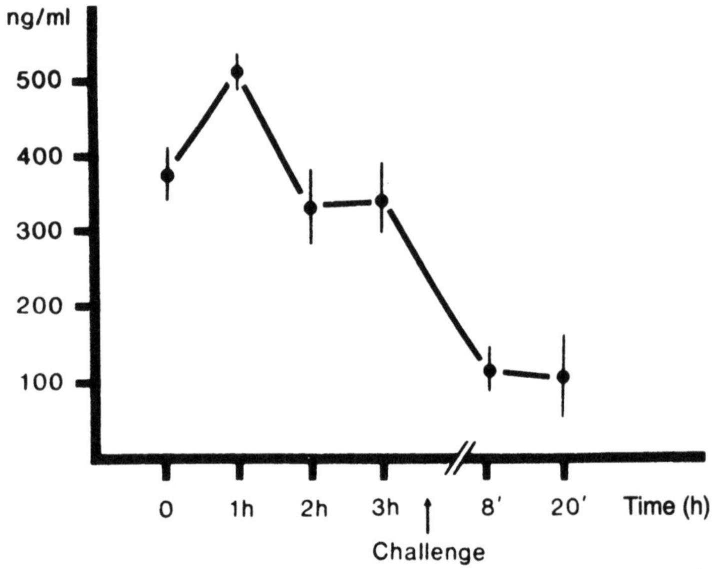

Fig. 7. Changes in the circulating antibody content in animals fed with the immunogen (HGG). A marked decrease could be observed during an observation time of 3 h. Antibody determination performed by radioimmunoassay

Table 4. Radioactively labelled circulating antibodies (250 mg) bound in different regions of the gut after enteral antigen application (% applied dosage in g)

	Duodenum	Jejunum	Ileum	Peyer's patches
Control group (n = 5)	0.015 ±0.005	0.012 ±0.003	0.017 ±0.002	0.012 ±0.002
Test group (n = 5)	0.032 ±0.005	0.028 ±0.006	0.030 ±0.004	0.029 ±0.005

then orally challenged. Blood flow was measured by radioactive microspheres in dogs. Activation of the complement system and release of histamine were studied in rabbits (Fig. 8).

An increase of blood flow could be ascertained in dogs (Fig. 9). The increase was particularly pronounced in the mucosa of the stomach, duodenum, jejunum and ileum in immunized animals after enteral antigen application [9]. The increase in blood flow stimulates not only secretion of digestive fluid [1] but may be associated with the liberation of gastrointestinal hormones. It was shown that gastrin was also released after oral antigen challenge in immunized animals, reaching a level which was almost ten times that which is normally found by a nutritional stimulus [10].

To investigate potential clinical consequences, e.g. desensitization, or decreasing circulating antibodies by antigen feeding, rabbits previously immunized against HGG were fed with HGG. During absoption HGG was intravenously given in addition.

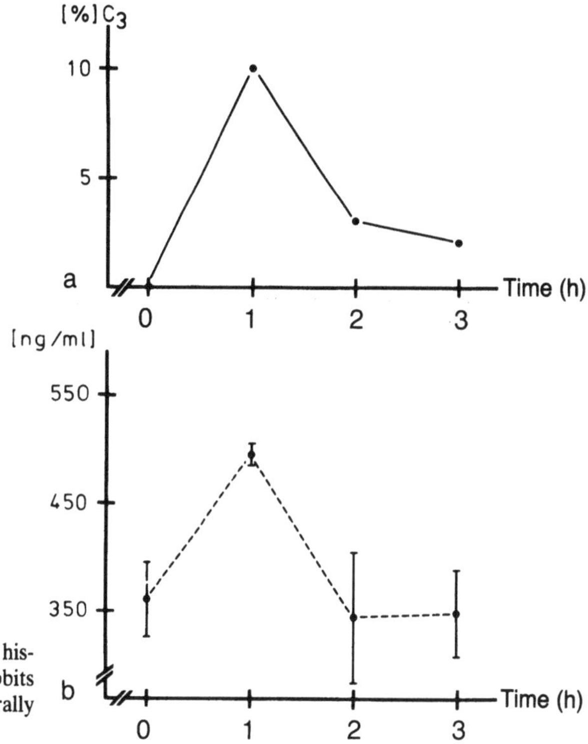

Fig. 8a, b. Complement **a)** and histamine **b)** increase in blood of rabbits immunized against HGG and orally treated with the antigen (HGG)

	Sensitised: Stomach	Sensitised: Duodenum	Sensitised: Jejunum	Sensitised: Ileum	Sensitised: Colon	Tolerant: Stomach	Tolerant: Duodenum	Tolerant: Jejunum	Tolerant: Ileum	Tolerant: Colon
Mucosa	↑	↑	↑	↑	–	–	–	–	↑	–
Muscularis	–	↑	↑	–	–	–	–	–	↑	–

Fig. 9. Changes in blood flow in various regions of the gastrointestinal tract after oral antigen challenge. *Arrows* indicate significant increases. Blood flow measured by microsphere technique

Table 5. Arterial pressure (mmHg) of rabbits immunized against human gammaglobulin (HGG) and fed with 1 g HGG during intravenous antigen exposure to 50 mg HGG; control animals also immunized but not fed with HGG

	Control value	10 Min	30 Min
Control animals	110 ± 10	40 ± 5	55 ± 8
Fed animals	105 ± 8	82 ± 8	110 ± 10

Changes in blood pressure were recorded as a clinical parameter of the degree of antigen-antibody reaction. Immunized animals without oral antigen challenge responded to intravenous antigen exposure with a deep and long-lasting decrease in blood pressure. Of all animals 50% died of circulatory shock, while all fed animals survived the intravenous antigen exposure. As shown in Table 5, fed animals showed only a slight decrease of blood pressure as compared with unfed controls. Long-term investigations demonstrate that the desensitization effect was not durable. At 24 h after oral challenge antibody concentrations in blood had similar values as prior to feeding. However, by repetitive and extensive feeding, concentrations of antibodies in blood remained permanently decreased [11]. The latter observations underline that immunological processes are important when digesting antigenic proteins. Another method for testing this hypothesis was employment of immunosuppression.

Influence of Immunosupression on Absorption of Proteins

For immunosuppression rats were intravenously given cyclosporin A (15 mg/kg) daily for 1 week. Peripheral lymphocyte counts were made to assess effectiveness of the procedure. The lymphocyte count was decreased by treatment to 50%. Absorption of HGG was tested in immunosuppressed animals in comparison with normal controls. Presence of intact HGG in serum was determined in fed animals by radial immunodiffusion with specific antisera. As shown in Table 6, immunosuppressed animals had a ten times higher absorption than normal control animals. In scanning electron micrographs of the surface of Peyer's patches, mucosa cells were largely normal, whereas M cells showed a marked decrease of microfolds. This may have caused changes in antigen recognition as a mechanism of the increased uptake of foreign proteins in the immunosuppressed animals. Thus, antigen recognition in the gut may be associated with inhibiting the absorption of high amounts of antigenic proteins.

Table 6. Human serum albumin in serum of rats after enteral application of 1 g HSA; control animals untreated, test animals treated with 15 mg/kg per day cyclosporin A over 1 week; serum albumin determined by immunodiffusion (mg/dl)

	Observation time					
	Before	1 h	2 h	3 h	4 h	5 h
Control animals (n = 10)	0	0	2.6 ±0.7	2.7 ±0.59	3.8 ±0.97	2.6 ±0.83
Test animals (n = 10)	0	6.2 ±2.8	15.1 ± 3.7	21.7 ± 5.0	25.7 ± 6.1	29.6 ± 6.8

Table 7. Absoption of human gammaglobin (HGG) in control animals and animals without Peyer's patches

	Absorbtion rate (% applied dosage, 100 mg)	Macromolekular	mg
Control	54%	5%	2.7
Animals without Peyer's patches	68%	8%	5.4

This hypothesis was further tested by resection of all visible Peyer's patches. After recovery of the animals absorption of HGG was studied. The absorption rates were significantly increased by the surgical reduction of the lymphoid tissue of the intestinal wall as shown in Table 7, suggestive of a decrease in antigen recognition in the gut.

In conclusion, absorption of macromolecules may be intimately involved in specific mechanisms of immune surveillance of the intestinal tract, particularly in the control of digestion of antigenic proteins.

References

1. Code CF (1968) Handbook of physiology. Williams and Wilkins, Baltimore
2. Brambell FWR (1966) The transmission of immunity from mother to young and the catabolism of immunglobulins. Lancet II: 7473–7475
3. Brambell FWR (1958) The passive immunity of the young mammal. Biol Rev 33: 488–493
4. Franks JJ, Takeda V, Reeve EB (1962) Preparation of autologous I-131-albumin for metabolic studies in man. L Lab Clin Med 60: 619–631
5. Seifert J (1976) Enterale Resorption großmolekularer Proteine bei Tieren und Menschen. Z Ernährungswiss [Suppl] 18: 1–70
6. Ouchterlony O (1962) Diffusion-in-gel methods for immunological analysis. Progr Allergy 6: 30–36
7. Seifert J (1983) Resorption großmolekularer Proteine und deren Wirkung auf das Immunsystem. Allergologie 6: 141–148
8. Seifert J, Hallfeld K, Eberle B, Krumbach J (1983) Changes of the immune response due to the absorption of antigenic proteins or peptides. Res Exp Med 182: 255–262
9. Seifert J (1984) Beeinflussung der Resorptionsrate großmolekularer Partikel. Allergologie 7: 258–262
10. Teichmann RK, Andress HJ, Gycha S, Seifert J, Brendel W (1983) Immunologische Reaktivität des Antrums zur Stimulation von Verdauungsprozessen. Langenbecks Arch Chir [Suppl]: 5–8
11. Seifert J, Ring J, Steininger J, Brendel W (1976) Influence of the immune response on the absorption of protein antigens. Nutr Metab 20: 195

Role of Immunology in Gastric Cytoprotection

R. K. TEICHMANN, E. PRATSCHKE, H. H. KRAEMLING, and H.-G. LIEBICH

A major pathophysiological principle of peptic ulcer treatment involves reduction of acid secretion by surgery (vagotomy or resection) and by medical therapy. Secretion of acid and pepsin plays a major role in the physiology of the stomach. A similar significance is attributed to these substances as aggressive factors in the pathogenesis of peptic ulcer disease [1]. As a defense against this action, however, mucosal cytoprotection resists digestion by acid and pepsin [2]; this is provided principally by mucus and bicarbonate secretion. Another important factor of cytoprotection is mucosal blood flow [3]. Both aggressive and cytoprotective functions are activated by ingestion of food.

Immunological Stimulation of Gastric Functions

Traditionally, stimulation of gastric secretion has been seen as ocurring in three phases: the cephalic, the gastric and the intestinal [1]. One aspect, however, has not hitherto been recognised: by ingestion of food the mucosa of the stomach comes in contact with substances which may be antigenic. These substances include not only food proteins but also bacteria and other material. Teichmann et al. [4–6] demonstrated for the first time that following systemic immunization, intragastric application of the antigen causes a marked release of serum gastrin together with an increase of local mucosal blood flow and mucus secretion. Gastrin is one of the major stimuli for gastric secretion [1].

Gastrin Release. Figure 1 shows serum gastrin release in controls and in test animals following immunization with the antigen after intragastric challenge. There was a significant increase of serum gastrin 5 min after the application of the antigen into the stomach in immunized animals. Serum gastrin remained elevated for 45 min. In controls there was no release of gastrin.

Gastrointestinal Blood Flow. Figure 2 shows changes of gastrointestinal blood flow following administration of antigen into the stomach of immunized animals [4, 6]. There was a significant increase of mucosal blood flow in the antrum at 10 min; a similar increase was found in the duodenal bulb.

Mucus Secretion. Electron-microscopy studies [8] revealed that 30 min after intragastric application of antigen the size of the secretory granules of mucus-producing epithelial cells had decreased by 45% (Fig. 3), indicating an increased mucus secretion into the lumen.

Surgical Research:
Recent Concepts and Results
Baethmann/Messmer (Eds.)

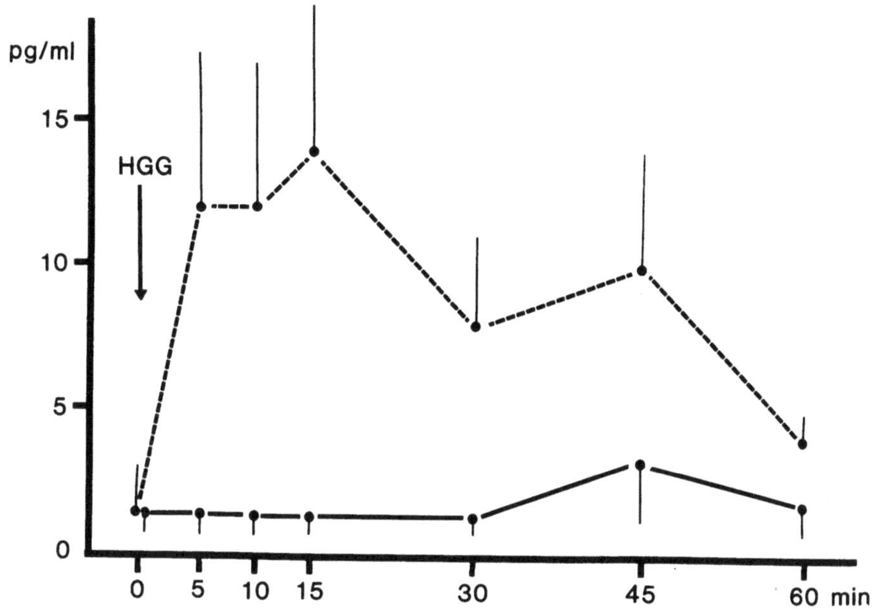

Fig. 1. Serum gastrin after intragastric administration of human gammaglobulin (1 g HGG/100 ml water) as antigen via a nasogastric tube in control (*solid line; n* = 6) and immunized dogs (*broken line, n* = 12). Immunisation was performed by weekly i. m. injections of 0.1 g HGG together with Freund's adjuvant until precipitating antibodies were detected by the Ouchterlony assay

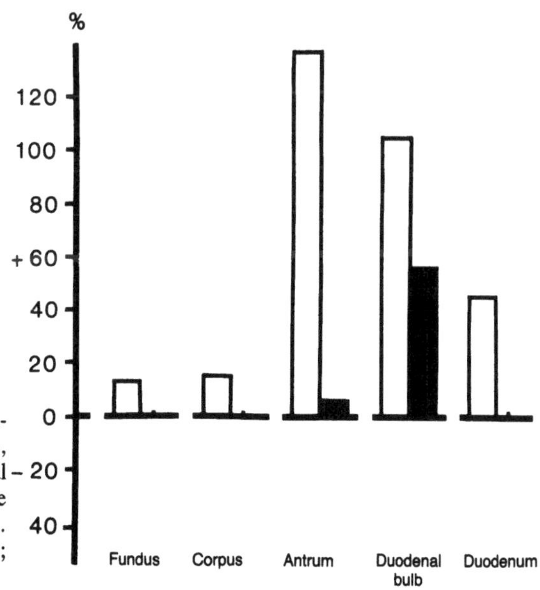

Fig. 2. Changes in blood flow (% of control) in the mucosa of fundus, corpus, antrum, duodenum and in the duodenal bulb measured by the microsphere technique [7] in immunised dogs (*n* = 5). *Unshaded bars,* 10 min after HGG; *shaded bars,* 60 min after HGG

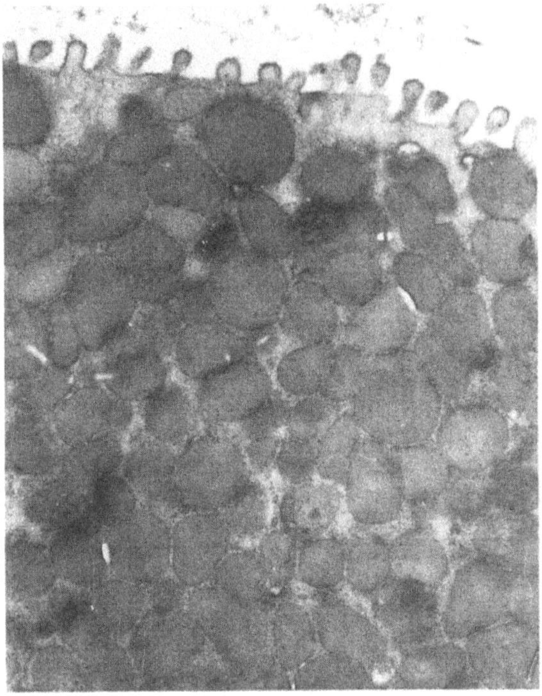

a

b

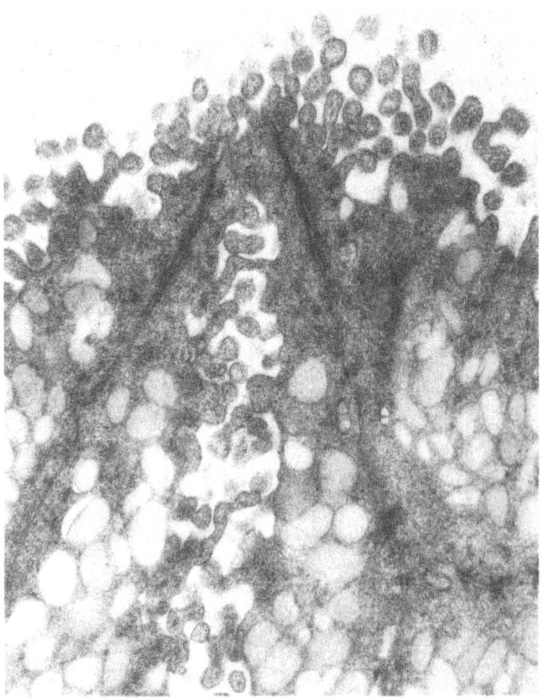

Fig. 3a, b. Electron-microscopy findings in mucus-producing epithelial cells of antral mucosa 30 min after intragastric application of antigen in controls **a)** and immunized dogs **b)**. Diameter of granules was assessed by calculating 1500 and 3000 granules, respectively, in controls (n = 3) and immunized dogs (n = 6) (× 30000)

Cellular Changes in the Mucosa. There was also an increase in mast cells and lymphoid cells in extra- and in intraepithelial spaces [4, 8]. These findings point to an involvement of immunocompetent cells in immunological stimulation.

The immunologically mediated gastrin release, increase of antral and duodenal blood flow and mucus secretion is a newly recognized mechanism of initiation of digestive processes in the stomach. It seems to stimulate the physiological cascade of digestion and represents a mode of stimulating gastric secretion during the gastric phase.

Evidence of Cytoprotection by Gastric Immunological Reactions

Blood Flow and Mucus Secretion. Obviously the immunological stimulation of gastric functions demonstrated by in vivo experiments elicits not only aggressive factors such as acid through the stimulation of gastrin, but also cytoprotective factors, for instance, an increase in local blood flow and mucus secretion.

Prostaglandin E_2. Regarding the immunological stimulation of digestive processes light microscopy also revealed degranulation of mast cells within the mucosa of the antrum [4, 8]. The atypical mast cell of the mucosa, as defined by Lorenz [10], produces 95% of histamine. Degranulation of these mast cells results in the release of histamine [9, 10] and leucotriene C4 [9]; both of which produced a significant release of prostaglandin E_2 from an isolated, vascularly perfused canine antrum [11] (Fig. 4). Prostaglandin E_2 is known to be a cytoprotective agent in the stomach [13].

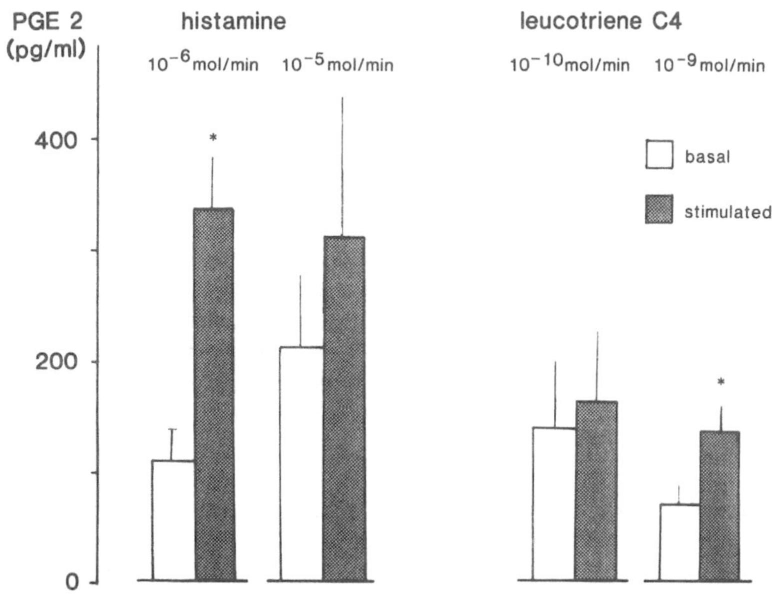

Fig. 4. Prostaglandin E_2 (PGE_2) release in vitro by histamine ($n = 4$) and leucotriene C4 ($n = 5$) [11] from an isolated, vascularly perfused canine antrum, modified from Makhlouf [12]. *Unshaded bars,* basal; *shaded bars,* stimulated; *asterisk,* $P < 0.05$ from basal

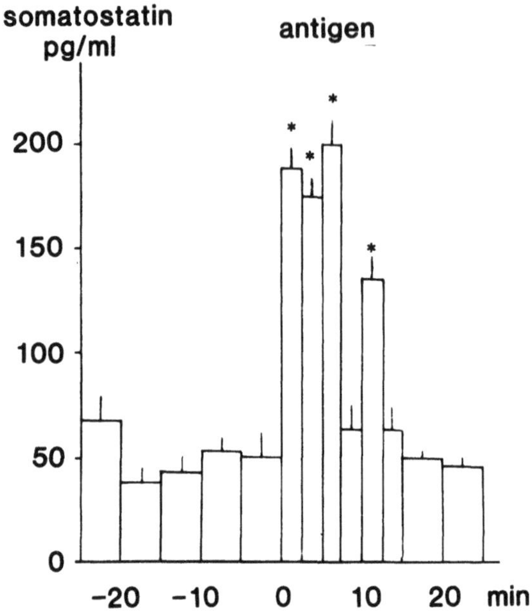

Fig. 5. Somatostatin release in vitro by antigen stimulation by 4-hydroxy-3-iodo-5 nitrophenyl, acetic acid (NIP) from antral mucosal slices of rats immunized with NIP (perfusion [14]). Determination of somatostatin was kindly provided by Dr. V. Schusdziarra, Department of Medicine, Klinikum Rechts der Isar, Technical University of Munich. *Asterisk*, $P < 0.05$ from basal

Somatostatin. Using an in vitro perifusion model [14] it could be demonstrated that the synthetic antigen 4-hydroxy-3-iodo-5 nitrophenyl acetic acid (NIP) releases gastrin in the antral mucosa of immunized rats [15]. Simultaneously there was a significant increase of somatostatin secretion from antral mucosal slices (Fig. 5). Somatostatin is known not only to inhibit serum gastrin, acid and pepsin secretion but also to stimulate gastric mucus production in humans [16]. Somatostatin may therefore also be cytoprotective for the gastric mucosa.

Ulcer Protection by Gastric Immunological Mechanisms

From in vivo and in vitro experiments it is thus demonstrated that the immunological stimulation of gastric functions releases gastrin and consequently acid but also induces the cytoprotective mechanisms of mucus secretion, increased blood flow and release of prostaglandin E_2 and somatostatin. The aim of the following experiments was to ascertain whether this stimulation may protect against ulcer formation. Two different models of experimental ulcers were used, alcohol-induced ulcerations and the Shay ulcer.

Alcohol-induced Ulcerations. Male Wistar rats (250–350 g) were systemically immunized with NIP. Ulcers were induced under anesthesia by application of 1 ml of absolute alcohol into the stomach [17]. In one group of animals the antigen NIP coupled to human gammaglobulin as carrier protein was introduced into the stomach 15 min prior to the alcohol. A control group received the carrier protein alone. One h after administration of alcohol, the length of the lesions was measured to calculate the

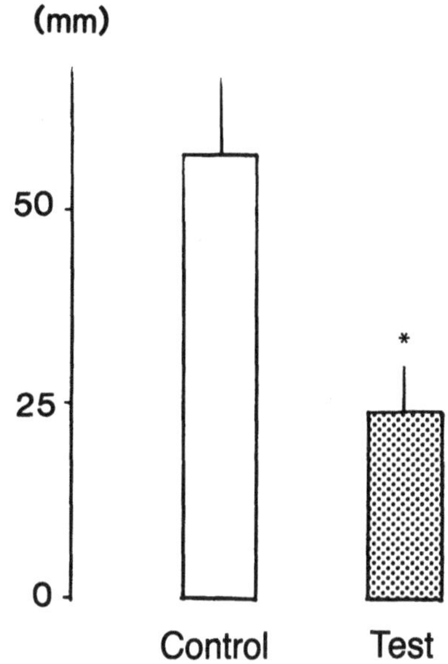

Fig. 6. Ulcer index following alcohol administration in controls (n = 12) and immunized test group (n = 12). *Asterisk*, $P < 0.02$

ulcer index [18]. The results are demonstrated in Fig. 6. Immunized rats had a significantly smaller extent of alcohol-induced lesions than controls [19]. This indicates that intraluminal immunological stimulation of the stomach significantly reduces the development of erosions. The finding provides the first evidence for an immunologically mediated ulcer protection.

Shay Ulcer. In order further to support the concept of immunological protection against ulcer, the Shay ulcer model [20] was applied. Male Wistar rats were immunized with NIP-ovalbumin. Under anaesthesia the pylorus was ligated. Thereafter the antigen NIP, coupled to human gammaglobulin, was administered into the stomach in one group; a second group of animals receiving only the carrier protein served as control. At 18 h after the operation the stomach was opened for evaluation of macroscopic lesions; these were defined as perforations, transmural ulcers or wall necrosis (more than 0.5 cm in diameter). Animals receiving the antigen showed a 52% reduction of lesions. Control rats had no lesions. This experiment confirms the findings obtained from the alcohol-induced ulcers regarding the reduction of ulcerative lesions following antigen-specific stimulation of gastric functions.

Conclusions

The immunological stimulation of gastric functions appears to be a physiological mechanism. The concomitant inrease during immune processes of mucosal blood flow, mucus secretion and release of ulcer-protective substances, such as somatostatin and prostaglandin E_2, may serve as a basis for the ulcer-protective effect. Thus far ulcer protection has been demonstrated in two animal models. The most interesting question is whether these immunological mechanisms of the gastric mucosa are also present in humans. This question must be addressed in future studies.

Acknowledgements. These studies were conducted in collaboration with Prof. Dr. Dr. h. c. W. Brendel and his colleagues of the Institute of Surgical Research, University of Munich, Kinikum Großhadern.

References

1. Grossman MI (1981) Regulation of gastric acid secretion. In: Johnson LR (ed) Physiology of the gastrointestinal tract. Raven, New York, pp 659–671
2. Allan AA (1981) Structure and function of gastrointestinal mucus. In: Johnson LR (ed) Physiology of the gastrointestinal tract. Raven, New York, pp 617–639
3. Carter DC (1980) Gastric mucosal barrier and mucosal blood flow. In: Fielding LP (ed) Gastrointestinal mucosal blood flow. Churchill Livingstone, Edinburgh, pp 206–216
4. Teichmann RK (1983) Vagale and immunologische Stimulation gastraler Funktionen. Habilitationsschrift, Ludwig-Maximilians-Universität, Munich
5. Teichmann RK, Andress HJ, Gycha S, Seifert J, Brendel W (1983) Immunologic mediated gastrin release. Gastroenterology 84 (2): 1333
6. Teichmann RK, Andress HJ, Gycha S, Seifert J, Brendel W (1983) Die immunologische Reaktivität des Antrums zur Stimulation von Verdauungsprozessen. Langenbecks Arch Chir [Suppl]: 5–8
7. Rudolph AM, Heymann MA (1967) The circulation of the fetus in utero: methods for studying distribution of blood flow, cardiac output and organ blood flow. Circ Res 21: 289–299
8. Steuer M (1985) Experimentell-morphologische Untersuchungen an der Tunica mucosa des Antrum pylori beim Hund. Inaugural Dissertation, Ludwig-Maximilians-Universität, Munich
9. Jarrett EE, Haig DM (1984) Mucosal mast cells in vivo and in vitro. Immunol Today 5: 115–118
10. Lorenz W, Schauer A, Halbach S, Calvoer R, Werle E (1969) Biochemical and histochemical studies on the distribution of histamine in the digestive tract of man, dog, and other mammals. Naunyn Schmiedebergs Arch Pharmacol 265: 81–100
11. Pratschke E (1986) Mediatoren der immunologischen Stimulation gastraler Funktionen: Experimentelle Untersuchungen am Beispiel der Gastrinfreisetzung. Habilitationsschrift, Ludwig-Maximilians-Universität, Munich
12. Makhlouf GM (1981) Peptide release in vitro. In: Bloom SR, Polak JM (eds) Gut hormones. Churchill Livingstone, Edinburgh, pp 154–159
13. Hawkey CJ, Rampton DS (1985) Prostaglandins and the gastrointestinal mucosa: are they important in its function, disease or treatment? Gastroenterology 89: 1162–1188
14. Hayes JR, Williams RH (1975) The effect on gastrin secretion of agents which increase the intracellular concentration of 3′, 5′-adenosine monophosphate. Endocrinology 97: 1210–1214
15. Krämling HJ, Teichmann RK, Demmel T, Merkle R, Enders G, Brendel W (1986) Antigen-stimulierte Gastrinfreisetzung im In-vitro-Modell (Mukosaperifusion). Acta Chir Austriaca 3: 333–334
16. Newman JB, Lluis F, Townsend CM Jr (1987) Somatostatin. In: Thompson JC, Greeley GH Jr, Rayford PL, Townsend CM Jr (eds) Gastrointestinal endocrinology. McGraw-Hill, New York, pp 286–299
17. Robert A, Nezamis JE, Lancaster C, Hanchar AJ (1979) Cytoprotection by prostaglandins in rats. Prevention of gastric necrosis produced by alcohol. HCL, NaOH, hypertonic NaCl, and thermal injury. Gastroenterology 77: 433–443
18. Takagi K, Okaba S (1968) The effects of drugs on the production and recovery process of stress ulcer. Jpn J Pharmacol 18: 9–18
19. Krämling HJ, Merkle T, Merkle R, Enders G, Teichmann R, Brendel W (1987) Immunologische Reaktivität des Magens – ein neuer Mechanismus der Ulkoprotektion. Langenbecks Arch Chir [Suppl] (in press)
20. Shay H, Komarov SA, Fels SS, Meranze D, Gruenstein M, Siplet H (1945) A simple method for the uniform production of gastric ulceration in the rat. Gastroenterology 5: 43–61

IV. Transplantation Immunology

Some Observations on Organ Transplantation

R. Y. CALNE

It is a pleasure and a privilege to participate in this Festschrift for Walter Brendel, who has been a friend and a colleague of mine since 1968.

Members of our respective departments have visited one another in Munich and Cambridge, and I have participated in all the winter immunology round tables with much pleasure and gratitude. A very instructive collaborative study, for instance, was conducted in Munich on dog-to-wolf liver xenografts, which benefited both departments.

Walter Brendel has been a beacon in surgical science for the past 30 years. The present healthy state of academic surgery in the Federal Republic of Germany is in large part due to his imagination and ceaseless endeavour. When he began his work, the Federal Republic was behind most other Western countries in surgical science; now German surgical research is of a high quality and is very productive. Many leading West German surgeons have worked in the Munich Institute and have benefited greatly from meeting basic scientists and learning the discipline of experimental methods.

Two years ago I had occasion to give the Lister Oration at the Royal College of Surgeons of England [5], and in my preparations I was struck by the similarity of Lister's studies towards safe surgery and the work of surgical transplanters in their early efforts to bring therapy to patients.

When Lister was beginning to grapple with surgical sepsis the work of Pasteur was brought to his attention, and the nascent science of bacteriology provided Lister with a platform on which to base his scientific clinical studies. He developed a practical method of killing bacteria so that they would not colonise wounds. His demonstration of the antiseptic technique of surgery and wound dressing was based on a small series of patients. Today his work would be regarded as unacceptable to any reputable scientific journal, as it did not consist of a randomised controlled trial with statistical assessment. Many of his contemporaries were sceptical of the results obtained, but facts gradually overcame rhetoric, as they always will in the end. Lister's life was punctuated with many disappointments, and there was a time when he was subjected to ridicule. He lost favour with Queen Victoria over experiments on animals. The Queen exerted quite inappropriate pressure on Lister to denounce medical research involving animals; in a very long and courteous letter of reply Lister ended with the following words:

I have myself often performed experiments upon the lower animals, and that, if I have been privileged in my professional career to do anything for the good of my fellow men, more is to be attributed to these experiments than to any other work in which I have been engaged.

Surgical Research:
Recent Concepts and Results
Baethmann/Messmer (Eds.)

Because of the opposition to vivisection in Britain, Lister went to France to perform important experiments. Lister's perseverance was eventually rewarded by recognition during his lifetime of the value of his work. Elective surgery became a safe and acceptable practice and opened the doors to a complete renaissance in surgery, with all the highly developed branches of the art owing a direct debt to the elimination of most operative sepsis.

Organ transplantation is a branch of surgery that is still young and bears some similarity to Lister's life work, albeit pale in reflection, on the control of surgical sepsis. When I was a medical student, terminal renal failure was a death sentence; all that could be done for the patient was to see to his or her comfort with sedative drugs. Liver and cardiac failure were similarly lethal, and even now with the best possible control some insulin-dependent diabetics become blind and develop renal failure. It is fortunate for these patients that surgeons considered their plight and conceived of the possibility of treatment by organ replacement. As a medical ward clerk working in Bright's old hospital, I remember once taking care of a young boy with terminal Bright's disease and asking the consultant physician whether the patient might be treated by a kidney transplant. He told me that such a procedure was impossible.

In the mid-1950s, however, Hume, a young surgeon in the department in Boston headed by Moore, transplanted a series of kidneys with the help of the nephrologist Merill; these had been taken from dead donors and were transplanted into patients with chronic renal failure [16]. Despite the lack of serious attempts at immunosuppression apart from small doses of steroids, some of these kidneys functioned for surprisingly long periods compared with the findings in animals, in which rejection of kidneys occurs between 7 and 10 days. The longest period of function in this clinical series was 5.5 months. Hume and Merrill felt that chronic uraemia may have contributed to the depressed allograft immunity. Shortly afterwards Murray et al. [21], working in the same institution, started a programme of transplanting kidneys between identical twins, using the iliac fossa technique developed by Kuss.

The success of the identical-twin transplants in restoring moribund patients to normal life was a great source of encouragement to the study of renal transplantation. Thus, as in the time of Lister, the clinical need for treatment of otherwise doomed patients was the spur to investigate a new form of treatment. Bacteriology was the new science on which Lister had based his work, and transplantation biology assumed an analogous role for organ transplantation.

Medawar and Gibson during the Second World War had defined the biological features of allograft rejection and had demonstrated this to be an immune process [10]. Experience of foreign tissue results in destruction of the graft and leaves the recipient with a specific memory of the graft, so that a second transplant from the same donor is destroyed more quickly than the first. Graft destruction is brought about by mononuclear cells, particularly lymphoid cells, which infiltrate the foreign tissue. In 1953, rejection of kidneys was shown by Dempster [9], working at the Buckston Browne Farm of the Royal College of Surgeons of England, and by Simonsen and colleagues [26] in Denmark, to be a process very similar to the rejection of skin grafts.

To prevent rejection without rendering the graft recipient extremely ill proved to be a difficult task. However, in work appropriately rewarded by the Nobel prize

Medawar and his colleagues showed that if transplantation antigens were presented to an individual in embryo or in the neonatal period before the immune response developed, these foreign proteins would be accepted by the individual as "self" products and not be reacted against.

My own interest in transplantation was reawakened by a lecture given by Medawar in Oxford in 1958. After showing photographs of tolerant white mice with black skin grafts and of black chickens with white feathers, he was asked by one of the students whether he could foresee any clinical application of his studies. "Absolutely none," he replied. Nevertheless, this was the first demonstration that allografts could be accepted permanently, and many investigators were stimulated by this work to try to prevent graft rejection. The most popular approach was to damage the reticulo-endothelial system with X-radiation but, although toxic, X-irradiation seldom prevented grafts from being rejected. Two successful cases, however, provided encouragement. These were recipients of kidney grafts from non-identical twins, one in Paris [15] and one at the Peter Bent Brigham Hospital [19].

I became disillusioned with X-irradiation following some early experiments on dogs in 1959. Later that year Schwartz and Dameshek [25] found that the anti-leukaemia drug 6-mercaptopurine would inhibit antibody formation in rabbits injected with human serum albumin, and that the effect persisted even after the drug had been stopped. After discussion with Porter it seemed to me that this agent might be useful in organ grafting; with enthusiastic support from Slome and Hopewell, I began experiments at the Buckston Browne Farm with kidney transplants in dogs. These showed that prolonged graft survival could occur; however, the results were not consistent [3].

A number of purine analogues synthesised by Hitchings and Elion in Burroughs Wellcome, Tuckahoe, New York, were then investigated at the Peter Bent Brigham Hospital in dogs with renal allografts and compared with 6-mercaptopurine [4]. Azathioprine, a derivative of 6-mercaptopurine, was found to be slightly more effective and this was the agent used in the first successful application of this experimental work in human kidney transplantation [22]. A most important addition was corticosteroids, which had been shown by Zukoski et al. [29] to prolong renal allograft survival in dogs and by Goodwin et al. [11] to reverse acute rejection of a human kidney graft. Many other agents were also investigated; the most useful was antilymphocyte globulin, prepared in animals and injected with human lymphocytes. This was first studied systematically by Woodruff and was developed for clinical use by Starzl and Brendel.

Each of these three agents, however, had undesirable side-effects. Azathioprine could cause marrow destruction and liver damage. Allergic reaction and thrombocytopaenia could follow antilymphocyte globulin treatment; potency also proved to vary from batch to batch. The worst side-effects were those due to corticosteroids. In order to avoid rejection high doses were sometimes necessary, which impaired wound healing and could cause aseptic bone necrosis, diabetes and disastrous stunting of growth and cushingoid changes in children.

With the emergence of tissue typing and cross-matching procedures it was possible to avoid the disaster of kidney grafting in specifically sensitised patients and to select donors on the basis of matching within a family. Tissue typing has flourished and has been responsible for major advances in human genetics, but it has not had a correspondingly favourable effect in selection of donor-recipient combinations from unrelated donors.

A totally unexpected finding was that prior blood transfusion from third-party blood donors, although sensitising some patients and making it difficult for them to receive a transplant from any source, rendered the remaining patients less likely to reject grafts. The mechanism of this blood-transfusion effect has not been clarified, and Opelz et al. [23], who made the original observation have recently been unable to confirm the effect [24]. This may be due to an active immunological reaction as well as to exclusion of bad responders.

Azathioprine and corticosteroids became the "sheet anchor" of immunosuppression and produced some remarkably good results, not only in the grafting of kidneys but also in that of hearts and of livers. Corticosteroids aggravate diabetes, and the results of kidney grafting in diabetics were poor; moreover, after some years kidney allografts in diabetics develop diabetic glomerulopathy. Liver transplantation, pioneered experimentally by Moore et al. [20] and Starzl el al. [27] and clinically by Starzl et al. [28], became a therapeutically valuable procedure. An interesting experimental finding in liver grafting has been the ability of the liver to survive in certain situations without rejection despite *no immunosuppressive treatment* being given [7, 17].

In spite of enormous strides in our understanding of transplantation immunology, application of this science to clinical practice has been difficult and disappointing. Medawar acknowledged that the surgeon "liberated transplantation immunology from the tyranny of the rodent with a skin graft."

Borel, working in the Sandoz Laboratories found that the cyclic peptide cyclosporin A had immunosuppressive effects in vitro and in vivo [2]. Investigation of this drug in animals with organ grafts showed that it was more effective than any other agent or combination of agents studied thus far [6, 12, 18]. Clinical application of cyclosporin A to organ grafting improved results of all organ transplants, but not without a penalty. The unpleasant side-effect in man is nephrotoxicity, which is in part reversible but in high doses may cause structural damage to the kidney [8]. One of the greatest advantages of cyclosporin A is that it can be used without steroids in addition.

The Future

For organ transplantation results to improve, more effective and less toxic immunosuppression is required, as are better methods of preserving the organs. There is hope that a non-nephrotoxic analogue of cyclosporin A may be developed. More discrete, safer and more effective antilymphocyte globulin preparations can be expected to result from development of monoclonal antibodies. We have been investigating a number of locally made monoclonal antibodies in Cambridge – the Campath series of monoclonals – which can be effective adjuncts to immunosuppression [13, 14].

Of course, advances in immunosuppression and organ preservation can only be brought about by experimentation, and this requires the use of animals, since in a civilised community experiments on humans would be intolerable. It is becoming increasingly difficult to perform experiments involving animals, and yet the community expects advances in medicine. It is sad that a small, militant and irrational minority can sway Government and public institutions, but, as noted above, in the last century even the Queen herself tried to do so. If a safe and effective immunosuppressive regimen were developed, there would be many new troubles resulting from this achievement. The demand for donor organs would become increased. Living donors can be used for kidney transplantation but not for that of most other vital organs. There is still difficulty in obtaining sufficient organs from cadaver donors, and if pancreas grafting became standard treatment for insulin-dependent diabetics, there would not be enough cadaver organs available, even if all suitable cases were utilised. Commercial and even criminal means might be used to procure organs. Our profession will need to be vigiliant to prevent unethical abuse of medical advances.

Perfect immunosuppression would also create a demand for transplantation of non-vital organs, and grafting of gonads could raise extraordinary ethical and legal debates. Looking further into the future, it may be possible to transplant organs from animals, although there will be a minority opposed to this and who would feel this to be wrong. Genetic engineering may enable proliferative culture of pancreatic β-cells, and even whole organs may eventually be grown in vitro.

An increasingly serious worry in modern medical advances is that of cost, and since the demands for medical resources are potentially unlimited, control is necessary. Whenever a new form of treatment is discussed in financial terms, for example liver grafting, comparisons are made with other needs in the health service, usually the care of the mentally ill and the aged, or the community in general, housing, schooling, public services and even armaments. These comparisons often have no meaning; the sick child dying of liver disease surely deserves as much compassion and financial support from the community as the child born with a malfunctioning brain, who will never be able to live in the community but may survive for a full life span.

The main theme in the professional work of Walter Brendel has been to apply laboratory study to the clinic. Organ transplantation is an example of such an application which is now accepted as therapy. I have suggested a similarity of this to the development of safe surgery pioneered by Lister. In the case of Lister it was one man's genius that changed surgery, whereas in organ transplantation many have been involved in its development. Nevertheless, patients who previously had no hope can now expect a good chance of effective treatment by organ transplantation that can restore them from a moribund state and allow them to become normal members of the community. We can anticipate a continual improvement in the results of organ transplantation, and we need to be prepared for the ethical and financial nettles that will have to be grasped as a result. The evolution of organ transplantation has been an extremely exciting endeavour and continues to have extraordinary interest for the scientifically minded surgeon, who will be engaged in the fascinating study of human biology linked to the objective of improving treatment for the sick.

I close with a quotation from Lord Lister in his graduation address delivered in Edinburgh in 1876:

... and truly if we have nothing but pecuniary rewards and worldly honours to look to; our profession would not be one to be desired, but in fact you will find it is attended with peculiar privileges second to none in intense interest and pure pleasures.

Some of the material in this article has been published in the *British Medical Journal* as a summary of the Lister Oration 1984.

References

1. Billingham RE, Brent L, Medawar PB, Sparrow EM (1954) Part I: Survival times of skin homografts exchanged between members of different inbred strains of mice. Proc R Soc Lond [Biol] 143: 143–158
2. Borel JF (1976) Comparative study of in vitro and in vivo drug effects on cell-mediated cytotoxicity. Immunology 31: 631–641
3. Calne RY (1960) The rejection of renal homograft inhibition in dogs by 6-mercaptopurine. Lancet i: 417–418
4. Calne RY (1961) Inhibition of the rejection of renal homografts in dogs by purine analogues. Transplant Bull 28: 445–461
5. Calne RY (1985) Organ transplantation from laboratory to clinic. Br Med J 291: 1751–1754
6. Calne RY, Rolles K, White DJG, Smith DP (1978) Prolonged survival of pig orthotopic heart grafts treated with Cyclosporin A. Lancet i: 1183–1185
7. Calne RY, Sells RA, Pena JR, Davis DR, Milland PR, Herbertson BM, Binns RM, Davies DA (1969) Induction of immunological tolerance by porcine liver allografts. Nature 223: 472–476
8. Calne RY, White DJG, Pentlow DB, Rolles K, Syrakos T, Ohtawa T, Smith DP, McMaster P, Evans DB, Herbertson BM, Thiru S (1979) Cyclosporin A: preliminary observations in dogs with pancreatic duodenal allografts and patients with cadaveric renal transplants. Transplant Proc XI: 860–864
9. Dempster WJ (1953) Kidney homotransplantation. Br J Surg 40: 447–465
10. Gibson T, Medawar PB (1943) The behaviour of skin homografts in man. J Anat 77: 299–310
11. Goodwin WE, Mims MM, Kaufman JJ (1962) Human renal transplantation. Trans Am Assoc Genitourin Surg 54: 116–123
12. Green CJ, Allison AC (1978) Extensive prolongation of rabbit kidney allograft survival after short-term cyclosporin A treatment. Lancet i: 1182
13. Hale G, Bright S, Chumbley G, Hoang T, Metcalf D, Munro AJ, Waldmann H (1983) Removal of T cells from bone marrow for transplantation: a monoclonal antilymphocyte antibody that fixed human complement. Blood 62: 873–882
14. Hale G, Waldmann H, Friend P, Calne R (1986) Pilot study of CAMPATH-1, a rat monoclonal antibody which fixed human complement, as an immunosuppressant in organ transplantation. Transplant Proc (in press)
15. Hamburger J, Vaysse J, Crosnier J, Tubiana M, Lalanne CM, Antoine B, Auvert J, Soulier JP, Dormont J, Salmon CR, Maisonnet M, Amiel J (1959) Transplantation d'un rein entre jumeaux non monozygotes après irradiation due receveur bon fonctionnement au quatrieme mois. Presse Medicale 67: 1771
16. Hume DM, Merrill JP, Miller BF, Thorn GW (1955) Experience with renal homotransplantation in the human; report of nine cases. J Clin Invest 34: 327
17. Kamada N, Davies HS, Roser B (1981) Reversal of transplantation immunity by liver grafting. Nature 292: 84–842
18. Kostakis AJ, White DJG, Calne RY (1977) Prolongation of the rat heart allograft survival by cyclosporin A. IRCS Med Sci 5: 280
19. Merrill JP, Murray JE, Harrison JP (1960) Successful homotransplantation of the kidney between non-identical twins. N Engl J Med 262: 1251–1260
20. Moore FD, Smith LL, Burnap TK (1959) One-stage homotransplantation of the liver following total hepatectomy in dogs. Transplant Bull 6: 103–107
21. Murray JE, Merrill JP, Harrison JH (1958) Kidney transplantation between 7 pairs of identical twins. Ann Surg 148: 343–359
22. Murray JE, Merrill JP, Dammin GJ (1964) Current evaluation of human kidney transplantation. Ann NY Acad Sci 120: 545
23. Opelz G, Terasaki PL, Graver B, Sasaki N, Langston M, Cohn M, Mickey MR (1979) Correlation between number of pretransplant blood transfusions and kidney graft survival. Transplant Proc 11: 145–147

24. Opelz G (for the Collaborative Transplant Study) (1987) Improved kidney graft survival in nontransfused recipients. Transplant Proc 19: 149–152
25. Schwartz R, Dameshek W (1959) Drug induced immunologic tolerance. Nature 183: 1682–1683
26. Simonsen M, Bremann J, Gammeltaft A, Jensen S, Jørgensen K (1953) Biological incompatibility in kidney transplantation in dogs. Acta Pathol Microbiol Scand 32: 1–35
27. Starzl TE, Bernhard VM, Cortes N, Benvenuto R (1959) A technique for one-stage hepatectomy in dogs. Surgery 46: 880–886
28. Starzl TE, Marchioro TL, Von Kaulla KN, Hermann G, Brittain RS, Waddell (1963) Homotransplantation in the liver of humans. Surg Gynecol Obstet 117: 659–676
29. Zukoski CF, Lee H, Hume DM (1960) The prolongation of functional survival of canine renal homografts by mercaptopurine. Surg Forum 11: 470–472

Clinical Developments and Current Immunological Research Approaches in Liver Transplantation

R. PICHLMAYR, and K. WONIGEIT

Introduction

It has only been within the last few years that liver grafting has gained world-wide interest and broad clinical application. The first phase of liver transplantation began 1967 with the first successful graft performed by T.E. Starzl in a child, and was followed by continous clinical employment of this procedure mainly by four centers (Denver/Pittsburgh, Cambridge, Hannover, Groningen) where, however, no more than 800 grafts were performed until 1983 [1, 2]. Since then more than 3000 liver transplants have been done in about 40 centers in Europe alone and an equal or even higher number in North America. The number of liver transplantations in Hannover and the distribution of the major groups are given in Fig. 1. During this development a marked improvement in results was achieved [3–7]. For some special indications and particularly in children, 1-year survival rates in the range of 80%–90% have been reached. For the majority of indication groups, however, the results are not so favorable and demonstrate that many problems still have to be solved. Although it is beyond any doubt that liver grafting is already a clinical treatment with high therapeutic value, its further development will depend very much on the success of current and future research activities in hepatology, organ preservation, evaluation of graft quality, and transplant immunology and immunosuppression.

Cyclosporin A in Liver Grafting: Therapeutic Potential and Problems

As in the transplantation of other organs the introduction of cyclosporin A marks a significant step forward in liver transplantation [8]. Its strong immunosuppressive potency combined with high selectivity for T-lymphocytes is particularly relevant in liver transplantation. Because liver grafted patients are more prone to infection than other transplant recipients, the lack of any adverse effect on bone marrow and phagocyte function is a very important advantage. On the other hand, its nephrotoxic and hepatotoxic effects are more disturbing after liver grafting than in other transplant patients. Furthermore, absorption and metabolism of cyclosporin A are dependent on the function of the liver and, thus, are affected by any dysfunction of the graft. Therefore, special protocols have been worked out for the use of cyclosporin A in hepatic transplantation [9, 10, 6]. Essential features are intravenous application during the first 2–3 weeks always combined with antihistamine prophylaxis (H1 and

Surgical Research:
Recent Concepts and Results
Baethmann/Messmer (Eds.)

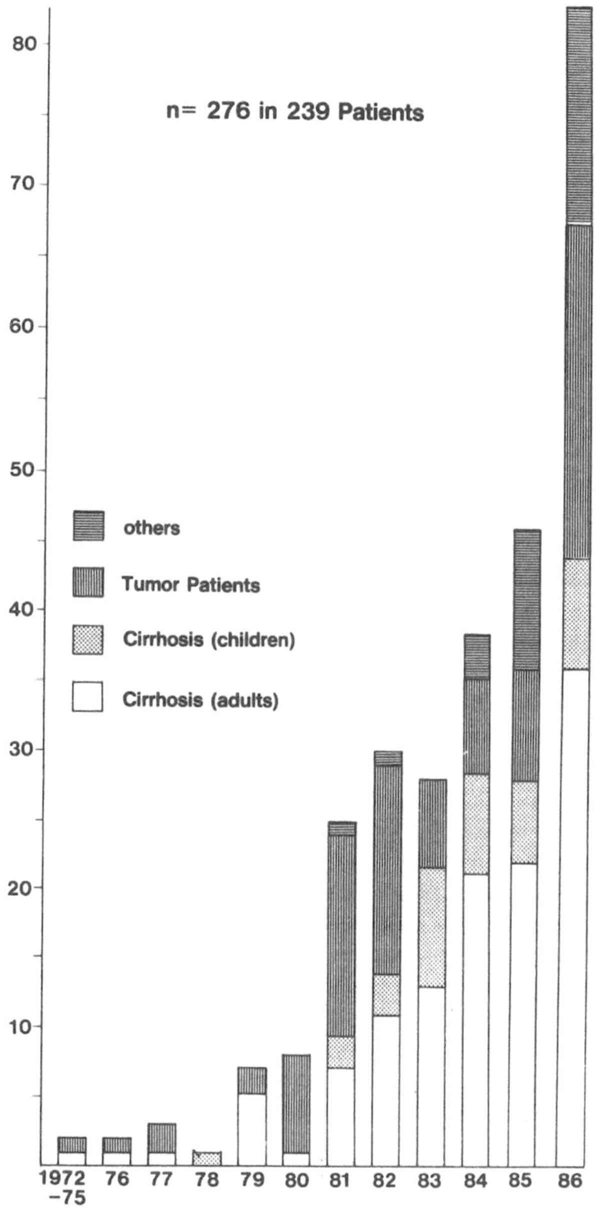

Fig. 1. Number of liver transplantations in Hannover 1972–1986: number of grafts performed per year and distribution by major groups

H2 receptor blockers), careful adaptation of the dose to blood levels, and individualized combinations with other immunosuppressants. Antihistamine prophylaxis is required to prevent anaphylactoid reactions to the solvent cremophor. To monitor drug level, methods should be used which determine unmodified parent drug and metabolites separately. The recent development of a new generation of radioimmunoassays (RIA) using monoclonal antibodies is a major step forward, which will permit a precise and detailed analysis of the drug level [11]. In patients with disturbed liver function, increased levels of drug metabolites have been observed. Misleading high blood levels were obtained with the conventional polyclonal RIA, detecting both cyclosporin A and many of its metabolites. As the metabolites have no or only a reduced immunosuppressive potential, this may increase the risk of rejection. Since little is known about the toxic effect of the metabolites, in the case of increased metabolite levels the dosage can not simply be increased. Improved immunosuppression has to be achieved by the addition of other drugs, such as azathioprine or antilymphocyte serum. Thus, immunosuppressive treatment in liver transplantation has to be tailor-made for each individual patient. In patients with well functioning grafts cyclosporin A combined with low-dose steroids is usually a very effective treatment with a low rate of adverse effects. In patients with disturbed graft function or an increased risk of toxicity resulting from impaired function of other organs, multiple drug regimens with no or only very reduced doses of cyclosporin A are preferred. In this situation drugs with even higher selectivity, such as monoclonal antibodies against T-lymphocytes, are important new approaches [6].

Surgical Improvements

In liver grafting further progress has also been accomplished recently. Three topics are particulary noteworthy. (a) The reintroduction of the portovenous and the venovenous bypass using a centrifugal pump technique which does not require heparinization. The circulatory status of the patient during the anhepatic phase is thus easier to control, and high venous pressure injuries to intestine and kidney are diminished. (b) Biliary tract complications have been further reduced by improved reconstruction techniques [4, 12, 13]. The most commonly used techniques are anastomoses between both common bile ducts or a choledochojejunostomy; in our experience the best procedure is a side-to-side choledocho-choledochostomy. (c) It has been realized that surgical skill is of utmost importance for all steps of this difficult operation. During explantation the preparation of the hepatic artery requires particular caution. In the recipient, complete hemostasis, in addition to the quality of the vascular and biliary anastomoses, is particularly important. It may take several hours to achieve this. Reoperations and the need for large amounts of blood transfusions reduce the chance for patient survival. Just as important as surgery is the anethesiological management, which is extremely demanding. In the case of complications or of an unclear course, an aggressive diagnostic approach with frequent and repeated controls is mandatory postoperatively in order to choose the correct treatment. The differential diagnosis of various states of postoperative graft dysfunction is still a major problem and should be a major objective of further research.

Evaluation of Donor Organ Quality

Evaluation of the quality of the potential donor liver is a great problem in liver transplantation. Perfect organ quality or severely altered liver function are recognized correctly in most instances. However, there is a wide spectrum of intermediate situations, which are difficult to evaluate. In light of the shortage of donor organs, it is essential that all acceptable grafts be used but this must not lead to an increased risk of using grafts without adequate function. Transplantation of a nonfunctioning liver is an event with an extreme risk for the patient. A research program in our group is devoted to this problem. A special combination of biochemical tests including, in particular, clearance of lidocain and its major metabolites after intravenous injection and other clearance methods help to assess graft quality [14]. In the desperate situation of transplantation of a nonviable liver, regrafting is the only procedure able to save the patient. This has to be done before severe extrahepatic complications occur, i.e., within 1–4 days after the first operation. To find a suitable donor organ within such a short period requires extensive cooperation between transplant centers and the willingness to share donor organs. Furthermore, it is necessary that the question of whether the liver fulfills the criteria for transplantation should be made clear in each cadaver organ donor.

Patient Selection Criteria

Indications for liver grafting are end stages of a great variety of liver diseases. The diagnoses of transplant patients in our center are given in Table 1. In many of the benign disorders the short-term course is difficult to predict when the patient has entered the end stage of the disease. This raises severe problems since the proper timing of a liver transplantation is an important prognostic factor. It has become obvious in the past that performance of this complex operation in a late, prefinal state of the disease is only occasionally successful and usually fails. On the other hand the chance of survival is high, i.e., up to 80%–9o% after 1 year, if transplantation is performed before the patient has reached the terminal stage with symptoms of multiorgan impairment (Fig. 2). It is an urgent but difficult task to define the most appropriate disease stage for transplantation in so-called benign liver diseases.

Another important aspect in the selection of recipients is recurrence of the original disease in the graft. According to our present experience patients with HBV or NANB posthepatitic cirrhosis can be transplanted successfully, although the long-term outcome is not yet clear. In patients with HBV infection passive immunization starting during the anhepatic phase of the transplant operation is important and may be able to prevent recurrence of the infection in some patients [15].

In recipients who have received a liver transplant because of irresectable liver tumors the recurrence rate is particularly high. But patients with long survival times demonstrate the potential offered by liver transplantation in this group as well. Establishing a prospective definition of tumor types and stages which permits successful treatment by transplantation is an important task and requires further work. The aim is treatment of all suitable patients at a time when the prognosis is still good.

Immunological Factors and Current Approaches in Research

As in other transplanted organs, rejection is also a central problem in liver transplantation. Clinical experience has not confirmed an immunological privilege of liver

Table 1. Liver transplantation in 239 patients (Nov. 25, 1972–Jan. 1, 1987)

Indication	Total (*n*)	Adults (*n*)	Children < 16 years (*n*)
Benign liver diseases	142	113	29
Postnecrotic cirrhosis		36	2
Acute/subacute hepatitis		9	–
Primary biliary cirrhosis		24	–
Secondary biliary cirrhosis[a]		3	1
Primary sclerosing cholangitis		9	–
Secondary sclerosing cholangitis		1	–
Alcoholic cirrhosis		10	–
Cirrhosis of other origin[b]		7	9
Extrahepatic biliary atresia		–	16
Alagille syndrome		–	1
Budd-Chiary syndrome		10	–
Other diseases[c]		4	–
Malignant liver tumors	86	83	3
Hepatocellular carcinoma		19	2
Hepatocellular carcinoma + cirrhosis		24	–
Cholangiocellular carcinoma		8	–
Cholangiocellular carcinoma + cirrhosis		2	–
Other primary liver tumors[d]		4	1
Bile duct carcinoma		18	–
Secondary liver tumors[e]		8	–
Hepatic-based metabolic diseases	11	5	6
Wilson's disease		3	–
Byler's disease		–	3
Alpha-1-antitrypsin deficiency		–	2
Hemochromatosis + hepatocellular carcinoma		1	–
Glycogenosis type I + adenoma		1	–
Crigler-Najjar-syndrome type I		–	1

[a] Caroli syndrome (1), polycystic liver disease (1), postoperative (2)
[b] cryptogenic cirrhosis (11), autoimmune hepatitis (1), cholangiodysplasia (3), neonatal hepatitis (1)
[c] Hemangiomatosis (1), polycystic liver disease (1), bile duct papillomatosis (1), postoperative liver failure (1)
[d] Hepatoblastoma (2), hemangioendothelioma (1), hemangiosarcoma (2)
[e] Colorectal carcinoma (3), carcinoid tumors (2), melanoma (2), teratoma (1)

grafts as observed in some animal models. A remarkable immunological peculiarity, however, is the increased resistance of the human liver against antibody-mediated hyperacute rejection. This permits successful transplantation despite a positive cross match and in ABO-incompatible combinations. Nevertheless, a "stormy course" appears to be more frequent in these situations. Although a clear antibody -mediated hyperacute rejection has not been described, acute cellular rejection is a frequent and severe problem. A new aspect of rejection which has been extensively studied by our group is the modification of major histocompatibility complex (MHC)-antigen expression during rejection and in other clinical complications. Another focus of our interest has been T-cell monitoring in patients with long-standing liver allografts.

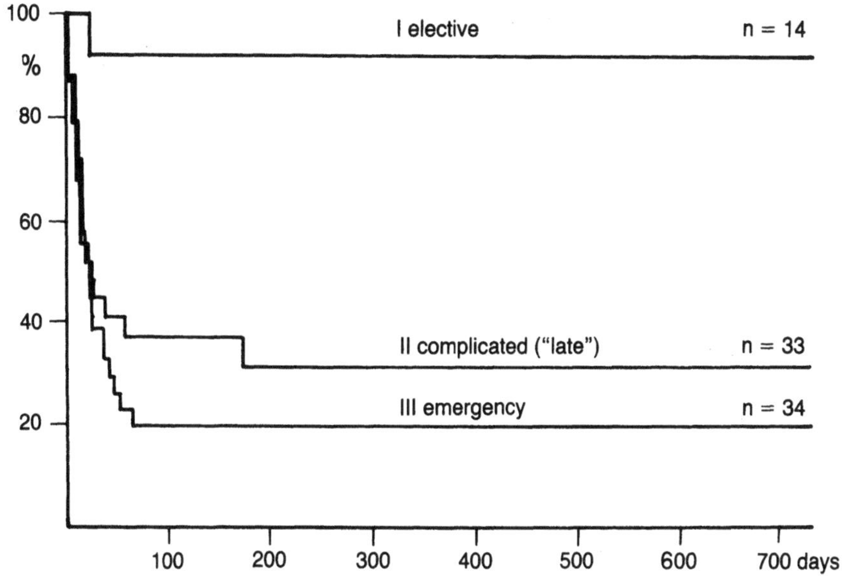

Fig. 2. Effect of the time of indication on the results of liver transplantation. In patients with end-stage cirrhosis ($n = 81$) transplanted in Hannover, satisfactory results could only be obtained if the recipient was still in an elective state (group I). Patients suffering already from multiorgan impairment (group II) or transplanted in coma (emergency state, group III) have a drastically reduced prognosis

MHC-Antigen Expression

The analysis of MHC-antigen expression in the liver is a new approach to study dynamic changes in the immunogenicity and immunological susceptibility of liver grafts. Monoclonal antibodies directed against monomorphic determinants of class I and class II MHC antigens and immunohistological procedures were used to study antigen expression on the different cell types of the liver [16]. In the normal liver class I antigens are present in all cells with the exception of hepatocytes, which express no or only very few class I molecules (Fig. 3a). Class II antigens are restricted to some endothelia, interstitial macrophages, dendritic cells, and Kupffer's cells. After transplantation different immunological states of the graft are associated with characteristic changes in antigen expression. During rejection episodes class I antigens become strongly expressed on all hepatocytes (Fig. 3). Of particular interest are changes in class II expression. Already during quiescence some bile ducts become class II positive; during rejection this is very much increased. In addition, hepatocytes in the infiltrated areas start to express class II antigens. A pattern similar to rejection may be seen in virus infections, in particular in cytomegalovirus hepatitis. The increased MHC-antigen expression is probably induced by lymphokines released from infiltrating cells. Gamma-interferon has been demonstrated to be a particularly effective inductor of class II antigen expression. The result of the antigen induction is a marked increase in susceptibility of the graft to the immune assault in the course of the

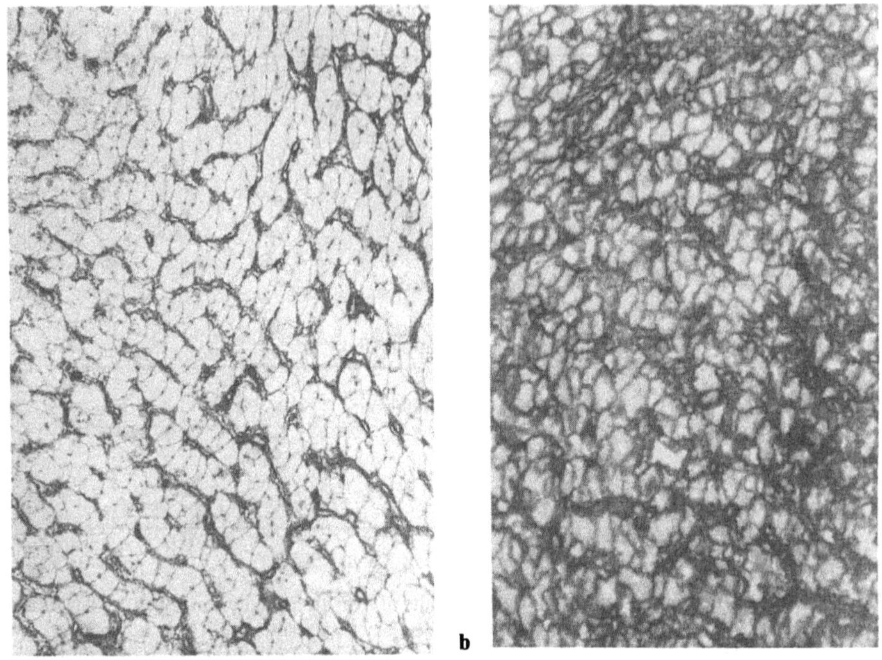

Fig. 3a, b. Immunohistological analysis of class I MHC expression in normal liver **a)** and during an acute rejection episode **b).** The normal liver tissue shown in *a* was obtained from the graft during the operation. Whereas Kupffer cells, endothelium, and interstitial cells are strongly class I positive, hepatocyte membranes are only weakly stained. In contrast, class I staining of hepatocytes in *b* is markedly increased. This section was prepared from a liver biopsy taken on day 10 during a moderate rejection episode. An indirect peroxidase staining procedure and the monoclonal antibody W 6/32 were used

rejection process (Fig. 4). Particular patterns of rejection, as the vanishing bile duct syndrome, could be elicited by induction of class II antigens in bile ducts. In case of class II incompatibility of the graft, de novo expressed class II antigens could serve as target antigens for the immune assault, or in the case of MHC compatibility, they could serve as restriction elements for T-lymphocytes directed against minor antigens, which may be predominatly expressed on bile ducts. Finally the marked de novo expression in viral infection could explain why these infections occasionally elicit acute rejection episodes despite a virally induced immunosuppression.

The up-regulation of MHC-antigen expression in all likelihood represents an amplification loop of the rejection process, which may explain the surprisingly dynamic nature of the effector phase of allograft rejection (Fig. 4). Increased density of some MHC antigens and de novo expression of others may not only render the graft more susceptible, but may also lead to the sensitization of additional lymphocyte clones reactive with the newly expressed determinants. Immunosuppresive therapy may interfere with this vicious circle at two different sites (Fig. 5). It may inhibit lymphokine release by eliminating or blocking sensitized T cells, but also inhibit increased MHC-antigen expression of the target cells. The latter mechanism may represent a powerful principle for new strategies of immunological intervention.

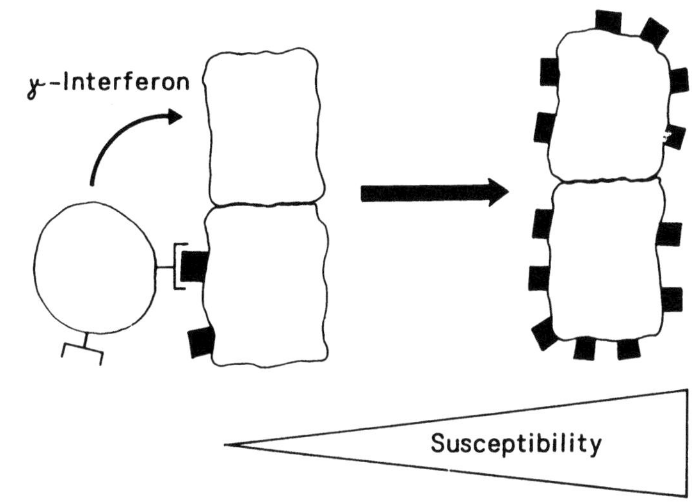

Fig. 4. Mechanism of the induction of increased MHC-antigen expression in rejecting grafts. During the effector phase of the rejection process specifically sensitized lymphocytes infiltrate the graft, recognize the incompatible antigens, and release lymphokines, in particular gamma-interferon. The latter induces increased transcription and translation of MHC antigens. This will lead to an increased density of antigens already present in the graft and also de novo expression of antigens normally not detectable. This leads to an increased susceptibility of the graft to antibody-mediated as well as to cellular effector mechanisms

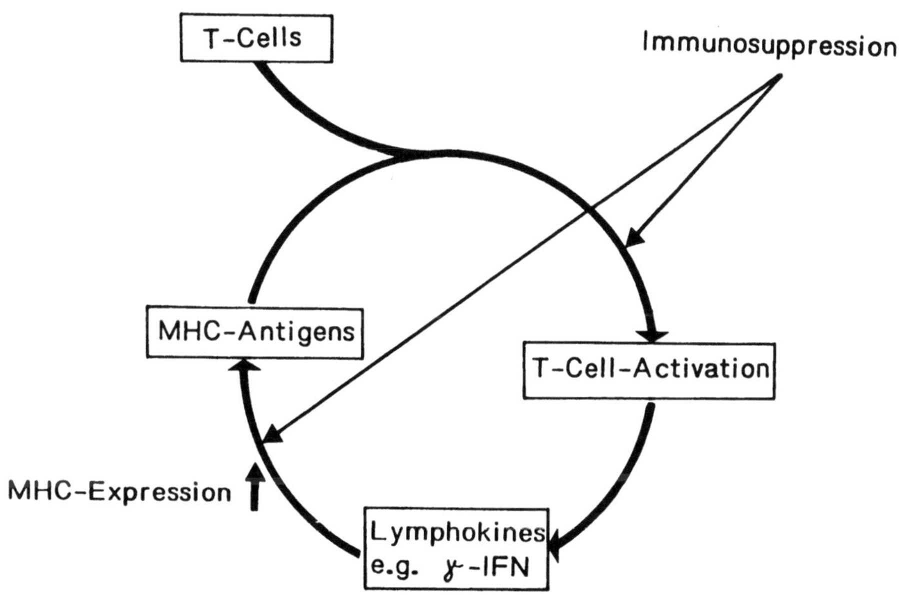

Fig. 5. Amplifying effect of increased MHC-antigen expression on the rejection process. The increased expression of MHC antigens leads not only to an increased susceptibility of the graft to the immune assault but may also be able to elicit sensitization to de novo induced antigens. This in turn will enhance infiltration of the graft and local lymphokine release. Thus, a vicious circle becomes established, which can only be interrupted by increased immunosuppressive therapy. Immunosuppressive treatment not only affects the infiltrating lymphocytes but also regulation of MHC antigen expression

T-Cell Monitoring in Patients with Long-Standing Liver Grafts

The amount of immunosuppressive treatment required to control rejection differs markedly from patient to patient in the early phase after transplantation and in the long-term course. This may in part be due to a reduction in immunogenicity of the graft caused by the replacement of donor dendritic cells by cells derived from recipient bone marrow and, of course, by the down-regulation of donor MHC expression to normal levels. In addition we have been able to demonstrate that the specific T-cell responsiveness of the donor can be markedly reduced. This is particularly true for donor specific cytotoxic T-cell responses, which can be completely abolished [17]. This phenomenon has now been confirmed widely and has been shown to develop not only in conventionally immunosuppressed patients but also under cyclosporin A.

Another important new approach to T-cell monitoring in transplant recipients is the phenotypical characterization of blood lymphocytes by monoclonal antibodies to T-cell differentiation antigens and flow cytometry. Peripheral blood lymphocytes of liver patients with long-standing grafts could be shown to contain increased numbers of cells expressing the CD8 differentiation antigen [18]. Since the $CD8^+$ subset is heterogeneous in function including cytotoxic, suppressor, and natural Killer cells, we have dissected the CD 8^+ subset of these patients by two-color fluorescence using additional monoclonal antibodies, which separate the $CD8^+$ cells in several subgroups. The results revealed that the increase in number of $CD8^+$ cells is caused by the expansion of a particular group of cells which express CD8 only in low concentration but coexpress the NK marker CD11 as well as the CD3/T-cell receptor complex. This unusual phenotype is present in normal individuals only in very small numbers. Further studies will have to clarify whether or not the expansion of this group of cells is associated with the described reduction in the donor specific cytotoxic T-cell reactivity.

Conclusions

Clinical liver transplantation is presently in a phase of dynamic development. The number of centers working in this difficult field and the number of transplants performed are rapidly increasing. Nevertheless, many problems are still unresolved and require intensive research activities. Major improvements can be expected from more refined methods to evaluate the function of the donor organ before transplantation, from better methods to define the most appropriate time of indication, and from further refined immunosuppressive treatment. A particularly new aspect of the immunology of liver transplantation is the dynamic nature of MHC-antigen expression in the graft. During rejection episodes and viral infections increased expression of both class I and class II MHC antigens can be observed. The detailed analysis of this phenomenon will provide new insights into the pathophysiology of the rejection process and may permit new approaches for therapeutic intervention.

References

1. Scharschmidt BF (1984) Human liver transplantation: Analysis of data on 540 patients from four centers. Hepatology 4: 95–101
2. Starzl TE, Iwatsuki C, van Thiel D, Gartner J, Zitelli B, Malatack J, Schade R, Shaw B, Hakala T, Rosenthal J, Porter K (1982) Evolution of liver transplantation. Hepatology 2: 614–636
3. Starzl TE, Iwatsuki S, Shaw BW, Gordon RD, Esquivel C (1985) Immunosuppression and other nonsurgical factors in the improved results of liver transplantation. Semin Liver Dis 5: 334–343
4. Calne RY, Williams R, Rolles K (1986) Liver transplantation in the adult. World J Surg 10: 422–431
5. Pichlmayr R, Neuhaus P (1985) Lebertransplantation. Chirurg 56: 211–215
6. Pichlmayr R, Ringe B, Lauchart W, Wonigeit K (1987) Liver transplantation. Transplant Proc 19: 103–112
7. Burdelski M, Schmidt K, Bernsau U, Galaske R, Hoyer PF, Brodehl J, Brölsch Ch, Neuhaus P, Ringe B, Lauchart W, Wonigeit K, Pichlmayr R (1986) Transplantation im Kindesalter, Wiener Med Wschr 98: 551–555
8. Starzl TE, Iwatsuki S, Shaw BW, Gordon RD, Esquivel C (1986) Liver transplantation in the ciclosporin era. Progr Allergy 38: 366–394
9. Wonigeit K, Brölsch C, Neuhaus P, Burdelski M, Schmidt E, Lang W, Pichlmayr R (1983) Special aspects of immunosuppression with cyclosporine in liver transplantation. Transplant Proc 15: 2586–2591
10. Wonigeit K (1985) Pharmakokinetik von Ciclosporin A und Bedeutung der Blutspiegelmessung für die Therapie. Internist 26: 534–542
11. Quesniaux V, Tees R, Schreier MH, Wenger RM, Donatsch P, van Regenmortl MHV (1986) Monoclonal antibodies to ciclosporin. Progr Allergy 38: 108–122
12. Starzl TE, Iwatsuki S, Esquivel C, Todo S, Kam I, Lynch S, Gordon RD, Shaw BW (1985) Refinements in the surgical technique of liver transplantation. Semin Liver Dis 5: 349–356
13. Neuhaus P, Brölsch C, Ringe B, Lauchart W, Pichlmayr R (1984) Results of biliary reconstruction after liver transplantation. Transplant Proc 16: 1225
14. Burdelski M, Lamesch P, Oellerich M, Raude E, Ringe B, Neuhaus P, Bortfeld S, Kämmerling C, Raith H, Westphal C, Worm M, Pichlmayr R (1987) Evaluation of quantitative liver function tests in liver donors. Transplant Proc (in press)
15. Lauchart W, Müller R, Pichlmayr R (1987) Immunoprophylaxis of hepatitis B virus reinfection in recipients of human liver allografts. Transplant Proc 19: 2387–2389
16. Steinhoff G, Wonigeit K, Ringe B, Lauchart W, Kemnitz J, Pichlmayr R (1987) Modified patterns of major histocompatibility complex-antigen expression in human liver grafts during rejection. Transplant Proc 19: 2466–2469
17. Wonigeit K, Bockhorn H, Pichlmayr R (1979) Posttransplant changes in specific precursor T-cell reactivity: comparison between liver and kidney allograft recipients. Transplant Proc 11: 1250–1255
18. Schwinzer R, Wonigeit K, Nashan B, Pichlmayr R (1987) Selective increase in $CD8^{+}$ $CD11^{+}$ cells in long-term liver allograft recipients. Transplant Proc (in press)

Has Eurotransplant Fulfilled Its Promise?

J. J. Van Rood

Everyone fortunate enough to have been involved in scientific research knows the excitement of obtaining a new finding or conducting an experiment that opens new vistas for further developments and possible applications. Enjoyment of life is at its peak when such excitement can be shared, preferably by a small group of scientists interested in the same topics. Nowadays there are many meetings for the exchange of research findings, but in the late 1960s when Walter Brendel began the tradition of the Round Table Symposia on Applied Immunology, this was certainly not the case. It was at these meetings that we presented our data on skin transplants and HLA matching data [1], the discovery of the DR serology [2, 3] and the impact of this on renal transplantation [4], CML nonresponsiveness developing posttransplantation [5], Ir genes in transplantation [6], and numerous other such findings. Much of what we presented dealt with the application of "basic" immunogenetics to "applied" clinical renal transplantation, most of this in the context of the Eurotransplant foundation which was initiated enthusiastically at the same time as the Round Table Symposia began [7].

Walter Brendel's 65th birthday seems a good opportunity to evaluate the extent to which the findings in "basic" science have indeed fulfilled their promise for the "applied" science of clinical renal transplantation. One of the goals of the Eurotransplant foundation, an international exchange organization for postmortem organs, has been the improvement of renal allograft survival by HLA matching. In this review we will focus on this aspect because it has been controversial from the beginning and has been repeatedly discussed during the Round Table Symposia. We will present first the immunogenetic evidence, translate this then to the clinical situation, and discuss finally some of the difficulties encountered when attempts are made to reach a concensus.

Matching for the "old Leiden" HLA Antigens

Figure 1 shows the results of a study by Van Hooff et al. [8] on a small group of patients given transplants in Eurotransplant's earliest years, who were typed for the old Leiden antigens, 4a, 4b, 6a, 6b, 6c, etc. The follow-up time is now over 17 years. In the first 12 years, there is a very clearcut and significant difference between patients well matched for these antigens and those who are poorly matched. After 12 years, there is a drop in graft survival among those patients who had received an identical

Surgical Research:
Recent Concepts and Results
Baethmann/Messmer (Eds.)

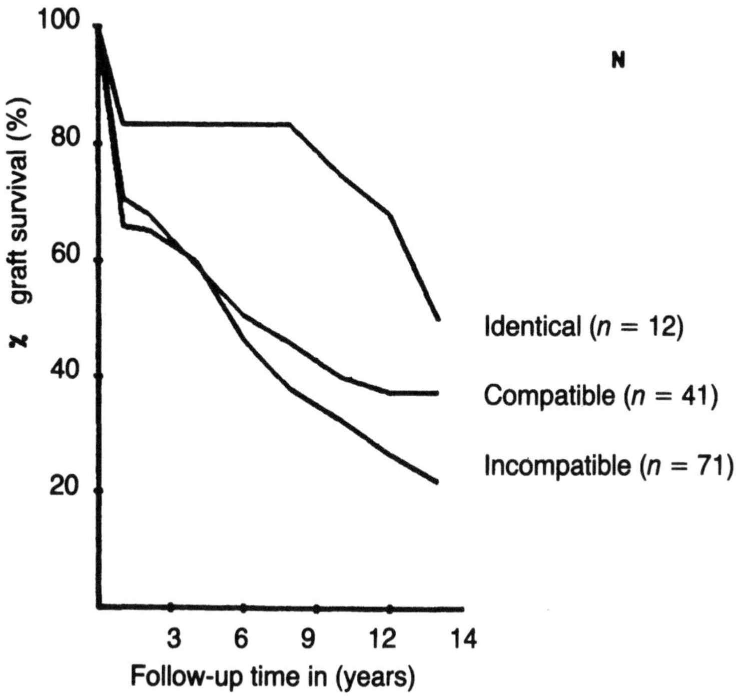

Fig. 1. Influence of matching for broadly reacting antigens on long-term kidney-graft survival, 1967–1972 ($n = 124$; $p = 0.033$) (Reprinted with permission from [8])

match. This was due to the death of two of the patients from "normal" causes. This confronts us with the reality that transplantation does not immortalize the patient.

Effect of HLA Matching on Graft Survival in a Single Center Study

This point is further illustrated in Fig. 2, which shows kidney graft survival and patient survival in a single center; this center was one of the first in Eurotransplant. The follow-up time is 14 years. Patient survival after 14 years is still over 60%. The middle curve shows functional graft survival, that is, taking into account only graft loss not due to patient death (14-year graft survival, 52%). The bottom curve shows overall graft survival (30% after 14 years). After 10 years, the line indicating functional graft survival remains horizontal because no grafts are lost due to rejection after this time. Whether this is because the rejection process has finally ceased is impossible to say but seems a priori unlikely in view of findings by other investigators. Matching data of this center are also available, but although the well-matched group does extremely well (90% at 5 years), the numbers are too small to draw any firm conclusions.

The effects of matching in two of the largest centers in Eurotransplant, however, are significant (Fig. 3); all patients received cyclosporin A. Figure 4 shows that a DR

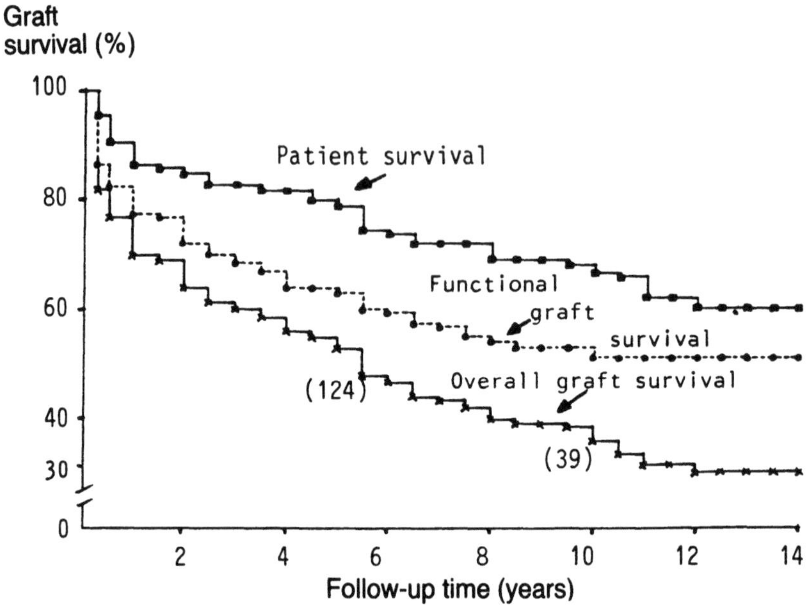

Fig. 2. Long-term graft and patient survival at the Rotterdam center, 1971–1973 (n = 278) (From E. van Steenberge, unpublished observations)

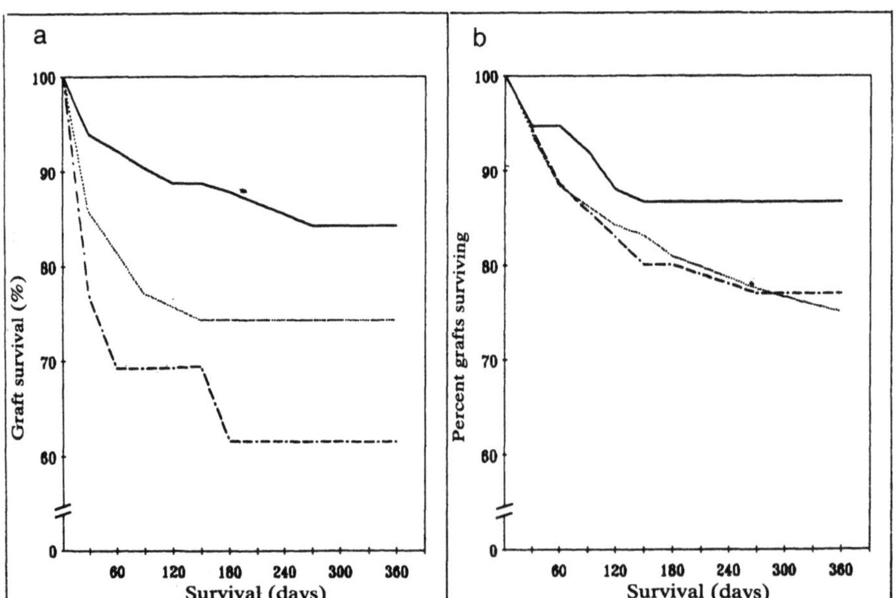

Fig. 3a, b. Influence of HLA-DR matching on survival of renal allografts treated with cyclosporin A in two single-center studies, **a** Center at Hannover; **b** center at Klinikum Großhadern, Munich. —, No HLA mismatch (**a** n = 165, **b** n = 75); ....., one HLA mismatch (**a** n = 111, **b** n = 95); –·–·–, two HLA mismatches (**a** n = 34, **b** n = 35) (unpublished observations)

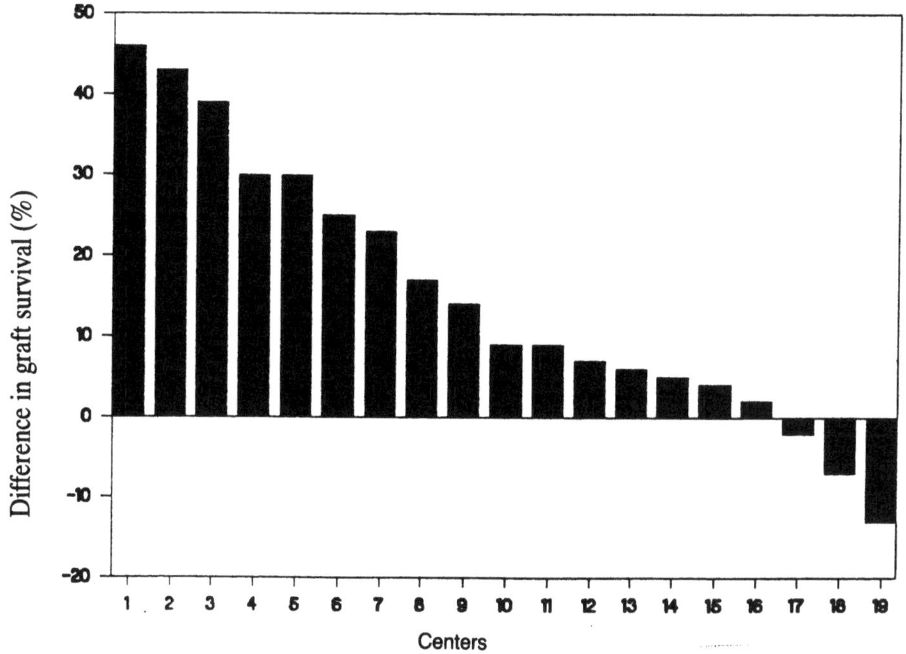

Fig. 4. HLA-DR matching in 19 study centers. Percentage differences in graft survival (at 1 year after transplantation) between the best and the worst HLA-DR matches

matching effect is found in almost all of the 19 centers in Eurotransplant that have performed a sufficient number of transplants to make a meaningful analysis possible. There are three centers in which such an effect is not found. Two of these have an overall graft survival of almost 95%. This may be due partially to patient selection. There is only one center (number 19) whose results are markedly different.

HLA Matching in Eurotransplant

Figure 5 shows the overall Eurotransplant data in three periods. In the earliest years of Eurotransplant (1968–1976) over 2500 patients received transplants (Fig. 5a); their follow-up time is now 17 years. The effect of matching HLA-A and -B is clear-cut ($p = 0.0001$). In the next period (1977–1981) over 4500 patients received transplants, of whom one-half ($n = 2291$) could be typed retrospectively for HLA-DR (Fig. 5b). The effect of matching is again highly significant. Note that after 10 years graft survival in the well-matched group is still 60%. For the last (the so-called, cyclosporin-A) period, the years 1982–1987 (Fig. 5c), the maximum follow-up time is 5 years. The number of transplants performed was over 5000. Graft survival in the well-matched group is over 70% after 5 years. The patients who received grafts mismatched for only one or two antigens also do well. Those patients who received a graft with some five or six mismatches have a graft survival of about 45% after 5 years.

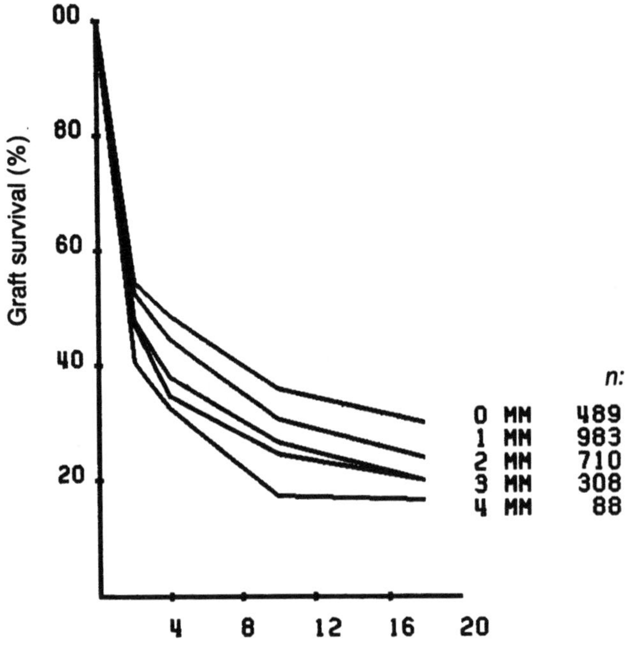

a

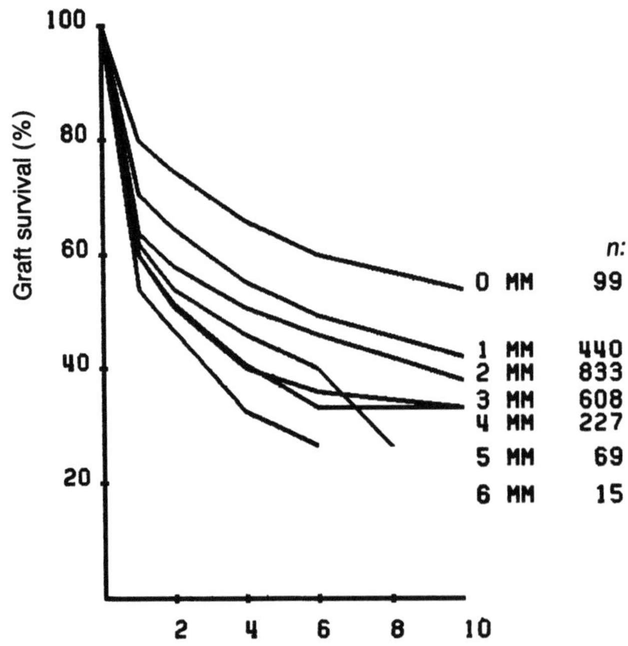

b

Fig. 5a–c. Influence of HLA-A, -B, and -DR matching on long-term graft survival. **a** HLA-A, -B, 1968–1976 ($n = 2578$; $p = 0.0001$); **b** HLA-A, -B, -DR, 1977–1981 ($n = 2291$; $p = 0.0000$); **c** HLA-A, -B, -DR ($n = 5752$; $p = 0.0019$). *MM*, number of HLA mismatches

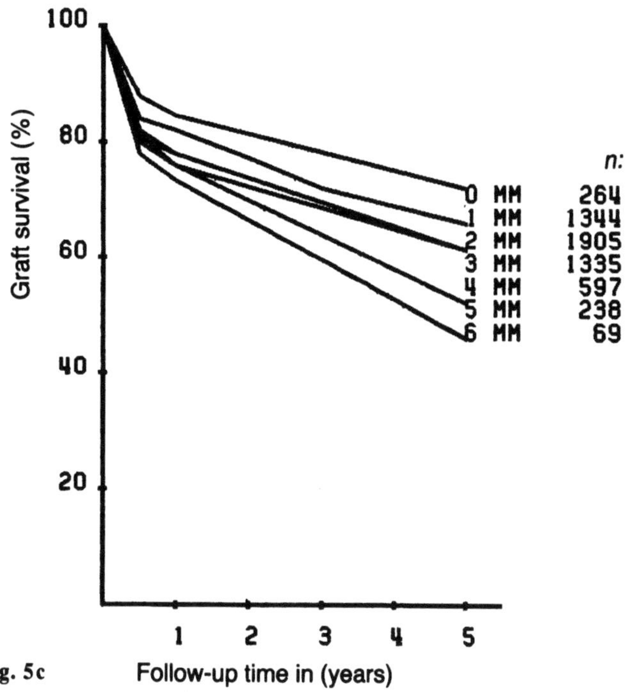

Fig. 5c

HLA Class I (HLA-A, -B) versus HLA Class II (HLA-DR) Matching

As illustrated in Table 1, the effect of HLA-A and-B matching did not influence renal allograft survival in the first 12 months, but it did do so after the first year. At this point the curves separate and the difference between well-matched and poorly matched grafts increases with time. In contrast, the effect of matching for HLA class II antigens (HLA-DR) on graft survival is already evident within the first 3 months after transplantation (Fig. 6). After the first year the effect of HLA-DR matching does not further increase, and the difference at 5 years is similar to that at 12 months. The bottom line of Table 1 shows that HLA-A, -B, and -DR matching have additive effects, resulting in a 30% difference of graft survival at 5 years posttransplantation between the well-matched and the poorly matched groups.

Table 1. Influence of HLA-A, -B, and -DR matching on graft survival at different time intervals after transplantation

Match	months posttransplantation		
	3	12	60
HLA-A, -B	–1%	–2%	12%
HLA-DR	10%	13%	14%
HLA-A, -B, -DR	9%	14%	30%

Figures give difference in graft survival between best and poorest match

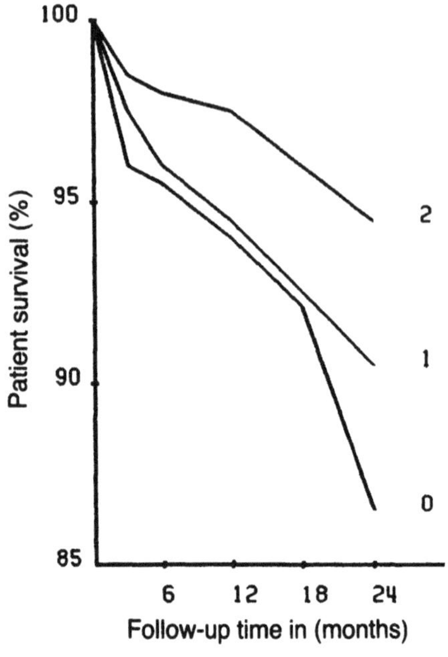

Fig. 6. Influence of DR matching and cyclosporin A on the survival of recipients of primary renal allografts, 1981–1985 (n = 3766; p = 0.000). O, no DR match (n = 357); 1, one DR match (n = 1989); 2, two DR matches (n = 1420)

Discussion

From these data we conclude that HLA-A, -B, and-DR matching has improved graft survival during Eurotransplant's operational history and that this effect is still evident even in the cyclosporin-A era. Apart from graft rejection there are additional penalties for not matching. For instance, the main reason for patients' becoming highly immunized (more than 85% panel reactivity) is graft rejection. Therefore, a poor match leads not only to a greater chance of rejection, but also to a greater chance of the patients' becoming highly immunized. This situation makes it very difficult to find a suitable donor for such patients.

Another problem for patients all over the world in need of a postmortem kidney is the shortage of kidneys available for transplantation. With 15000 kidneys transplanted worldwide, the loss of kidneys due to mismatching translates to over 1000 wasted annually. This could be prevented to a large extent by reliable matching. The third penalty has been identified by Birkeland [9]. Patients who receive mismatched grafts run a significantly greater chance of getting a malignant disease than do patients who receive a well-matched graft.

The greatest penalty of all of course occurs when the patient dies. As shown in Fig. 6, this chance is significantly increased in patients who received an HLA-DR mismatched graft [10]. All patients have received transfusion, were treated with cyclosporin A, and received an unrelated first transplant. After 3 years there is not only a significant difference in graft survival but also in patient survival. We conclude that the unnecessary transplantation of HLA-DR mismatched grafts places the patient's life at risk.

Table 2. Effectiveness of matching for HLA of cyclosprin A treated first unrelated renal grafts ($n = 3750$)

	Percentage graft survival at 1 year posttransplantation		Poolsize required for match		
Match	Best match	Worst match	30%[a]	60%	90%
HLA-DR	87	82	20	40	*500*[b]
HLA-A -DR	87	78	500	*4000*[b]	10^4
HLA-B -DR	88	76	500	*4000*[b]	10^4
HLA-A, -B, -DR	91	73	10^4	>>	>>

[a] Chance of finding an identical recipient for a given donor
[b] Attainable in Eurotransplant
Overall survival at 1 year, 84%

This conclusion is based on the fact that a pool of 500 or more potential recipients can guarantee 90% of recipents a graft fully identical in terms of DR (Table 2). Such a pool is easily attainable both in Western Europe and the USA. Table 2 further shows that by matching for HLA-A and -DR or HLA-B and -DR the difference of graft survival at 1 year posttransplantation between best and worst matches is further increased, and that it is maximized for HLA-A, -B, -DR identical matches. With a waiting list of about 6000 patients (the actual situation in Eurotransplant) only about 20%–30% of the patients can hope for an HLA-A, -B, -DR identical graft but over half of them could have an HLA-A and -DR, or HLA-B and -DR identical one.

This brings us back to the question, "Has Eurotransplant fulfilled its promise?" The answer is a whole-hearted "Yes!" Not only have hundreds of patients received well or better-than-average matched grafts, but the lives of many have been saved. Whether the application of immunogenetics in the clinic after the arrival of even more effective immunosuppressive regimes will be of the same importance remains to be seen.

The lesson from the introduction of cyclosporin A should, however, not be forgotten. During the euphoria caused by the effectiveness of cyclosporin A as an immunosuppressant, many patients received a graft with a poorer HLA match than was necessary. Later, it could be shown that such patients would have benefitted significantly from a better HLA match, but this was then unfortunately too late. We are convinced that discussions at further Round Table Symposia on Applied Immunology will help to prevent this from happening in the future.

References

1. Jonker M, Hoogeboom J, van Leeuwen A, Koch CT, Blussé van Oud Alblas A, Persijn GG, Frederiks E, van Rood JJ (1979) Experimental skin grafting in man. Transplant Proc XI: 607–610
2. Van Leeuwen A, Schuit HRE, van Rood JJ (1973) Typing for MLC (LD). II. The selection of non-stimulator cells by MLC inhibition tests using SD-identical stimulator cells (MISIS) and fluorescence antibody studies. Transplant Proc V: 1539–1542
3. Van Rood JJ, van Leeuwen A, Keuning JJ, Blussé van Oud Alblas A (1975) The serological recognition of the human MLC determinants using a modified cytotoxicity technique. Tissue Antigens 5: 73–79

4. Persijn GG, Gabb BW, van Leeuwen A, Nagtegaal A, Hoogeboom J, van Rood JJ (1978) Matching for HLA antigens of A, B and DR loci in renal transplantation by Eurotransplant. Lancet i: 1278–1281
5. Goulmy E, Persijn GG, Blokland E, D'Amaro J, van Rood JJ (1981) CML studies in renal allograft recipients. Transplantation 31: 210–217
6. Hendriks GFJ, D'Amaro J, Persijn GG, Schreuder GMTh, Lansbergen Q, Cohen B, van Rood JJ (1983) Excellent renal allograft prognosis with DRw6 positive donors in the face of HLA-DR mismatches. Lancet ii: 187–189
7. Van Rood JJ (1967) A proposal for international cooperation in organ transplantation: Eurotransplant. In: Curtoni ES et al. (eds) Histocompatibility Testing 1967. Williams and Wilkins, Baltimore, pp. 451–458
8. Van Hooff JP, van Leeuwen A, Paul LC, Leunissen KML, Lecomte C, D'Amaro J, Cohen B, Alexandre GRJ, van Rood JJ (1985) The influence of matching for broadly reacting antigens on long-term kidney graft survival. Transplant Proc XVII: 2205–2206
9. Birkeland SA (1983) Malignant tumours in renal transplant patients. Cancer 51: 1571–1575
10. Van Rood JJ (1987) Prospective HLA typing is helpful in cadaveric renal transplantation. Transplant Proc XIX: 139–143

Hematological Cytology in Organ Transplantation

C. Hammer, and C. Lersch

Introduction

Modern organ transplantation, with its access to a wide repertoire of immunosuppressive therapies, needs new sophisticated, sensitive, and fast methods both for monitoring immunological events concerning grafts after transplantation and for their successful treatment.

Immunological mechanisms leading to rejection episodes are largely unknown and can often not be clearly distinguished from viral and bacterial infections. Cells infiltrating the allografts include: T cells of CD4 and CD8 phenotypes, monocytes, macrophages, B cells, plasma cells, natural killer cells, cells with potential for antibody-dependent cell-mediated cytotoxicity, neutrophils, basophils and eosinophils. The CD4 and CD8 subclasses of T cells are able to trigger rejection by direct cytotoxic mechanisms or by release of lymphokines and recruitment of accessory cells such as monocytes and macrophages. Activated lymphocytes produce gamma-interferon which induces MHC expression on somatic cells. MHC expression possibly determines vulnerability to vascular rejection. While CD4 effector cells attack cells with the class II MHC, CD8 effectors are directed against class I – incompatible grafts [1]. Analysis and functional characterization of the infiltrating cells would allow investigation of the origin of these lymphocyte populations, their recruitment from lymphoid organs, e. g., spleen and lymph nodes, and their possible autonomous sensitization and proliferation in the graft itself.

Analysis of effector cells and also "bystander" cells from the graft would furnish massive information when compared with circulating populations of lymphoid cells. It would allow the differentiation of systemic and localized events. Parenchymal organs such as liver and kidney can easily be approached using biopsies, while cytology gives access to pancreas, lung, and kidney, with their additional secretory functions. Cells infiltrating cardiac and liver transplants during rejection are able to leave the graft and return into the circulating blood; they thus offer a distinct means for a cytoimmunological monitoring.

Principles of Hematological Cytology

Methods

As graphically depicted in Fig. 1, inflammatory cells isolated from grafts, peripheral blood, and other body fluids are spread onto slides by a cytocentrifuge (α) and stained

Surgical Research:
Recent Concepts and Results
Baethmann/Messmer (Eds.)

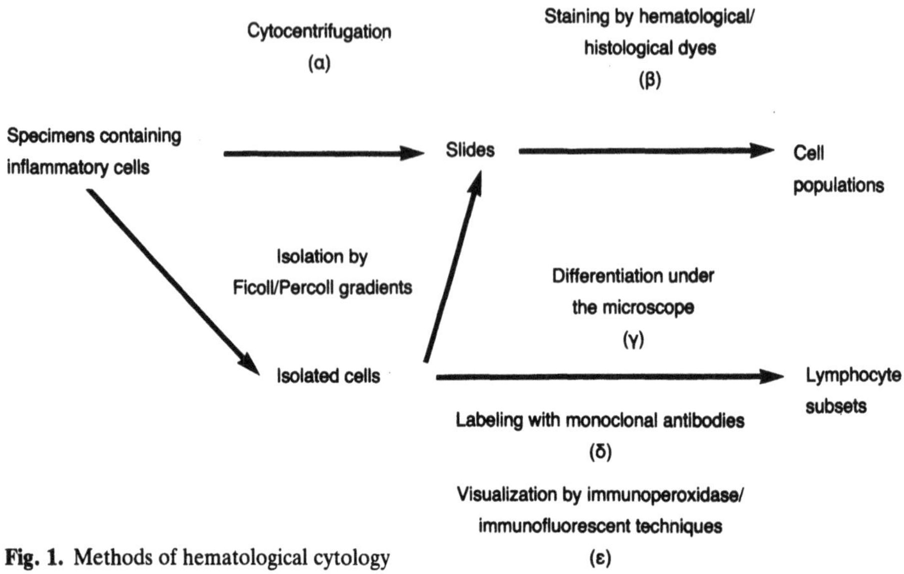

Fig. 1. Methods of hematological cytology

by various dyes (β). Percentages of different cell populations can be evaluated under the light microscope (γ). For further determination of lymphocyte subsets, isolated cells are incubated with monoclonal antibodies (δ). Using immunoperoxidase or immunofluorescent techniques (ε) a visualization of labeled cells is possible. Inflammatory cells in biopsies are identified in sections after staining by monoclonal antibodies or histological dyes.

Marker Cells For Inflammatory Events

The most alarming cells, those indicating acute inflammatory events in the grafts, are (a) lymphoblasts and activated lymphocytes and (b) cells of the monocyte-macrophage series. Cytological monitoring in organ recipients is of major importance for an early diagnosis using these cells in grafts, peripheral blood, or other body secretions. Lymphoblasts are large cells (15–25 μm in diameter) with a dark basophilic cytoplasm and a perinuclear bright zone when stained according to the Pappenheim method. The "large" nuclei contain 4–6 prominent nucleoli. Lymphoblasts are normally found in bone marrow and lymphopoietic tissues and are precursor cells of lymphocytes. It is not yet proven, whether lymphoblasts invade grafts during inflammation or originate from lymphocytes already resting in the grafts. Activated lymphocytes are cells intermediate between lymphocytes and lymphoblasts, they are twice as large as normal lymphocytes (6–8 μm in diameter) and have a basophilic cytoplasm and a round nucleus. Macrophages are very large phagocytic cells (25–40 μm in diameter) with vacuoles, granules, a foamy greyish-blue cytoplasm, and a typical nucleus. They invade the organ from the surrounding tissue or are blood-borne. Macrophages remove graft detritus during progressive rejections and ischemic lesions.

Acute Rejections

During acute rejections inflammatory cells accumulate in the graft. The intensity of inflammation associated with rejection can be quantified from fine needle aspirates and expressed as an increment [2], or from the peripheral blood and expressed as an activation index [3]. In core biopsies the severity of rejection is defined by the extent of edema and by the nature and number of infiltrating cells.

Infections

VIRAL INFECTIONS. During certain generalized viral infections an inversion of the ratio of CD4- to CD8-positive lymphocytes is observed [4]. In addition, large granular lymphocytes (LGLs) comprising 70% of natural killer cells increase in number in peripheral blood and in the graft during the infections [5]. Only cytomegalovirus, herpesvirus, and Ebstein-Barr virus induce such phenomena; other common viruses obviously do not. Serological methods and virus isolation from a recipient are still the method of choice for diagnosis of viral infection [11].

BACTERIAL OR FUNGAL INFECTIONS. The diagnosis of bacterial or fungal infections by cytological methods is possible. An increase of juvenile granulocytes in the mononuclear concentrates is one sign of infection by these organisms. The isolation and cultivation of bacteria or fungi from the recipient, however, is still the most reliable method. Chemiluminescence activity of phagocytes measured in peripheral blood or aspirates of grafts supports the cytological diagnosis of microbial infections [3]. Criteria for the differential diagnosis of acute rejections, viral infections, and microbial infections are depicted in Table 1.

Table 1. Characteristic changes during inflammatory events in patients who have received transplants

	Acute rejection	Viral infection	Microbial infection
Lymphoblasts, activated lymphocytes	+ to +++	++	+
Inversion of CD4/CD8 ratio	–	+ to +++	–
Large granular lymphocytes	+	+++	(+)
Juvenile granulocytes	+	(+)	+++
Monocytes	+++	+	++
Chemiluminescence, activity of phagocytes	+	–	+++

Cytology in Different Grafts

Types of specimens which can easily be obtained from recipients and prepared for cytological differential diagnosis are summarized in Table 2.

Table 2. Cytological monitoring of acute rejections and infections in organ transplants

	Specimens			
Organs	Peripheral blood	Biopsies	Fine needle aspirates	Body fluids
Kidney	+	+++	+++	Urine
Liver	+++	+++	+++	(Bile)
Heart	+++	+++	–	–
Pancreas	+	++	+	Pancreatic juice, urine
Lung	++	+++	+	Sputum, lavage fluid
Bone marrow	+++	++	–	–
(Bowel)	(++)	(+)	(+)	Bowel juice (feces)

Kidney

Fine needle aspiration cytology (FNAC) from kidneys has become an indispensable method for postoperative monitoring of kidney grafts. FNAC allows (a) early diagnosis of inflammatory events and acute tubular necrosis in kidney grafts, (b) staging of an acute rejection by the increment method [2], (c) monitoring of successful immunosuppression during acute rejection, and (d) ascertaining drug toxicity (under certain conditions). FNAC should be repeated in 3-day intervals during the first 6 weeks after transplantation, since most severe acute rejections occur during this period. FNAC consists of a differentiation of inflammatory cells, such as lymphoblasts, activated lymphocytes, macrophages, plasma cells, LGLs, monocytes, granulocytes, lymphocytes, and parenchymal cells (e.g., endothelial and tubular cells), together with an evaluation of lymphocyte subsets by monoclonal antibodies. Typical morphological changes in tubular cells – damaged nuclei, vacuoles, cytoplasmic inclusions, erythrophagocytosis – occur during Cyclosporine but not during Azathioprine therapy [6]. During viral infections CD8-positive lymphocytes are predominant in grafts, as compared to acute cellular rejections [4]. The CD4/CD8 ratio is inversed and stands at below 0.8 [5]; in addition, LGLs significantly increase with virus infections.

Urinary sediment cytology is a less specific but noninvasive method for postoperative graft monitoring [7]. Tubular cells, collecting duct cells, and inflammatory cells are counted in cytocentrifuge preparations of the urine sediment. Acute rejection and acute tubular necrosis are associated with an increasing number of tubular-, collecting duct-, and inflammatory cells. Differential diagnosis between these events seems to be difficult.

Clinical data, such as creatinine, urea and β^2 microglobulin levels in peripheral blood, urine production, and levels of neopterins in peripheral blood and urine, are still the most frequently used parameters for routine kidney graft monitoring. For exact differential diagnosis of inflammatory events affecting graft function, FNAC and the more invasive core biopsies are necessary. Cytological monitoring in the peripheral blood of patients has proven to be an inappropriate method, since large numbers of inflammatory cells are excreted in the urine.

Liver

Inflammatory cells associated with rejections of infections in liver graft recipients can be found in histological specimens, fine needle aspirates, peripheral blood, and perhaps also in the bile. Biopsies are the most valuable approach to receive a clear diagnosis of graft rejection or infection but may be difficult and dangerous due to concomitant coagulopathy and hypervascularity of the transplanted liver. During rejections a rapid disappearance of interlobular bile ducts associated with a dense portal infiltrate of mononuclear cells and severe central lobular cholestasis is typical.

FNAC enables the monitoring of intragraft inflammatory events by an incremental method [8]. Lymphoblasts and lymphocytes dominate in the beginning of rejection, resulting in an elevated intragraft CD4/CD8 ratio. Blood eosinophilia and fever are frequently associated with the onset of rejection. Degenerative changes in parenchymal cells and cholestasis are seen in fine needle biopsy specimens during rejection. Lymphoblasts and activated lymphocytes in the peripheral blood of liver transplant recipients are recorded during inflammatory events. A differential diagnosis is possible when using the criteria summarized in Table 1. The usefulness of cytoimmunological monitoring of liver grafts as reported for heart-transplanted patients is under investigation [9].

Useful clinical data can be obtained by daily physical examination, determination of serum enzymes (transaminases, alkaline phosphatase, lactic acid, and dehydrogenase), bilirubin, and prothrombin time, and identification of inflammatory blood cells. In future, analysis of inflammatory cells in the bile, obtained by endoscopy, may be desirable.

Heart

In 1973 Caves et al. [10] reported on the percutaneous transvenous endomyocardial biopsy in human heart recipients. This method has proven to be reliable for (a) early diagnosis of acute rejections, (b) grading of the inflammation, and (c) control of a successful immunosuppressive therapy. In 1984 Hammer et al. [11] first described the cytological and immunological monitoring (CIM) of Cyclosporine-treated heart recipients. This method allows the reduction of the frequency of invasive endomyocardial biopsy after cardiac transplantation by 70%.

Quick monitoring requires only 75 μl heparinized peripheral blood [9]. After separation over a Ficoll-microgradient the mononuclear cells are differentiated in a cytocentrifuge smear. The number of lymphoblasts and activated lymphocytes defines the "activation index." This scoring index makes a grading of inflammatory events possible. Further differention can be performed by the phenotypic analysis of lymphocytes, using an indirect immunofluorescence technique (Table 1) and by measuring the chemiluminescence activity of monocytes and polymorphonuclear cells.

Clinical information on the course of rejection may be obtained by frequent analysis of surface electrocardiograms, intramyocardial electrograms [14], two-dimensional echocardiography [12], daily urinary neopterin evaluation [13], and monitoring of enzymes. At present CIM together with two other noninvasive methods are required for effective postoperative monitoring of heart recipients. Introducing CIM for timing of the endomyocardial biopsy has significantly reduced the number of biopsies during a patient's clinical stay from 15 to 4. Yet, CIM does not totally replace the endomyocardial biopsy.

Pancreas

Exocrine secretions of transplanted pancreas obtained either by a catheter after pancreatico – enteric anastomosis [15] or by using the bladder as conduit after pancreatico – vesical anastomosis can be analyzed. Pancreatic juice cytology is an appropriate method for the diagnosis of graft rejection [16]. Urine amylase, neopterins, and the amount of pancreatic juice and lactate dehydrogenase [16] are reliable markers for rejection in addition to serum insulin, glucose, and C-peptide levels. Using these parameters can reduce the number of pancreas graft biopsies.

For the monitoring of renal-pancreatic transplants from the same donor, markers for kidney graft rejections can additionally be taken into account. In experimental studies FNAC of the pancreas has not been feasible. And since inflammatory cells are excreted by the pancreas via juice, CIM of peripheral blood is of minor importance for diagnosis of acute rejection.

Lung

Lungs are transplanted almost exclusively as heart-lung allografts. Postoperative monitoring is therefore performed as described above for heart-transplanted patients. In addition, transvenous, transbronchial, and open lung biopsies after thoracotomy can be performed in order to diagnose inflammatory events in lung tissues. Chest roentgenograms are very useful for an early diagnosis of lung infiltrations.

The bronchoalveolar lavage (BAL) allows cytologists to obtain inflammatory cells from transplanted lungs. In experimental studies a decreased number of total cells and macrophages and an increased proportion of lymphocytes was found in BAL fluids [17] during rejection episodes. Cytological examination of BAL fluid seems to be even more important for an early diagnosis of heart-lung rejections since Prop et al. [19] demonstrated that the lymphoid tissue transplanted together with the lung is an important stimulus making the unmodified rejection of lungs more vigorous than that of hearts. Cytoimmunological analysis of peripheral white blood cells has proven to be of help for postoperative monitoring of lung allografts [18]. This should be performed in the manner described for heart allografts. Infections induce increased chemiluminescence activity of free lung cells [18].

Bone Marrow

After bone marrow transplantation monitoring of urinary neopterin excretion [20] and of inflammatory cells – lymphoid blast cells, LGLs, and small lymphocytes – in the liver, skin, and later also in the blood [21] seems to be useful for the early detection of graft-versus-host disease or infection. An increase of chemiluminescence activity of peripheral blood cells is an early indication of successful bone marrow transplantation [22].

Bowel

Histological monitoring of small-intestinal allografts has been accomplished by daily biopsies of stomas [23]. Increased monocyte procoagulant activity and an index of monocyte/macrophage immune activation are additional parameters for graft rejection. Data on the monitoring of inflammatory cells in the peripheral blood and the excrements during intestine rejection are as yet insufficient.

Conclusion

Cytoimmunological monitoring enables transplant surgeons to diagnose early inflammatory complications in allograft recipients. Cells indicating such events can be obtained by biopsies or fine needle aspirates from grafts. Secretions of kidney, liver, pancreas, lung, and perhaps also bowel grafts can be analyzed for these inflammatory cells. Rejections of heart, liver, and lung grafts are diagnosed by monitoring peripheral blood cells. Differential diagnosis distinguishing acute rejections or infections can be made by analyzing chemiluminescence activity of phagocytes or phenotypes of white blood cells (Table 1). Cytological examination in organ transplantation helps considerably to reduce the number of invasive biopsies and to increase the reliability of the postoperative follow-up of patients.

References

1. Hall BM (1987) Cellular infiltrates in allografts. Transplant Proc 19: 50–56
2. Häyry P, von Willebrand E (1981) Monitoring of human renal allograft rejection with fine-needle aspiration cytology. Scand J Immunol 13: 87–97
3. Lehmann M, Lersch C, Krombach F, Osterholzer G, Hammer C, Kemkes BM, Klanke D (1987) Cytoimmunological monitoring and chemiluminescence of peripheral blood phagocytes in heart recipients. Langenbecks Arch Chir (Suppl Chir Forum): 211–215
4. Stadler J, Koller C, Hammer C, Weber B, Land W, Castro LA, Brendel W (1985) Monitoring of viral infections after renal transplantation by fine needle aspiration biopsy and monoclonal antibodies. Transplant Proc 17: 168–170
5. Dendorfer U, Hammer C, Schleibner S, Hillebrand G, Stoffner D, Nguyen LH, Koller C, Gokel YM, Land W (1985) Comparison of renal transplant cytology with histological findings. Transplant Proc 18: 2584–2585
6. Weber B, Welte M, Stadler J, Koller C, Hammer C, Land W, Castro L, Hillebrand G, Schleibner S, Csapo C, Brendel W (1985) Detection and differentiation of pathologic changes in nonrejecting kidney grafts. Transplant Proc 17: 120–121
7. Klima G, Spielberger H, König P, Margreiter R (1985) Fine needle aspiration biopsy and urinary sediment cytology in renal allograft recipients. Transplant Proc 17: 2083–2084
8. Lautenschlager J, Höckerstedt K, Scheinin TM, Häyry P (1984) Aspiration cytology of liver transplants. Preliminary experience in man. In: Kreis H, Droz (eds) Renal Transplant Cytology. Wichtig Editore, Milan, pp 173–178

9. Lersch C, Hammer C, Plahl M, Lehmann M, Reichenspurner H, Reichart B (1985) Differential diagnosis between rejection and infection arising in the peripheral blood in heart transplant recipients. Langenbecks Arch Chir (Suppl Chir Forum): 179–181
10. Caves PK, Stinson GB, Billinghamm E, Shumway NE (1973) Percutaneous transvenous endomyocardial biopsy in human heart recipients. Ann Thorac Surg 16: 325
11. Hammer C, Reichenspurner H, Ertel W, Lersch C, Plahl M, Brendel W, Reichart B, Überfuhr P, Welz A, Kemkes BM, Reble B, Functius W, Gokel M (1984) Cytological and imunologic monitoring of Cyclosporine-treated human heart recipients. Heart Transplant 3: 228–232
12. Reichenspurner H, Kemkes BM, Haberl R, Angermann Ch, Weber M, Osterholzer G, Anthuber M, Steinbeck G (1987) Frequency analysis of surface electrocardiogram and two-dimensional echocardiography for noninvasive diagnosis of rejection after heart transplantation. Transplant Proc 19: 2552–2553
13. Margreiter R, Fuchs D, Hauser A, Huber C, Reibnegger G, Spielberger KM, Wachter H (1983) Neopterin as a new biochemical marker for diagnosis of allograft rejection. Transplantation 36: 650–653
14. Wahlers T, Haverich A, Schäfer HJ, Fieguth HG, Frimpong-Boateng K, Hermann G, Borst HG (1987) The intramyocardial electrogramm (IMEG): a reliable marker of allograft rejection (Ry) in orthotopic heart transplantation (H-Tx) Transplant Proc 19: 1059
15. Brattström C, Tyden G, Malmborg AS, Lundgren G, Öst L, Groth CG (1987) Studies of the exocrine secretion of segmental pancreatic grafts with reference to the diagnosis of rejection and to the penetration of drugs into the pancreatic juice. Transplant Proc 19: 2332–2335
16. Steiner E, Klima G, Niederwieser D, Königsrainer A, Herold M, Margreiter R (1987) Monitoring of pancreatic allograft by analysis of exocrine secretion. Transplant Proc 19: 2336–2338
17. Schäfers HJ, Haverich A, Dammenhayn L, Takayama T, Wahlers T, Worch K, Kemnik J (1987) The role of bronchoalveolar lavage in diagnosing pulmonary rejection after heart-lung-transplantation. Transplant Proc 19: 2551
18. Hoefter E, Reichenspurner H, Krombach F, Kemkes BM, Fiehl E, Kugler C, Ertl W, Osterholzer G, König G, Gokel JM, Hammer C (1987) Morphology and function of free lung cells following combined hetero-orthotopic heart-lung transplantation in the dog. Transplant Proc 19: 1045–1048
19. Prop J, Kuijpers K, Nienwenhuis P, Wildevuur CPH (1985) Why are lung grafts rejected more vigorously than heart grafts? Heart Transplant 4 (suppl 2): 143
20. Volin L, Jansson SE, Trupeinen U, Pomoell UM, Ruutu T (1987) Urinary neopterin in bone marrow recipients. Transplant Proc 19: 2651–2654
21. Renkonen R, Leszczynski D, Wangelt A, Häyry P (1987) Characteristics and functions of inflammatory cells isolated from acute graft-versus-host disease target organs after bone marrow transplantation in the rat. Transplant Proc 19: 2689
22. Toivanen A, Nikoskelainen J, Lilius EH, Salmi TT, Kätkä K, Pelliniemi TT, Mäki AL, Rajamaki A (1987) Peripheral blood chemiluminescence as an early indicator of successful bone marrow transplantation. Transplant Proc 19: 2745–2746
23. Cohen Z, Silverman R, Levy G, Wassef R, Langer B (1987) Clinical small intestinal transplantation using Cyclosporine A and methylprednisolone. Transplant Proc 19: 2588–2590

Towards an Understanding of the Immunosuppressive Effect of Cyclosporin A*

H. WAGNER, D. KABELITZ, and K. HEEG

Introduction

The setting during which we first became confronted with the biological effect of cyclosporin A was that of Axams, Austria, the location chosen for the annual Round Table Symposium on Applied Immunology, organized by Prof. W. Brendel and his associates. The hallmark of these meetings has been a felicitous combination of science and joyful recreation at skiing snowy mountain slopes. Most importantly, the relaxed atmosphere during long evenings has allowed discussion of work still in progress. It was during such an evening session that Calne showed a slide depicting an apparently healthy dog jumping over a fence. This slide documented an aspect of the impressive results obtained as early as 1977 [1] by the English group in assaying the immunosuppressive effect of cyclosporin A in dogs receiving a kidney allograft. A report given concomitantly by Borel on the effect of cyclosporin A in various model systems [2] further stirred our interest and induced us to study the immunosuppressive action of cyclosporin on our own. The prime question we wished to answer was how cyclosporin inhibits T-lymphocyte dependent allograft rejection. We have concentrated on the mixed lymphocyte response, the in vitro correlate of in vivo allograft responses.

T-T cell Interactions During in Vitro Cytotoxic Allograft Responses

Since cyclosporin A was shown to prevent allograft rejection in vivo, attempts have been made to analyze its mode of action in vitro. Recent progress in the analysis of T-cell mediated cytotoxic responses towards allogeneic stimulator cells, seen by many as a valid in vitro model of allograft rejection, has revealed a cascade of cellular interactions ultimately yielding cytotoxic T-lymphocytes (CTL). CTL rather than delayed-type hypersensitivity responses [3] are thought to mediate the allograft rejection process. In simple terms, the induction of alloreactive CTL requires several important steps in addition to antigen recognition. First, class II MHC-reactive CD4 T cells provide the main source of helper T cells capable of secreting the T-cell growth factor interleukin 2, (Il-2), while class I MHC-reactive CD8 T cells are the main

* This work was supported by the SFB 322.

Surgical Research:
Recent Concepts and Results
Baethmann/Messmer (Eds.)

source of precursors of cytoxic T Cells (i. e., CTL) with reactivity towards class I MHC antigen. Second, upon recognition of antigen by Ia^+ macrophages with the subsequent production and release of interleukin 1 (IL-1) T helper cells secrete IL-2. Third, precursors of CTL become activated by antigen recognition and subsequently express high-affinity (biologically active) receptors for IL-2 (IL-2 receptors). Fourth, IL-2 mediates clonal amplification (growth) of activated CTL. And finally, T suppressor cells are activated to become capable of down-regulating and controlling CTL activation.

Cyclosporin Impairment of Lymphokine Secretion

From work by Borel and associates it was clear that cyclosporin (Cs) interferes at an early stage during T-cell activation in vitro. Since in the murine mixed lymphocyte reaction (MLR) growth of activated CTL is dependent on the availability of IL-2, we postulated that Cs may preferentially inhibit secretion of IL-2 from IL-2 producer T cells. Indeed, we demonstrated that addition of Cs to T-lymphocytes, stimulated with alloantigen in murine MLR, effectively suppressed the production of IL-2 [4]. Subsequently similar results were obtained in a human [5] and in a guinea pig [6] allogeneic MLR system. In addition we noted [4] that even upon addition of IL-1 to Cs-treated cultures, T helper cells remained refractory in terms of their ability to secrete IL-2. These findings were confirmed in the human MLR [7]. While initial studies demonstrating the effect of Cs on IL-2 production were obtained in a *primary* sensitization protocol, independent work has revealed that Cs also effectively inhibits IL-2 secretion in *secondary* responses of primed lymphocytes [8]. Essentially these results corroborate data obtained in vivo [9]. Thus, Cs may be effective in suppressing the allograft response of sensitized individuals.

From the literature it is known that the inhibitory effect of CsA upon lymphokine secretion of activated T (helper) cells is not only restricted to IL-2, but also includes the production of IL-3 [10], interferon [11], and migration-inhibitory factor [12]. In the case of IL-2 it has been shown that CsA selectively blocks the induction (or production) of IL-2 mRNA while leaving constitutive processes unchanged [13]. Whether this mechanism explains CsA-mediated inhibition of other lymphokines is at present unclear.

Inhibition of Primary Sensitization

T-cell activation can be defined rather narrowly as that series of events which are required to induce IL-2 responsiveness, i. e., expression of high-affinity (functional) IL-2 receptors. Once functional IL-2 receptors are expressed on T cells, CsA does not impair IL-2 mediated growth [4]. Initial studies by Larsson [14] provided evidence that one mechanism of the immunosuppressive effect of Cs is to block acquisition of IL-2 responsiveness, i.e., IL-2 receptor expression during primary activation of T cells. Using a limiting dilution system to quantify the frequency of murine CTL precursors reactive toward alloantigens, we noted that up to 80% of resting CTL-p are sensitive to the immunosuppressive effect of Cs [15]. Thus, even though exogenous

IL-2 is provided, the vast majority of antigen-reactive CTL precursors are blocked by Cs from developing IL-2 responsiveness, that is, from expressing functional IL-2 receptors. Similar results have been obtained in the human system [16]. It should be noted that in the murine model system at lower doses of Cs (100 ng/ml) the addition of high doses of exogenous IL-2 resulted in significant levels of CTL activity [4]. This type of data suggests that, depending on the concentration of Cs used, antigen-reactive CTL are induced, but clonal expansion does not take place because IL-2 producer T cells are effectively blocked at this concentration of Cs [4]. In fact, recent data obtained in the human system indicate that T cells of some individuals may be resistant up to the level of 1000 ng/ml Cs in terms of inhibition of IL-2 receptor expression [16].

One apparent paradox also needs to be discussed here. The availability of monoclonal antibodies capable of recognizing IL-2 receptors (i. e., TAC) has allowed direct analysis of the effect of CsA upon IL-2 receptor expression of T cells. Several investigators have noted that Cs did not, in fact, inhibit the expression of IL-2 receptors (as detected serologically), yet the same cells remained refractory to the growth-promoting effect of exogenous IL-2 [17, 18]. This paradox may be explained in view of very recent data [19]. Thus high-affinity IL-2 receptors represent a two-chain stucture, an alpha (p 75) chain noncovalently linked to a beta (p 55) chain. Since the monoclonal antibody used for studying IL-2 receptor expression recognizes an epitope only on the beta chain, and since transfection of cDNA of the beta chain induces only low-affinity IL-2 binding, the possibility exists that CsA blocks the expression of the alpha chain of the IL-2 receptor.

Evidence for Cyclosporin Receptors

Two major sites of action of Cs have thus far been discussed: inhibition of lymphokine secretion and inhibition of the sequence of events required for resting T cells to develop responsiveness to IL-2. Findings on these address consequences of the effect of Cs yet obviously do not explain how Cs initiates its effects. At least three directions of investigations appear to be promising. First, a 17-KD protein termed cyclophilin has been identified in the cytoplasmic fraction of cells which binds Cs [20]. Second, there is evidence that Cs acts via the prolactin receptor, thus inhibiting the polyamine biosynthetic pathway [21]. In line with this conclusion is the finding that Cs inhibits the induction of ornithine decarboxylase within 4 h following mitogen stimulation of T cells. Third, Cs appears to bind to calmodulin, thus preventing calcium-dependent cytoplasmic activation events [22]. The way in which Cs influences a number of subcellular events is at present being intensively investigated.

Epilogue

A substantial amount of good luck contributed to the fact that over the years we have been members of the "Axams family," meeting here many scientists from various disciplines and from a variety of backgrounds. We feel that not serendipity but the mastermind of Walter Brendel provided the chance as early as 1978 to discuss with

Borel and Calne the interesting immunosuppressive functions of Cs. Walter Brendel's strong belief that research endeavors are successfully initiated when scientists of different disciplines mix in a relaxed atmosphere such as that provided in Axams has rewarded us with becoming involved in the analysis of the immunosuppressive effect of Cs. The authors use this occasion to wish Walter Brendel "good luck" for the future.

References

1. Calne RY, White DJG (1977) Cyclosporin A – a powerful immunosuppressant in dogs with renal allografts. IRCS Med Sci 5: 595
2. Borel JF, Feuer C, Magnee C,Stähelin H (1977) Effects of the new anti-lymphocyte peptide cyclosporin A in animals. Immunology 32: 1017–1025
3. Loveland BE, Hogarth PM, Ceredy RN, McKenzie IFC (1981) Cells mediating graft rejection in the mouse. I. Lyt-1 cells mediate skin graft rejection. J Exp Med 153: 1044-1052
4. Bunjes D, Hardt C, Röllinghoff M, Wagner H (1981) Cyclosporin A mediates immunosuppression of primary cytotoxic T cell responses by impairing the release of interleukin 1 and interleukin 2. Eur J Immunol 11: 657–661
5. Hess AD, Tutschka PJ, Pu Z, Santos GW (1982) Effect of cyclosporin A on human lymphocyte response in vitro. IV. Production of T cell stimulatory growth factors in CS treated primary MLR cultures. J. Immunol 128: 360–365
6. Dos Reis GA, Shevach EM (1982) Effect of cyclosporin A on T cell function in vitro: the mechanism of suppression of T cell proliferation depends on the nature of the T cell stimulus as well as the differentiation state of the responding T cell. J Immunol 129: 2360–2366
7. Hess AB, Tutschka PJ, Santos GW (1983) Effect of cyclosporin on the induction of cytotoxic T lymphocytes: role of interleukin 1 and interleukin 2. Transplant Proc 15: 2248–2251
8. Andrus L, Lafferty KJ (1981) Inhibition of T cell activity by cyclosporin A. Scand J Immunol 15: 449–453
9. Shulak JA, Monson D, Shelby J, Carry RJ (1983) Abrogation of second-set rejection with cyclosporin. Transplantation 36: 289–293
10. Lafferty KJ, Borel JF, Hodgkin P (1983) Cyclosporine A: models for the mechanism of action. Transplant Proc 15: 2242–2246
11. Reem GH, Cook LA, Vilcek J (1983) Gamma interferon synthesis by human thymocytes and T lymphocytes inhibited by cyclosporin A. Science 221: 63–64
12. Thomson AW, Moon DK, Nelson DS (1983) Suppression of delayed type hypersensitivity reactions and lymphokine production by cyclosporin A in the mouse. Clin Exp Immunol 52: 599–604
13. Krönke M, Leonard WJ, Depper JM, Arya SK, Wong-Stahl F, Gallo RC, Waldmann TA, Greene WC (1984) Cyclosporin inhibits T cell growth factor gene expression at the level of mRNA transcription. Proc Natl Acad Sci USA 81: 5214–5217
14. Larsson EL (1980) Cyclosporin A and dexamethasone suppress T cell responses by selectively acting at distinct sites of the triggering process. J Immunol 124: 2828–2833
15. Heeg K, Deusch K, Solbach W, Bunjes D, Wagner H (1984) Frequency analysis of cyclosporin sensitive cytolytic T lymphocyte precursors. Tansplantation 38: 532–536
16. Kabelitz, D, Zanker B, Zanker C, Heeg K, Wagner H (1987) Human cytotoxic T lymphocytes. III. Frequency analysis of CS sensitive alloreactive CTL-p. Immunology 61: 57–62
17. Miyawaki T, Yachie A, Ohzeki S, Nagaoki T, Taniguchi N (1983) Cyclosporin A does not prevent expression of TAC antigen, a probable TCGF receptor molecule on mitogen stimulated human T cells. J Immunol 130: 2737–2742
18. Solbach W, Heeg K, von Steldern DU, Röllinghoff M, Wagner H (1985) On the partial suppression of IL-2 receptor expression and the prevention of lectin-induced blast formation by cyclosporin A. Clin Exp Immunol 60: 501–508
19. Smith KA (1987) The two-chain structure of high affinity IL-2 receptors. Immunol Today 8: 11–13

20. Handschuhmacher RE, Hardong MW, Rice J, Drugge RJ (1984) Cyclophilin: a specific cytosolic binding protein for cyclosporin A. Science 226:544–547
21. Russel D, Kibler R, Matrisian L, Larsson D, Poulos B, Magun B (1985) Prolactin receptors on human T and B lymphocytes: antagonism of prolactin binding by cyclosporin. J Immunol 134: 3027–3031
22. Colombani PM, Robb A, Hess AD (1985) Cyclosporin A binding to calmodulin: a possible site of action on T Lymphocytes. Science 228: 337–339

V. General Immunology

Host Antigen-Presenting Cells and the Induction of In Vivo Allograft Reactivity

L. BRENT, and R. A. SHERWOOD

Introduction

It is generally accepted that most antigens stimulate T-lymphocytes only after they have been taken up and presented by various kinds of cells (antigen-presenting cells, APC) that include macrophages, dendritic cells and Langerhans' cells [4, 17, 22, 25]. Whether antigens must be internalized and processed in some way before they can act as immunogens on the cell surface of APC is still debated; the majority view is that this is a necessary prerequisite, but some [8] have argued against this. Most studies on antigen presentation have made use of proteins or other well-defined molecules, whereas alloantigens have received less attention, and then, in the main, by in vitro techniques. For example, it has been shown in the murine primary mixed lymphocyte reaction that glass-adherent, Ia-positive cells provide the dominant stimulatory effect [14] and that purified responder lymphocytes require the participation of donor dendritic cells (DC) (see [23]). However, the additional presence of *host* DC can greatly enhance such responses (J. Goodacre, P. Bedford and S. C. Knight, personal communication). Likewise, the generation of cytotoxic T-lymphocytes has been shown to depend on the presence of either stimulator or responder APC [6].

In vivo studies have focussed mainly on the role of donor APC. Thus, Knight et al. [9] induced host-versus-graft responses in parental-strain mice by the inoculation of small numbers of F_1 hybrid DC into the footpads, and Boog et al. [3] found that female mice from an H-Y non-responder strain rejected syngeneic male skin grafts following the injection of male DC. Finally, Lechler and Batchelor [12] carried out experiments involving renal allografts in rats, and as they are highly relevant to our own studies we shall summarize their data below.

Enhanced long-surviving (AS × Aug) F_1 hybrid kidneys that had been resident in antigen/antibody-treated AS recipients were retransplanted to normal AS secondary hosts. Such grafts are thought to lose class II antigen-bearing passenger cells during their sojourn in the enhanced primary hosts, and, indeed, in this particular strain combination many of these kidneys survived upon retransplantation. The concomitant inoculation of the secondary hosts on the day of retransplantation with a variety of cells derived from the donor strain revealed that small numbers of donor dendritic cells prepared from the spleen were highly effective in triggering an acute rejection response in the secondary hosts against the retransplanted kidneys. These workers therefore suggested that class II MHC-bearing cells, principally dendritic cells, provide the most important immunogenic signal to allogeneic host lymphocytes, thus

Surgical Research:
Recent Concepts and Results
Baethmann/Messmer (Eds.)

initiating rejection. They further suggested that in other circumstances a second route of allosensitization might be operative via antigen presentation by host cells.

We therefore devised a murine model that has enabled us to examine the role of host APC in the generation of a response against skin allografts [18, 19].

In Vivo Assay

The cell transfer assay has been described in detail elsewhere [18]. In brief, CBA (H-2^k) mice were injected intraperitoneally with 5×10^4 allogeneic spleen cells (SC), usually from the BALB/c (H-2^d) strain. Soon after this activation with alloantigens, spleen and peritoneal cells (SC and PC, respectively) were prepared from these primary (1°) hosts. Following the removal of T-lymphocytes from these cell populations by treatment with an anti-Thy 1.2 monoclonal antibody and guinea pig complement the cells were transferred intraperitoneally to syngeneic (CBA) secondary (2°) hosts. Three days later the latter were given BALB/c skin grafts and their survival times were carefully established following removal of the bandages 7 days after transplantation. In this situation, an accelerated rejection of grafts would be indicative of the transfer of donor alloantigens with the 1° host cells. Accelerated rejection was always judged by direct comparison with grafts transplanted concurrently to normal CBA mice (negative controls), and in each experiment the efficacy of 1° host activation was ascertained by the direct transplantation of BALB/c skin to a few members of the 1° host pool, 6 days after the inoculation of the activating donor strain cells (positive controls).

Results were routinely analysed by the nonparametric Wilcoxon (Mann-Whitney) summed-ranks test.

Results

Cell Transfer 3 Days After Activation

We initially chose a 3-day interval between activation and cell transfer because alloantigen presentation to lymphocytes, if it happens at all, would have to occur well before the first signs of sensitization become evident. This proved to be well founded (see below). The results of a typical experiment (Table 1) show that the 1° host SC and PC induced a markedly faster graft rejection compared with the negative controls; indeed it was comparable to that induced in the actively sensitized 1° hosts themselves. Although most of our analytical work has been confined to the BALB/c→CBA strain combination, similar results have been obtained in a variety of other strain combinations.

The donor cells used in the activation of 1° hosts and the number of 1° host cells transferred (see Table 1) were based on cell titration studies, which showed that these were the minimum numbers required for consistently positive results.

Table 1. Typical cell transfer experiment carried out 3 days after primary-host activation[a]

Group	Activation of 1° hosts	Transfer to 2° hosts	Number of mice	MST[b] (days)	*p* value
A	None[c]	None	8	10	
B	BALB/c SC[d]	None	5	< 7	< 0.01
C	BALB/c SC	5×10^7 SC[e]	7	< 7	< 0.01
D	BALB/c SC	3×10^6 PC[e]	8	< 7	< 0.01

[a] CBA 1° hosts were activated by an intraperitoneal injection of 5×10^4 BALB/c SC. Three days later SC and PC were harvested, depleted of T-lymphocytes and transferred into untreated 2° hosts. The latter were tested 3 days later with a BALB/c skin graft

[b] Median survival time

[c] Untreated, negative controls given a BALB/c skin graft

[d] Activated positive controls

[e] T-cell depleted

Specificity of Sensitization by Cell Transfer

The specificity of the cell transfer phenomenon was tested as follows. CBA 1° hosts were activated with BALB/c cells, and SC or PC were transferred into CBA 2° hosts. The latter were divided into subgroups that received either BALB/c or third-party C57BL/10 (H-2^b) skin grafts. Provided that there was no significant antigenic overlap between the BALB/c and C57BL/10 strains, one would expect the C57BL/10, but not the BALB/c, grafts in this experiment to show normal survival times, and this proved to be the case [18]. The sensitization brought about by cell transfer was therefore specific for antigens of the donor strain.

Mechanism of the Sensitization Phenomenon

There are three possible explanations to account for the sensitization of 2° hosts.

Adoptive Transfer with T-Lymphocytes? The fact that all 1° host cells were routinely depleted of T-lymphocytes by exposure (twice in succession in the case of SC) to an anti-T cell antibody and complement virtually rules out the possibility of an adoptive transfer with T-lymphocytes. Even if 1%–2% of T cells had survived the treatment, this would be well below the level required to sensitize adoptively. In any case, 3 days is far too early for the generation of sensitized T cells, and T-cell enrichment at this time interval, with a consequent reduction of antigen-presenting cells, failed to bring about sensitization. The fact that our T-cell depletion protocol was effective was indicated by our failure to transfer sensitivity adoptively with T-depleted SC taken 10 days after activation, i.e. at a time when SC would normally be expected to contain specifically sensitized lymphocytes.

We are therefore confident that adoptive transfer of sensitivity plays no role in our model.

Transfer of Contaminating Donor Cells? It could be argued that the 1° host cells included some of the BALB/c cells used for activation, thus accounting for the accelerated rejection of skin grafts. Such an explanation would reduce our findings to the realm of the trivial.

There are several strong arguments against this, however. First, we have shown the number of cells used for activation of 1° hosts – 5×10^4 – to be only just over the threshold required for direct sensitization. Even on the assumption (which is clearly incorrect) that all donor cells were resident in the spleens and body cavities of the 1° hosts at 3 days, each of these two compartments would not contain a sufficient number of T-depleted donor cells to give rise to the consistent pattern of accelerated rejection. Second, transfer of 1° SC 3–4 hours after activation, i. e. at a time when it would be reasonable to expect donor cells to survive in tissues of the 1° hosts, failed to sensitize. Third, a substantial proportion of allogeneic cells are known [13] to be eliminated within a few hours after inoculation. Fourth, in order further to minimize the possibility of donor-cell contamination, we used frozen and thawed donor SC for the activation of 1° hosts. Although such preparations are less immunogenic than viable cells and had to be prepared from relatively large numbers of cells (10^7), accelerated rejection of 2° hosts was nevertheless achieved. Direct antigen transfer was here most unlikely because this kind of material would be cleared very rapidly and metabolized. Fifth, activation could be brought about by the transplantation of BALB/c skin grafts to one side of the thorax; both the draining lymph-node cells and SC, but not PC, sensitized 2° hosts, the former when transferred on days 3 and 5 and the latter on day 5 (Table 2). Here contamination of the transferred cells with free and immunogenic donor antigen is virtually impossible, especially for the SC.

Finally, and of the utmost importance in the context of our discussion, was the demonstration that present in the 1° SC and PC on day 3 were large cells that carried both host *and* donor class II MHC antigens, but none that carried solely donor antigens. This is considered in more detail below.

Do Antigen-Presenting Cells from the Donor Spleen Play a Role? Because Lechler and Batchelor [12] have provided evidence in a rodent kidney transplantation model for the hypothesis that host lymphocytes are primed via the direct presentation of alloantigens by donor dendritic cells, we have examined this possibility in our model.

Table 2. Transfer of primary host cells 5 days following their activation with an allogeneic skin graft[a]

Group	Activation of 1° hosts	Transfer to 2° hosts	Number of mice	MST[b] (days)	p value
A	None[c]	–	7	10	
B	BALB/c skin graft[d]	–	5	< 7	< 0.01
C	BALB/c skin graft[d]	5×10^7 SC[e]	8	< 7	< 0.01
D	BALB/c skin graft[d]	3×10^6 PC[e]	7	10	NS[f]
E	BALB/c skin graft[d]	5×10^6 LNC[e]	8	7½	< 0.02

[a] CBA primary host cells were harvested five days following activation with a BALB/c skin graft. Following their T-cell depletion the cells were transferred intraperitoneally into CBA 2° hosts and the latter tested 3 days later with BALB/c skin grafts
[b] Median survival time
[c] Untreated, negative controls given a BALB/c skin graft
[d] Skin-graft activated positive controls
[e] T cell depleted
[f] Not significant

Table 3. Activation of primary hosts with allogeneic spleen cells depleted of class II positive cells[a]

Group	Activation of 1° hosts	Transfer to 2° hosts	Number of mice	MST[b] (days)	*p* value
A	None[c]	–	8	11.5	
B	BALB/c SC[d]	–	5	< 7	< 0.01
C	BALB/c SC[d]	5×10^7 SC[e]	9	< 7	< 0.01

[a] CBA primary hosts were activated intraperitoneally with 5×10^4 BALB/c SC that had been depleted of class II positive cells by a double treatment with anti-class II monoclonal antibody and complement. Three days later T-cell depleted SC and PC were harvested and transferred into CBA 2° hosts. These were tested with a BALB/c skin allograft 3 days later
[b] Median survival time
[c] Untreated, negative controls
[d] BALB/c SC depleted of class II positive cells
[e] T-cell depleted

When donor cells were inoculated into 1° hosts after they had been depleted of either plastic-adherent cells (L. Brent and R. A. Sherwood, unpublished material) or of all cells bearing class II MHC antigens (using an antibody directed against BALB/c class II antigens plus complement; Table 3), sensitization of 2° hosts was not in the least impaired. It may therefore be concluded that donor APCs are not important in our model and may not be playing any role whatever.

Presentation of Donor Alloantigens by Host Cells

If none of the above explanations are valid, we are left with only one alternative. i. e. that host APC acquire and present donor alloantigens to the T cells of 2° hosts. Direct evidence in support of this stems from an examination of histocompatibility antigens present on the surface of activated 1° host cells. Thus, SC or PC obtained 3 days after activation were first treated with an anti-I-A^d (anti-donor) antibody, followed by a rabbit anti-mouse IgG FITC antibody (green fluorescence), and then with an anti-I-A^k (anti-host) antibody directly conjugated with rhodamine (red fluorescence). Cells carrying both host and donor antigens, i. e. our putative APC, would fluoresce in both colours under UV light. On the other hand, any donor cells that had sneaked through would fluoresce green only.

The results of this analysis are shown in Table 4. Approximately 50% of SC and 70% of PC were large cells carrying host class II antigens. Of these, 10%–12% expressed, additionally, donor class II antigens. We postulate that these cells are host APC that have taken up donor antigen and present it to the lymphocytes of the 2° hosts, thus initiating the accelerated rejection of skin grafts. These data have been confirmed by the use of a cell analyser (in preparation). Significantly, we have never succeeded in identifying cells in the 3-day population that carried only donor class II antigens, thus lending strong support to our contention that our results are not caused by contaminating donor-strain cells.

Table 4. Immunofluorescent analysis by double-labelling of class II antigens on primary-host SC and PC 3 days after activation

Antibody	Mean number of cells Counted[a]	Fluorescent[b]	% Fluorescent
A. Spleen cells			
RAM IgG FITC[c]	116 (3)	3 ± 2.0	2.5
Anti-I-A^k TRITC	400 (8)	189 ± 25.2	47.3
Anti-I-A^d + RAM IgG FITC	200 (4)	21 ± 2.2	10.5
Anti-I-A^d + RAM IgG FITC then anti-I-A^k TRITC[d]	433 (4)	44 ± 3.7	10.2
B. *Peritoneal cells*			
RAM IgG FITC[c]	273 (3)	3 ± 0.6	1.1
Anti-I-A^k TRITC	300 (6)	209 ± 9.6	70.0
Anti-I-A^d + RAM IgG FITC	200 (3)	23 ± 3.5	11.5
Anti-I-A^d + RAM IgG FITC then anti-I-A^k TRITC[d]	500 (3)	62 ± 3.9	12.5

[a] Numbers in parenthesis indicate the number of experiments on which the mean figures are based
[b] ± Standard error of mean
[c] Rabbit anti-mouse IgG-Fc specific antibody conjugated with FITC
[d] Cells were first exposed to the anti-I-A^d (donor, BALB/c) monoclonal antibody, followed by RAM IgG-Fc specific antibody conjugated to FITC; cells were then incubated with the anti-I-A^k (host, CBA) monoclonal antibody directly conjugated with TRITC, and fixed

Nature of the Antigen-Presenting Cell

We have already shown [18, 19] that the cells responsible for the cell transfer phenomenon belong to the macrophage/dendritic cell population, for 1° host cells 3 days after activation lose their capacity for sensitization if the cells that adhere to plastic are removed from them. Because both macrophages and dendritic cells adhere to plastic over a 3-h incubation period, this experiment does not permit us to distinguish between these two cell types. However, recent experiments in which dendritic cells were removed by lysis with a specific antibody (33D1, kindly supplied by Dr. R.M. Steinman) and complement show very clearly that sensitization is wholly, or at least in large measure, attributable to this cell type. Experiments are in progress in which purified dendritic cells are used for transfer.

Is Presentation of Histocompatibility Antigens Confined to Any One Class of Alloantigen?

Using appropriate strains of mice we have examined the ability of host APC to present either class I or class II MHC antigens. It is clear [18] that both types of antigen can be presented in our model. For example, spleen cells from CBA 1° hosts activated with donor cells that differed only by class I antigens induced accelerated rejection in 2° hosts to donor-strain skin grafts. The same was found to be true for donors and recipients differing only for class II antigens. Whereas the latter observation was expected, the former was not and is of considerable interest in relation to the transplantation of organs partially depleted of class II bearing cells and of cultured pancreatic islets (see Discussion).

A further surprise came when we looked into the question of whether minor histocompatibility antigens can be presented in this way. Some experiments indicating that this may not be the case have already been published [18], but we have explored this further by varying some of the parameters using the strain combination, C3H ($H\text{-}2^k$ + C3H minors) → CBA ($H\text{-}2^k$ + CBA minors). In particular, we have increased the interval between activation and cell transfer from 3 to 6 or 9 days and used larger cell numbers in the transfer. Neither of these strategies has resulted in the induction of accelerated rejection. Whilst there are other possibilities yet to be examined, we have had to come to the tentative conclusion that minor histocompatibility antigens are not presented by host APC in this experimental model (see Discussion).

Discussion

We hope to have demonstrated that alloantigens can be presented to great effect by host cells which bear the hallmark of dendritic cells, although we have not yet fully excluded macrophages as participants. The fact that we have so far failed to sensitize 2° hosts with purified DC 3 days after activation is a matter of some concern, and this continues to receive our attention. It is quite possible that this failure reflects not so much on the DC themselves as on the method available for their isolation [21]. Because it involves incubation at 37 °C for 24–30 h (splenic DC become non-adherent to plastic surfaces after an initial period of adherence, and this enables one to separate them from macrophages), it is possible that alloantigens acquired during the activation stage are either lost, attenuated or rendered less immunogenic during the culture period. A time-course study (R. A. Sherwood and L. Brent, unpublished) has revealed that there is, in fact, a relatively narrow window of antigen presentation; sensitization occurred on days 1, 2, and 3, but not on day 5 or subsequently. We are currently looking at cells (both whole spleen and DC) taken at these intervals for the expression of donor antigens, and our preliminary finding (S. R. Lyall, R. A. Sherwood and L. Brent, unpublished) is that in whole spleen cells (which are prepared much more rapidly) donor antigens are present throughout the window of presentation. It will be interesting to see whether the same is true for isolated DC, or whether there are quantitative changes. If macrophages are involved at all it can only be at a relatively trivial level or in a synergistic form, for the removal of DC from 1° host cells, using a specific anti-DC antibody and complement, completely prevented the cells from sensitizing 2° hosts. Although the 33D1 antibody is thought to be highly specific, it is possible that it bound to a subpopulation of macrophages that can present alloantigens; this is being investigated.

Our overall conclusion is strongly supported by experiments in which 3-day 1° host splenic and peritoneal cells were exposed to either an anti-host or an anti-donor class II monoclonal antibody without complement. Such cells failed to bring about accelerated rejection of skin allografts. This is further proof of our hypothesis that the antigen-presenting cells in this model are host cells carrying donor antigens. Inhibition with anti-donor antibodies might be brought about either by modulation (e.g.

internalization) of donor antigens or simply by antigen masking; inhibition with anti-host antibodies could be due to molecular interference, or it could be taken to indicate that alloantigen presentation is restricted to host class II molecules.

We have stated our reasons above for believing that the transfer effect cannot be ascribed to active sensitization by donor strain APC or other donor cells bearing class II antigens. Our conclusion that donor antigens are taken up by and presented to host lymphocytes is therefore at variance with the results of Lechler and Batchelor [12], which indicate that in a kidney allograft model *donor* APC (in the form of dendritic cells) appear to activate host lymphocytes directly without the intervention of host APC. These workers showed that enhanced rat kidney allografts retransplanted to untreated secondary hosts survived unless the recipients were given 10^4–10^5 splenic DC from normal rats of the donor strain on the day of retransplantation. Because a similar effect was not obtained with 0.1 ml blood (calculated to be the amount of donor blood in a kidney transplant), and because 5/6 kidneys retransplanted to secondary hosts given 2×10^6 cells enriched for B-lymphocytes accepted their grafts, these authors argued that donor DC did not merely act as immunogen but as APC. However, larger volumes of donor blood (0.5 ml) did bring about rejection crises in 4/4 retransplanted kidneys, and two of these were in fact acutely rejected. No attempt was made to assess the effect of inoculating DC prepared from animals of the host strain. Hence, although Lechler and Batchelor demonstrated a far greater efficiency of sensitization by donor DC compared with other donor-cell types, one cannot rule out entirely the possibility that in their experiments the donor DC acted as ultra-efficient immunogens that activated host APC as in our model. Allogeneic DC can be expected to be good immunogens by virtue of their very large surface area and, hence, a potentially far greater number of cell surface class II molecules than in B cells or even in macrophages; further, the dramatically convoluted nature of the DC membrane may contribute not only to the cells' ability to present extraneous antigens but also to activate host APC with respect to MHC antigens. These problems could be clarified if we had more accurate information on the cell surface area of DC compared with other cell types and the number of class II molecules per cell; we are currently examining these parameters.

It should be pointed out that Lechler and Batchelor [12] have drawn attention to the fact that retransplantation of enhanced rat kidneys to normal syngeneic secondary hosts is not successful in every strain combination, and they suggest that, in such cases, rejection is brought about by the presentation of donor antigens by host APC ("second route of sensitization"). This would be in accord with the data presented here.

Apart from our own data [18, 19, present article] in vivo evidence for the presentation of histocompatibility antigens by host cells has been presented by others. In particular, rabbit corneal allografts were rejected when the adjacent host tissue and the grafts themselves became infiltrated with host cells of the macrophage/dendritic lineage following the deliberate induction of vascularization and inflammation [26]. Further, it has been observed that rat renal allografts undergoing acute rejection are infiltrated by large, Ia-positive, non-phagocytic cells of host origin,bearing a striking morphological resemblance to DC [7].

Our data concerned with the class of histocompatibility antigen presented by host APC raises some interesting questions. We are puzzled by our inability, so far, to show that minor antigens can be presented in our experimental model, especially as it is perfectly possible to bring about the accelerated rejection of minor-incompatible skin grafts by direct inoculation, 6 days before grafting, of 5×10^4 minor-incompatible spleen cells. It seems likely that our lack of success is due to limitations of our model rather than an inherent defect of minor antigen presentation, and several parameters of the transfer system remain to be analysed.

That class II antigens can be presented by host cells is not so very surprising in view of the fact that these antigens are well known to be critically important in the induction of alloresponses. Our results showing that the presentation of class I antigens on their own is sufficient to bring about graft rejection not only support our contention that donor cells carrying class II antigens are not necessarily required, but also suggest that, despite the observations of Lechler and Batchelor [12], attempts to deplete organ allografts of class II bearing passenger cells may not necessarily lead to a significant reduction in their vulnerability to host responses.

This raises two issues. First, it has recently been shown [1] that rat renal allografts actively enhanced by the prior transfusion of 1 ml donor blood undergo an early phase of increased class I and class II MHC expression equivalent to or in excess of that seen in allografts undergoing acute rejection. The fact that enhanced kidneys, which were also infiltrated with various host effector cells such as cytotoxic T cells, survived is a clear indication that whatever immunosuppressive mechanisms are operative in these hosts override the immunogenic stimulus of these antigens. It is, however, relevant that enhanced kidneys examined 100 days after transplantation revealed levels of class I and class II antigens characteristic of normal kidneys (i.e. very little class II). Although the retransplanted kidneys in the experiments of Lechler and Batchelor [12] were removed from their primary hosts 4 weeks after transplantation, it is possible that MHC expression in these kidneys had already reverted to normal, thus minimizing the possibility of antigen presentation by host APC.

Second, our data cannot, on the face of it, be reconciled with the finding that murine pancreatic islet allografts lose their immunogenicity following tissue culture [10, 2, 5] or by removal of dendritic cells by treatment with a specific antibody and complement [5]. Whilst both forms of treatment evidently lead to the removal of class II bearing passenger cells, our data would suggest that the remaining class I antigens should, nevertheless, be taken up by host APC and thus presented to host T cells. Were this the case, long-term survival of islets could not be expected. However, the following factors need to be taken into account:

1. There does not appear to be universal agreement about the survival of cultured pancreatic islets.
2. It has been reported that murine pancreatic islet allografts from donors differing from hosts in only class I antigens are rejected [27]; here, presumably antigen presentation by host cells is operative. The same is clearly true for the generation of cytolytic T-lymphocytes following culture of splenic responder cells with allogeneic hepatocytes, which do not possess class II antigens [20].
3. The strenght of class II antigen response against islets varies greatly in different strain combinations, presumably reflecting the amount of class II antigen present; in some, even non-cultured islet allografts incompatible for either class I or II antigens are not always acutely rejected [15].

4. The removal of class II positive cells from pig pancreatic islets, using an anti-class II monoclonal antibody bound to ricin toxin, failed to prevent the acute rejection of the islets [16].
5. Cultured human islet allograft transplantation has so far yielded very poor results [24].
6. Evidently the survival of cultured murine pancreatic islets, when it occurs, depends to some degree on the induction of specific hyporesponsiveness in the hosts [11], and Lafferty et al. believe that this is brought about by the generation of enhancing antibodies that owe their existence to antigen presentation by host APC.

Overall, then, the situation concerning islet allografts is far from clear. Much would depend on the precise level of class I antigens present in cultured or passenger cell-depleted islets, and there is at present a dearth of information on this vital point. Whilst we believe that in vivo antigen presentation of alloantigens is an important step in the initiation of graft rejection, this by no means excludes the possibility that, in some circumstances, donor APC are involved.

Addendum

We are delighted to be able to contribute to this Festschrift in honour of Professor Walter Brendel. L. B. has known him for some 17 years and has greatly admired his skill and flair in developing immunology at the Institute of Surgical Research in Munich, as well as his manifold and important contributions to surgical research. The geniality with which he has presided over the annual Round Table Discussions on Applied Immunology, begun almost 20 years ago, has been a vital factor in making these symposia such enjoyable and much sought-after events.

Acknowledgements. This work has been supported by the Medical Research Council, and we are pleased to acknowledge assistance from St. Mary's Hospital Joint Standing Research Committee.

References

1. Armstrong HE, Botton EM, McMillan I, Spencer SC, Bradley JA (1987) Prolonged survival of actively enhanced rat renal allografts despite accelerated cellular infiltration and rapid induction of both class I and class II MHC antigens. J Exp Med 164: 891–907
2. Bartlett ST, Naji A, Silvers WK, Barker CF (1984) Evidence that major histocompatibility complex restriction is involved in the survival of cultured endocrine allografts in mice. Transplant Proc 16: 851–853
3. Boog CJP, Kast WM, Timmers H, ThM Boes J, DeWaal LP, Melief CVP (1985) Abolition of specific immune response defects by immunisation with dendritic cells. Nature 318: 59–62
4. Chesnut R, Grey HM (1981) Studies on the capacity of B cells to serve as antigen-presenting cells. J Immunol 126: 1075–1079
5. Faustman DL, Steinman RM, Gebel HM, Hauptfield V, Davie JM, Lacy PE (1984) Prevention of rejection of murine islet allografts by pretreatment with anti-dendritic cell antibody. Proc Natl Acad Sci USA 81: 3864–3862

6. Golding H, Singer A (1984) Role of accessory cell processing and presentation of shed H-2 alloantigens in allospecific cytotoxic T lymphocyte responses. J Immunol 133: 597–605
7. Ishikura H, Natori T, Aizawa M (1985) Host origin dendritic cells in acutely rejected rat renal allografts. Transplant Proc 17: 875–879
8. Klein J, Walden P (1986) Antigen presentation: paradigm lost? Prog Immunol 6: 212–220
9. Knight SC, Mertin J, Stackpoole A, Clark J (1983) Induction of immune reesponses *in vivo* with small numbers of veiled (dendritic) cells. Proc Natl Acad Sci USA 80: 6032–6035
10. Lafferty KJ, Prowse SJ, Simeonovic CJ, Warren HS (1983) Immunobiology of tissue transplantation: a return to the passenger leukocyte concept. Annu Rev Immunol 1: 143–173
11. Lafferty KJ, Gill RG, Babcock SK, Wang Y (1986) Active and passive antigen presentation: its role in the induction of tissue immunity and allograft tolerance. Prog Immunol 6: 1040–1054
12. Lechler RI, Batchelor JR (1982) Restoration of immunogenicity to passenger cell-depleted kidney allografts by the addition of donor strain dendritic cells. J Exp Med 155: 31–41
13. McNeilage LJ, Heslop BF (1980) Lymphocyte homing in syngeneic and unsensitised MHC compatible allogeneic hosts. I. Evidence for both syngeneic self-recognition and early killing of allogeneic cells. Cell Immunol 50: 58–70
14. Minami M, Shreffler DC (1981) Ia-positive stimulator cells are required in primary, but not in secondary, mixed leukocyte reactions against H-2K and H-2D differences. J Immunol 126: 1774–1779
15. Morrow CE, Sutherland DER, Steffes MW, Najarian JS, Bach FH (1983) H-2 antigen class: effect on mouse islet allograft rejection. Science 219: 1337–1339
16. Mullen Y, Shiogama T, Ozawa A, Leonard JE, Papoian T, Tsunoda T, Terada M, Motojima K, Brown J (1987) Immunogenicity and viability of class II immunotoxin-treated pig islet cells. Transplant Proc 19: 934–936
17. Schuler G, Romani N, Steinman RM (1985) A comparison of murine epidermal Langerhans cells with spleen dendritic cells. J Invest Dermatol 85: 99s–106s
18. Sherwood RA, Brent L, Rayfield LS (1986) Presentation of alloantigens by host cells. Eur J Immunol 16: 569–574
19. Sherwood RA, Brent L, Rayfield LS (1987) Major histocompatibility complex antigens are presented by murine host accessory cells. Transplant Proc 19: 239–241
20. So SKS, Wilkes LM, Platt JC, Ascher NC, Simmons RL (1987) Purified hepatocytes can stimulate allospecific cytolytic T lymphocytes in a mixed lymphocyte-hepatocyte culture. Transplant Proc 19: 251–252
21. Steinman RM, Guthinov B, Witmer MD, Nussenzweig MC (1983) Dendritic cells are the principal stimulators of the primary mixed leukocyte reaction in mice. J Exp Med 157: 613–627
22. Steinman RM, Inaba K, Schuler G, Witmer M (1986) Stimulation of the immune response: contributions of dendritic cells. In: Steinman RM, North RJ (ed) Mechanism of host resistance to infectious agents, tumours and allografts. Rockefeller University Press, New York, p 71
23. Steinman RM, Inaba K, Schuler G, Witmer M, Koide S, Flechner E, Bhardwaj N, Young JW (1986) The role and mechanism and action of dendritic cells in transplantation immunity. Prog Immunol 6: 1013–1021
24. Sutherland DER, Kendall D (1985) Clinical pancreas and islet transplant registry report. Transplant Proc 17: 307–311
25. Unanue ER (1984) Antigen presenting function of the macrophage. Annu Rev Immunol 2: 395–428
26. Williams KA, Mann TS, Lewis M, Coster DJ (1986) The role of resident accessory cells in corneal allograft rejection in the rabbit. Transplantation 42: 667–671
27. Zhu XY, Sutherland DER, Steffes MW, Morrow CE, Gores PF, Najarian JS, Bach FH (1985) Rejection of mouse islet allografts according to donor and recipient genotype. Transplant Proc 17: 425–427

Immunogenetics of Chronic Arthritis in Childhood

E. D. ALBERT, and S. SCHOLZ

Introduction

In recent years most inflammatory rheumatic diseases both of adults and of children have been shown to be related to the genetic system of histocompatibility antigens (HLA). However, diseases associated with HLA are not restricted to rheumatic disorders, and a large number of widely differing diseases have been found to be related to one or more alleles of the HLA system. These include: ankylosing spondylitis, Behçet's syndrome, de Quervain's thyroiditis, acute lymphocytic leukemia, idiopathic hemochromatosis, psoriasis, juvenile diabetes mellitus, celiac disease, Graves' disease, myasthenia gravis, autoaggressive hepatitis, rheumatoid arthritis, juvenile chronic arthritis, nephrotic syndrome, multiple sclerosis, narcolepsy, lupus erythematosus, scleroderma, IgA deficiency, and C21-hydroxylase deficiency. The fact that so many genes, strongly influencing such a large number of widely differing diseases, are mapped in this very limited space of the human genome, suggests that a common principle could be involved in the pathogenesis of many of these disorders.

The purpose of this study is briefly to review the findings on HLA associations in rheumatic diseases of childhood and to discuss the biological significance of these associations. This requires, first, a brief outline of the genetic organization and the known physiological functions of the HLA gene cluster on chromosome 6.

Genetic Organization and Function of the HLA Region

The genetic organization of the HLA system is shown in Fig. 1. HLA-linked genes are subdivided into three structurally and functionally distinct groups: class I, class II, and class III. Class I genes HLA-A, -B, and -C (a considerable number of additional class I gene loci exist, the products of which have not yet been defined) code for the classical transplantation antigens expressed on the surface of all nucleated cells. The class I molecule consists of an α-chain with its three immunoglobulin-like domains (α1, α2, and α3), an intramural part, and a cytoplasmic tail. This α-chain is anchored in the cell membrane and forms a dimer with β2 microglobulin which is coded for on chromosome 15. Class I antigens are recognized in conjunction with antigen by the T-cell receptor of cytotoxic T-lymphocytes and therefore form the target for self-recognition. The action of cytotoxic T cells against autologous cells which either are infected, are chemically modulated, or show malignant transformation is considered one of the most important functions of immunological surveillance.

Surgical Research:
Recent Concepts and Results
Baethmann/Messmer (Eds.)

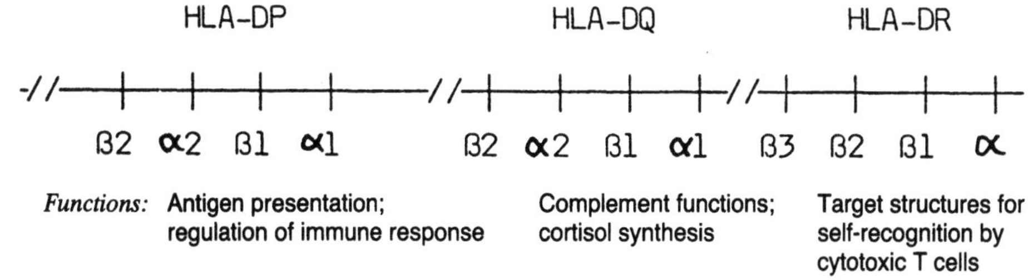

Fig. 1. Genetic Organization of the HLA Complex on Chromosome 6

Gene products of class I genes (DR, DQ, and DP) show a restricted tissue distribution; they are expressed on B-lymphocytes, macrophages, monocytes, and immunologically active cells in various tissues, e. g., Langerhans' cells in the skin and Kupffer cells in the liver. The class II molecule consists of a dimer of an α- and a β-chain, both of which are coded in the HLA region and consist of two extracellular domains (α1 and α2 or β1 and β2), an intramural part, and a cytoplasmic tail. The two chains are noncovalently bound, so that a functional class II molecule is dependent upon close structural "compatibility" between the two chains. The noncovalent binding between α- and β-chains allows the occurrence of dimers which are formed by α- and β-chains from the two different haplotypes. This formation of hybrid antigens adds considerably to the already existing polymorphism of class II molecules. It is conceivable that hybrid antigens may have immunological functions which differ slightly from those of α-β-dimers coded for by the same haplotype [12, 17]. Class II molecules are recognized in conjunction with antigens on the surface of macrophages/monocytes by the T-cell receptor of helper-inducer T cells.

In the class III region of the HLA chromosome we find genes for the complement components C4, Bf, and C2, as well as those for hydroxylase. C2 and C4 are important factors in the classical pathway, while Bf is the proactivator of C3 in the alternate pathway of complement activation. Their immunological importance is best documented by the observation of severe lupus-like syndromes in the rare cases of genetic deficiency of C2 or of C4 [41]. It is not clear whether the C21-hydroxylase gene is of immunological importance; however, it is quite conceivable that this enzyme, which plays a key role in cortisol metabolism, may even in the heterozygote form of C21-hydroxylase deficiency influence the immunological reactivity of a given individual. Thus there is no a priori reason to exclude genes located in the class III region of the HLA linkage group from consideration as primary disease-susceptibility genes, as it has recently been demonstrated that in lupus erythematosus the same type of deficiency for C4A has been found in several ethnic populations [27].

HLA Associations of the Clinical Subgroups of Juvenile Chronic Arthritis

Juvenile chronic arthritis (JCA) [39], formerly designated juvenile rheumatoid arthritis, includes a number of different diseases which can be distinguished on the basis of

Table 1. HLA Associations with Subgroups of Juvenile Chronic Arthritis

Clinical subgroup	HLA association
Juvenile spondylitis	B27, DR5 (?)
Early-onset pauciarticular JCA	HLA-DRw8, DR5, A2
Polyarticular-onset, rheumatoid factor positive JCA	HLA-DR4, DR1
Polyarticular JCA, rheumatoid factor negative JCA	HLA-DRw8(?), DR4(?)
Systemic-onset JCA	DR4
Juvenile psoriatic arthritis	B27

such factors as the following: disease onset, disease course, number and pattern of joints involved, the presence of rheumatoid factor, antinuclear antibodies, the presence of extra-articular disease (e.g., acute or chronic iridocyclitis, acute or chronic gastrointestinal disease, and psoriasis), family history, and the presence of certain HLA markers. Although it is very well possible to diagnose typical cases belonging to each of the subgroups of JCA, the considerable overlap between the different diseases frequently makes diagnosis difficult, particularly early in the course of the disease. This overlap and the existence of heterogeneity even within the subgroups may be responsible for the sometimes conflicting results of investigations into the association with HLA antigens. A summary of the HLA-association data in JCA is given in Table 1.

Juvenile Spondylitis (Juvenile Spondylarthropathy, Juvenile Ankylosing Spondylitis)

This subgroup of JCA is characterized by (a) pauciarticular onset in predominantly male patients with an older age at onset (around 9 years), (b) frequent family history of ankylosing spondylitis [6] affecting predominantly larger joints of the lower limbs, and (c) occurrance of acute iridocyclitis during follow-up. Sacroiliitis, the most important sign of ankylosing spondylitis, is seldom found in childhood, but may be observed on the average some 6 years after disease onset [6] without necessarily leading to backpain. 90% of patients belonging to this subgroup show presence of HLA-B27 [6, 32]. It is therefore generally agreed that juvenile spondylitis is the childhood manifestation of ankylosing spondylitis, showing the same genetic background, i.e., HLA-B27, as the latter in adults.

Although the systematic study of a suffiently large group of patients testing for all HLA-A, -B, -C, and DR markers has not been performed, there is evidence that HLA alleles other than HLA-B27 may also play a role in this subgroup. Schuchmann et al. [35] found a significant increase of HLA-A2; this is interesting, as this same antigen has been found associated with the JCA of the pauciarticular-onset type [8, 29]. Similarly, we found that among 44 patients with juvenile spondylitis (all B27-positive) the antigen DR5 was present in 39% as compared to 25% in controls [35]. This finding, if confirmed, indicates a possible interaction of several different HLA-linked disease-susceptibility genes in JCA.

Early-Onset Pauciarticular JCA

This subtype of JCA [31, 30] is characterized by an early onset (before age 6), affecting no more than 4–5 joints, with the frequent presence (in up to 80% of cases) of antinuclear antibodies, and with a high frequency of chronic iridocyclitis. It is probably due to a high representation of this particular subtype in the series of Stastny et al. [37] and of Suciu-Foca et al. [40] that these studies noted a different genetic background in juvenile rheumatoid arthritis (as it was called at that time) than in rheumatoid arthritis of the adult. The antigens DR5 and DRw8 were found in increased frequencies, while the antigen DR4, which is highly associated with adult rheumatoid arthritis, was only rarely found. Results of a multicenter study, organized within the framework of the Ninth International Histocompatibility Workshop, confirm that early-onset pauciarticular JCA is strongly associated with DR5 and DRw8 as well as with HLA-A2 [8].

It has been shown that the association with HLA-A2, on the one hand, and that with DR5 and DRw8, on the other, are independent of each other. Regarding the association with the latter, the possibility must be investigated that there could be an interaction between the two disease-susceptibility alleles associated with DR5 and DRw8, as has been observed in juvenile diabetes for the heterozygote combination of DR3 and DR4 [34]. The analysis of this multicenter study has shown [8] that the number of DR5/DRw8 hererozygotes among patients is only slightly (not significantly) greater than the number expected on the basis of the gene frequencies of DR5 and DRw8 in these patients. Thus, there is as yet no compelling evidence for a possible interaction between DR5 and DRw8 in JCA pathogenesis. It should, however, be pointed out that available data are by no means sufficient to exclude such a possibility.

In some reports the association with DRw52 specificity has been noted [8, 28]. Among caucasians the DRw52 specificity includes all individuals positive for DR3, DR5, DRw6, and DRw8; it is therefore not surprising that this specificity should be increased in frequency, since two of the included DR alleles are increased (DR5 and DRw8), and the other two are not clearly decreased. If one assumes that the association with the broadly distributed allele DRw52 is primary and that the association with DR5 and DRw8 is secondary, one cannot explain why, of the four alleles included in DRw52 in the normal population, the very rare antigen DRw8 is the most strongly increased, while the other, more frequent alleles are not so increased. Present evidence therefore does not favor primary association with supertypic DRw52 specificity.

Since the mode of onset of JCA is one of the important criteria for classification, it has been investigated whether there could be a special association with any of the various types of onset of JCA. The results of this analysis [3, 8] show that HLA alleles associated with this subtype of JCA (HLA-A2, DR5, and DRw8) are approximately equally distributed in the groups of monoarticular onset in both large and small joints. It has been noted, however, that the allele DR4 is completely absent in patients with monoarticular onset.

A similar analysis was performed relating to the course of the disease in patients, with a minimum observation time of 5 years. Again, the frequency of JCA-associated alleles (HLA-A2, DR5, and DRw8) did not vary significantly between the group of persistent pauciarticular disease (1 – 4 joints involved during the observation period), the group of extended pauciarticular disease (4 – 9 joints involved), and the group with a polyarticular pattern (more than 9 joints involved). Again, DR4 was absent in the persistent pauciarticular group, very rare (0.05% gene frequency) in the extended pauciarticular group, and of normal frequency in the polyarticular pattern group [3].

Polyarticular-Onset, Rheumatoid Factor-Positive JCA

This relatively rare subgroup of JCA has a clinical picture very similar to that of adult rheumatoid arthritis: symmetrical involvement of small and large joints, osseous erosions, and subcutaneous nodes [5]. Immunogenetic investigations of this subtype of JCA have shown an association with DR4, very similar in extent to the DR4 association with rheumatoid arthritis of the adult [13, 15, 16].

It has recently been recognized that in adult rheumatoid arthritis, besides the association with DR4, there is also a (somewhat weaker) association with DR1 [1]. The data here were recently reanalyzed, and it was found that also in rheumatoid factor-positive polyarticular JCA there is an increased frequency of DR1, although this increase is not statistically significant. It therefore appears that rheumatoid factor-positive polyarticular JCA is both clinically and genetically identical to adult rheumatoid arthritis. An interesting observation was made by Nepom et al. [28], investigating DR4-homozygous children with rheumatoid factor-positive polyarticular-onset JCA. They found that the DR4-associated D-region antigens LD40 and Dw4 were present in heterozygous state in 9 out of 10 patients. This may indicate the possibility of a heterozygote effect involving, most likely, the HLA-DQ region.

Polyarticular-Onset Rheumatoid Factor-Negative JCA

This subgroup of JCA probably still represents a quite heterogeneous group of diseases. Although it is far more common than the rheumatoid factor-positive subtype, there have not been enough patients investigated in relation to HLA. One study [9] has reported an increase in DR1, which would be in keeping with the results in adult seronegative RA [11, 33]. More recent data from Allan and Ansell [5] provide information about the existence of a particularly aggressive form of seronegative arthritis in teenagers which may be associated with DR4. On the other hand, it seems that the cases with earlier onset and milder course could be associated with DRw8 [21]. Obviously a great deal of work is still needed in order to clarify the immunogenetic situation of this subgroup.

Systemic-Onset JCA

Systemic-onset JCA is characterized by the classic triad of arthritis, fever, and rash; it is frequently also accompanied by lymphadenopathy, hepatosplenomegaly, signs of cardiac, cerebral, and hematological involvement, and generalized growth retardation [5]. It is quite likely that systemic-onset JCA consists of a heterogeneous group of different diseases. Various HLA associations, based on small groups of patients, have been postulated [18, 19, 20, 24]. In the largest group of patients reported thus far ($n = 84$), there was a moderate association with DR4: 46% in patients versus 26% in controls [21]. This is in line with the findings of Miller et al. [24], who also found a significant increase in DR4.

Systemic-onset JCA frequently leads to the development of amyloidosis. An immunogenetic basis for this complication, however, has not been found [5].

Juvenile Psoriatic Arthritis

Psoriatic arthritis in childhood is particularly difficult to diagnose, as the arthritis frequently precedes skin manifestations by many years [36]. Important criteria for diagnosis are asymmetric joint distribution isolated dactylitis of fingers or toes, nail-pitting, and a family history of psoriasis with or without arthritis [5].

Surprisingly, in this relatively little-studied group of patients those antigens highly associated with psoriasis vulgaris (Cw6, B13, B 17, B16, and B37) have not been found, while the markers B27 and Dr1 show a moderate increase in frequency [21]. Although there is a slight linkage disequilibrium between B27 and DR1, the increase of DR1 cannot be entirely due to this disease, because DR1 is found in 46% of patients and B27 in only 22%.

Family Studies

Since families in which two or more siblings are affected with JCA are very rare, we have been able to collect data on only 19 such families [8]. The distribution of HLA haplotypes in the affected sibling pairs shows that 13 pairs share both paternal HLA haplotypes, 4 share one, and only 2 share no parental haplotype [3]. These data indicate that susceptibility to JCA is linked to HLA and – since none of these sibling pairs are homozygous for any of the disease-associated alleles – that in the majority of the cases both paternal haplotypes contribute to disease susceptibility. We therefore conclude that there must be a number of different HLA-linked alleles which can convey disease susceptibility in JCA [34]. This conclusion is also supported by the finding of the association with several different HLA alleles in a number of the clinical subgroups of JCA.

Involvement in Disease Susceptibility of Several Different Alleles of the HLA-D Region

We began with the observation that the presence of HLA-DR2 haplotype has a protective function against the development of juvenile diabetes [34]. We have demonstrated that besides the alleles DR3 and DR4, which are positively associated with susceptibility to juvenile diabetes, there are other alleles which are not neutral with respect to disease susceptibility. While the presence of DR2 and/or DR5 is protective, the DR1 haplotype may be seen as "permissive" for the development of juvenile diabetes [1].

The same type of analysis has been performed with the data of the multicenter study on JCA [8]. The results show that the alleles DR3 and DRw6 are much more frequent among patients with pauciarticular early-onset JCA than one would expect if these were neutral with respect to disease susceptibility. Thus, DR3 and DRw6 may also be regarded as "permissive" toward this subgroup of JCA. On the other hand, DR4 occurs much less frequently than expected and could therefore be assumed to have a "protective" function against this subtype of JCA. Taking into consideration the results of the analysis of type of onset and the evolution of the disease, one could interpret these data as indicating that the presence of DR4 in patients with JCA would tend to influence the clinical picture toward a more polyarticular disease with a more aggressive clinical course. These considerations are in agreement with the observation in adult patients with ankylosing spondylitis that the presence of DR4 is associated with the involvement of peripheral joints [22].

Mechanisms

In the discussion of possible mechanisms of HLA-linked disease genes we would like to stress two important points which are relevant for almost all HLA-associated diseases, but particularly for rheumatic disease. First, as documented by analyses of multicase families and, more directly, by studies of discordant pairs of monozygotic twins, it is clear that HLA-linked disease genes function as susceptibility genes. Here disease occurs only if genetically susceptible individuals meet the appropriate environmental activation factors (e.g., viral or bacterial infections). Second, disease susceptibility involves one or more alleles of the HLA system, although it may also include other genetic factors which may or may not be linked with HLA.

Class I Associated Susceptibility Genes (A2, B27)

Presently available data do not allow one to ascertain whether the products of disease-susceptibility genes are identical to HLA antigens, whether they represent as yet undetected, closely linked MHC products, or whether they are gene products of entirely different but closely linked genes. The known immunological functions of MHC antigens however, make it very likely that in the case of at least some HLA-associated diseases susceptibility genes are identical with HLA genes.

Since MHC class I antigens are the target for self-recognition by cytotoxic T-lymphocytes in the elimination of infected, chemically modulated, or malignant cells, it is conceivable that allelic variation of these antigens could be the genetic basis for autoimmune reactivity, triggered in rare cases by an unusual set of environmental circumstances (e.g., gastrointestinal infection). We therefore speculate that the A2- and B27-associated susceptibility to rheumatic diseases in childhood could involve a misled or overshooting reaction of cytotoxic T cells against autologous cells modified by bacterial products.

Class II Associated Susceptibility Genes (DR5, DRw8, DR4)

The presentation of antigen in the initiation and regulation of immune response is dependent upon the presence of HLA class II molecules, which are recognized together with the antigen by the T-cell receptor of helper-inducer T cells. It is conceivable, therefore, that allelic variation of class II antigens and, even more, the formation of hybrid antigens by two chains coded for on different haplotypes can quantitatively or qualitatively change the immune response. This includes also the possibility of an occasional dysfunction (too much or too little immune response) triggered by an unlucky set of environmental circumstances (e. g., infection with one or more types of virus leading to an autoimmune attack against autologous tissues).

T-Cell Receptor Repertoire

Since T-cells must in the process of their maturation learn to recognize self-histocompatibility antigens, and since this learning process must in some way involve somatic mutations, it has been speculated that the nature of self-histocompatibility antigens (i. e., the presence of one or another allele) could strongly influence the development of the T-cell repertoire of a given individual. It may therefore be hypothesized that certain class I or class II genotypes provide for a defect in the T-cell repertoire, which could lead to the type of autoimmunity observed in rheumatic diseases.

Regulation of Expression of MHC Molecules

It is conceivable that disease susceptibility may be related to quantitative variation of the expression of normal HLA genes. Specific infections could, for example, lead to an inappropriate expression of HLA class II genes in certain tissues, leading to inappropriate presentation of autologous antigens and thereby to autoimmune processes. Since the regulation of expression of HLA molecules is suspected to be, at least in part, coded for in the nontranslated regions flanking HLA genes, analysis of HLA-disease association at the level of the DNA is now extended to these regions.

Finally, it should be stressed that the possible mechanisms discussed here are not mutually exclusive. Indeed, the very strongly variable expression of rheumatic diseases would suggest quite a complex nature of the underlying genetic basis for disease.

References

1. Albert ED, Scholz S (1979) Immunogenetic implications in rheumatic diseases. Acta Rheum 3: 121–127
2. Albert E, Scholz S (1987) Immunogenetics and rheumatic disease. Clin Exp Rheumatol 5 (suppl 1): 29–34
3. Albert E, Ansell BM (1987) Immunogenetics of juvenile chronic arthritis. Scand Rheumatol (in press)
4. Alexander EL, Bias WB, Arnett FC (1981) The coexistence of rheumatoid arthritis with Reiter's syndrome and/or ankylosing spondylitis: a model of dual HLA-associated disease susceptibility and expression. J. Rheumatol. 83: 398–404

5. Allen RC, Ansell BM (1986) Juvenile chronic arthritis – clinical sub-groups with particular relationship to adult patterns of disease. Postgrad Med J 62: 821–826
6. Ansell BM (1978) Heberden Oration 1977: Chronic arthritis in childhood. Ann Rheum Dis 37: 107
7. Ansell BM, Clemens LE (1982) HLA in chronic arthritis in childhood. In: Dawkins RL, Christiansen ET, Zilko TJ (eds) Immunogenetics in rheumatology. Excerpta Medica, pp 164–166
8. Ansell BM, Albert ED (1984) Juvenile chronic arthritis, pauciarticular type. In: Albert ED, Baur MP, Mayr WR (eds) Histocompatibility testing 1984. Springer, Berlin Heidelberg New York pp 368–374
9. Arnaiz-Villena A, Gomez-Reino JJ, Gamir ML, Regueiro JR, Vicario JL, Gomez-Reino FJ, Alonso A, Fernandez-Dapica MP, Irigoyen MV, Mateo I, Zea A (1984) DR, C4 and Bf allotypes in juvenile rheumatoid arthritis. Arthritis Rheum 27: 1281
10. Balogh Z, Gyodi E, Petranyi G, Meretey K, Bozsoky S (1982) HLA-DR antigens in juvenile chronic arthritis. J Rheumatol 9: 448
11. Bardin T, Legrand L, Naveau B, Marcelli-Barge A, Debeyre N, Lathrop GM, Poirier JC, Schmid M, Ryckwewaert A, Dryll A (1985) HLA antigens and seronegative rheumatoid arthritis. Ann Rheumat Dis 44: 50
12. Charron D, Lotteau V, Turmel P (1984) Hybrid HLA-DC/DS antigens, molecular evidence for gene trans-complementation. In: Albert ED Baur MP, Mayr WR (eds) Histocompatibility testing 1984. Springer, Berlin Heidelberg New York, pp 539–543
13. Clemens LE, Albert ED, Ansell BM (1983) HLA studies in IgM rheumatoid factor positive childhood arthritis. Amer Rheum Dis 42: 431–434
14. Clemens LE, Albert E, Ansell BM (1985) Sibling pairs affected by chronic arthritis of childhood: evidence for a genetic predisposition. J Rheumatol 12(1): 108–113
15. Forre O, Dobloug JH, Hoyeraal HM, Kass E, Thorsby E (1982) HLA-antigens in rheumatoid arthritis and juvenile rheumatoid arthritis: increased frequency of the HLA-DRw4 antigen only in seropositive patient groups. Adv Inflam Res 3: 195–201
16. Forre O, Dobloug JH, Hoyerall HM, Thorsby E (1983) HLA antigens in juvenile rheumatoid arthritis: genetic basis for the different subtypes. Arthritis Rheum 26: 35–38
17. Germain RN, Bentley DM, Quill H (1985) Influence of allelic polymorphism on the assembly and surface expression of class II MHC (I a) molecules. Cell 43: 233–242
18. Gershwin ME, Opelz G, Terasaki PI, Castles JJ, Gorman TA (1977) Frequency of HLA-Dw3 in juvenile chronic arthritis. Tissue Antigens 10: 330–336
19. Glass DN, Litvin DA (1980) Heterogeneity of HLA associations in systemic onset juvenile rheumatoid arthritis. Arthritis Rheum 23: 796–799
20. Glass D, Litvin DA, Wallace K (1980) Early onset pauciarticular juvenile rheumatoid arthritis associated with human leukocyte antigen DRw5, iritis, and antinuclear antibody. J Clin Invest 66: 426–429
21. Hall PJ, Berman SJ, Laurent MR, Briggs DC, Venning HE, Leak AM, Bedford TA, Ansell BM (1986) Genetic susceptibility to early onset pauciarticular JCA: a study of HLA and complement markers in 158 British subjects. Ann Rheum Dis 45: 464–474
22. Miehle W, Schattenkirchner M, Albert ED, Bunge M (1985) HLA-DR4 in ankylosing spondylitis with different patterns of joint involvement. Ann Rheum Dis 44: 39–44
23. Miller ML, Glass DN (1981) The major histocompatibility complex antigens in rheumatoid arthritis and juvenile arthritis. Bull Rheum Dis 31: 21–25
24. Miller ML, Aaron S, Jackson J (1985) HLA gene frequencies in children and adults with systemic onset juvenile rheumatoid arthritis. Arthritis Rheum 28: 146–150
25. Moore TL, Oldfather JW, Osborn TG, Dorner RW, Wayne Scheridan P, Weiss TD, Zuckner J, Rodey GE (1984) HLA antigens in black and white patients with juvenile arthritis: associations with rheumatoid factor, hidden rheumatoid factor, antinuclear antibodies and immune complex levels. J Rheumatol 11: 2
26. Morling N, Hellesen C, Jakobsen BK, Platz P, Ryder LP, Svejgaard A, Thomsen M (1981) HLA-A, B, C, D, DR-antigens and primed lymphocyte typing (PLT) defined DP-antigens in juvenile chronic arthritis. Tissue Antigens 17: 433–441

27. Naito S, Kong FH, Hawkins BR, Mehra NK, Serjeantson SW, Hammond MG (1986) Joint-report: HLA and disease: SLE. In: Aizawa M (ed) HLA in Asia-Oceania 1986. Hokkaido University Press, Sapporo, Japan, pp 354–365
28. Nepom BS, Nepom GT, Mickelson E, Schaller JG,. Antonelli P, Hansen JA (1984) Specific HLA-DR4 associated histocompatibility molecules characterize patients with seropositive juvenile rheumatoid arthritis. J Clin Invest 74: 287–291
29. Oen K, Petty RE, Schroeder ML (1982) An association between HLA-A2 and juvenile rheumatoid arthritis in girls. J Rheumatol 9: 916–920
30. Petty RE, Cassidy JT, Sullivan DB (1973) Clinical correlates of antinuclear antibodies in juvenile rheumatoid arthritis. J Pediatr 83, 386
31. Schaller JG, Johnson GH, Holborrow EJ, Ansell BM, Smiley WK (1974) The association of antinuclear antibodies with the chronic iridocyclitis of juvenile rheumatoid arthritis (Still's disease). Arthritis Rheum 17: 409
32. Schaller JG (1979) The seronegative spondyloarthropathies of childhood. Clinic Orthop 143: 76
33. Schiff B, Mizrachi Y, Orgad S, Yaron M, Gazit E (1982) Association of HLA-Aw31 and HLA-DR1 with adult rheumatoid arthritis. Ann Rheum Dis 41: 403–404
34. Scholz S, Albert ED (1983) HLA and diseases: involvement of more than one HLA linked determinant of disease susceptibility. Immunol Rev 70: 79–88
35. Schuchmann L, Albert ED, Michels H, Renz K (1984) Differenzierung der juvenilen chronischen Arthritis (JCA) – diagnostische Bedeutung der HLA-Assoziationen. Klin Pädiatr 196: 355–359
36. Shore A, Ansell BM (1982) Juvenile psoriatic arthritis: an analysis of sixty cases. J Pediatr 100: 529
37. Stastny P, Fink CW (1979) Different HLA-D association in adult and juvenile rheumatoid arthritis. J Clin Invest 63: 124–130
38. Stastny P (1980) Joint report: rheumatoid arthritis: In: Terasaki PI (ed) Histocompatibility testing 1980. The Regents of UCLA, pp 681–687
39. Still GF (1897) On a form of chronic joint disease in children. Med Chir Trans 80: 47. Reprinted in 1941, Arch Dis Childhood, 16: 156
40. Suciu-Foca N, Jacobs J, Godfrey M, Woodward K, Khan R, Reed E, Rohowsky C (1980) HLA-DR5 in juvenile rheumatoid arthritis confined to few joints. Lancet ii: 40
41. Tappeiner G, Hintner H, Scholz S, Albert E, Linert J, Wolff KJ (1982) Systemic lupus erythematosus in hereditary deficiency of the fourth component of complement. J Am Acad Dematol 7(1) 66–79

Anaphylaxis and Anaphylactoid Reactions

J. Ring

Cases of fatal hypersensitivity reactions have been described in the history of medicine for several thousand years [44, 62]. However, it was only in 1902 that Richet and Portier conducted their experiments on the yacht of the Prince of Monaco, describing and naming this dramatic condition "anaphylaxis" – distinguishing the phenomenon from "prophylaxis" achieved by repeated injection of biological materials [39].

Definitions

Anaphylaxis represents the maximal variant of an immediate-type allergic reaction involving the whole organism. In anaphylaxis allergen contact takes place mostly in the blood (after injection or oral ingestion of the allergen); however, intense contact with the skin or mucous surfaces can also elicit anaphylaxis.

The term anaphylaxis has been used variably

a) to describe the clinical syndrome of an acute systemic reaction following allergen exposure,
b) to define an immunological pathologic mechanism, more specifically, to define an IgE-mediated reaction.

In most allergy textbooks anaphylaxis is defined as immunologically mediated acute systemic reaction with certain typical symptoms (see below). Thus, the purely clinical term *"anaphylactoid reaction"* is needed to describe an incompatibility reaction resembling the symptoms of classical anaphylaxis, irrespective of the pathologic mechanisms involved [43, 44]. Since many anaphylactoid reactions are elicited by drugs, it seems justified to provide definitions commonly used in the description of adverse drug reactions (Table 1). It should be stressed that some of these definitions are treated differently in the literature [3, 10, 25, 44, 62, 63].

Pseudoallergic reactions are hypersensitivity reactions with clinical symptoms of an allergy that are induced by nonimmunological mechanisms [19, 44]. Pseudoallergic reactions must be distinguished from true allergies as well as from other incompatibility phenomena, such as toxicity and pharmacological intolerance reactions, the symptoms of which correspond to the expected pharmacological effect (Fig. 1). Once it is possible to establish or to rule out an immunological mechanism, an anaphylactoid reaction can be further classified as either anaphylaxis or a pseudoallergic anaphylactoid reaction.

Surgical Research:
Recent Concepts and Results
Baethmann/Messmer (Eds.)

Table 1. Definitions

Intoxication	:	Adverse reaction due to poison
Allergy	:	Immunological hypersensitivity
Intolerance	:	Hypersensitivity to normal pharmacological dosis
Idiosyncrasy	:	Nonimmunological hypersensitivity (unrelated to pharmacological effect)
Pseudoallergy	:	Nonimmunological hypersensitivity with allergy-like symptoms
Anaphylaxis	:	Immunologically mediated immediate allergic reaction
Anaphylactoid reaction	:	Incompatibility reaction with the clinical symptoms of anaphylaxis (irrespective of the pathologic mechanism involved)

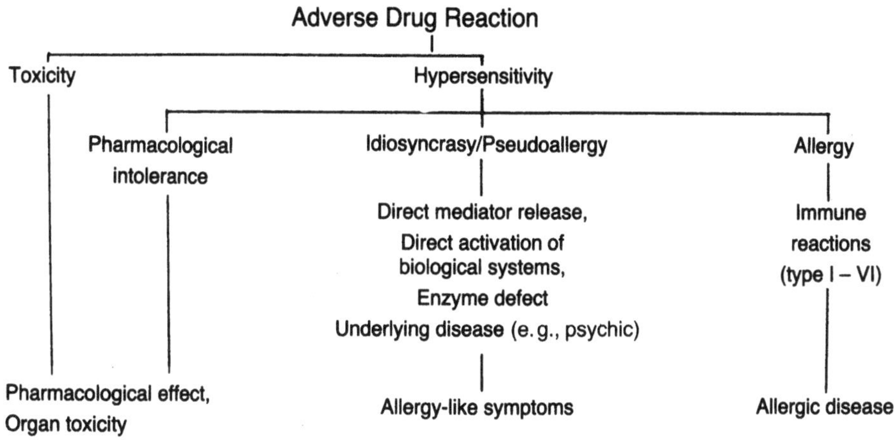

Fig. 1. Classification of various forms of drug-induced adverse reactions

Clinical Symptoms

The clinical symptoms of anaphylaxis represent a syndrome involving many organs. Most commonly the reaction begins with skin involvement (pruritus, flush, urticaria, or angioedema); itching in the pharynx or paresthesia of the palm may be early symptoms. In the respiratory tract sneezing or rhinorrhea may precede dyspnea or bronchospasm and lead to cyanosis or respiratory arrest. Frequently the gastrointestinal tract is involved, with subjective symptoms such as nausea and cramping (uterus cramps may also occur); in severe cases defecation or diarrhea can complicate the situation. Cardiovascular involvement may consist of early tachycardia, changes in blood pressure (sometimes initial rise and only later hypotension), arrhythmia, shock, or cardiac arrest. A grading scale for the intensity of clinical symptoms has proved valuable (Table 2). There are, however, a variety of other signs and symptoms occurring in anaphylactoid reactions, including sweating, headache, disorientations. In severe cases loss of consciousness may be the first sign. Despite immediate and correct therapy, fatal outcomes have been described [4, 24, 62].

Table 2. Grading of anaphylactic/anaphylactoid reactions according to severity of clinical symptoms

	Symptoms			
Grade	Skin	Abdomen	Respiratory tract	Cardiovascular system
I	Pruritus Flush Urticaria Angioedema			
II	Pruritus Flush Urticaria Angioedema (not mandatory)	Nausea Cramping	Rhinorrhea Hoarseness Dyspnea	Tachycardia (> 20 beats/min) RR change (> 20 mmHg systolic) Arrhythmia
III	Pruritus Flush Urticaria Angioedema (not mandatory)	Vomiting Defecation Diarrhea	Laryngeal edema Bronchospasm Cyanosis	Shock
IV	Pruritus Flush Urticaria Angioedema (not mandatory)	Vomiting Defecation Diarrhea	Respiratory arrest	Cardiac arrest

Modified from Ring and Meßmer [42]

Pathologic Findings

Autopsy studies in cases of fatal systemic anaphylaxis sometimes show pulmonary hyperinflation or pulmonary edema; in many cases, however, no pathologic findings are demonstrable. This holds true especially for IgE-mediated reactions [4, 24, 62]. Endoscopic examination of the gastric mucosa can show hemorrhagic lesions [37]. Sometimes eosinophile infiltration is seen around the bronchi [62]. Swelling of liver, spleen, and intestine may also be observed. In cases of IgG-mediated immune-complex anaphylaxis pulmonary hemorrhage and fibrinoid deposits are found in the lung [38, 43, 53]. Studies on cardiac alterations during anaphylactoid reactions show electrocardiographic changes (T flattening or inversion, supraventricular arrhythmias, bundle branch blocks, etc.) in a high percentage of patients [7, 9, 32, 54, 61, 64]. There have been reports of myocardial infarction following anaphylactoid reactions [32, 43, 61, 64].

Eliciting Agents

The most important elicitors of anaphylactoid reactions are the drugs and foods listed in Table 3. Among the drugs known to induce anaphylactoid reactions, xenogeneic proteins (such as hyperimmune sera, antilymphocyte globulin, etc., monoclonal

Table 3. Eliciting agents of anaphylactoid reactions

Specific drugs
Additives in drugs and foods
Specific foods
Occupational substances (e.g., latex)
Animal venoms
Aeroallergens
Contact urticariogens
Physical agents (cold, heat, UV irradiation)
C1-inactivator deficiency
Systemic mastocytosis
Exercise
Seminal fluid
Echinococcal cyst
"Summation-anaphylaxis"
Idiopathic (?)

antibodies, live vaccines), protein hormones (insulin, ACTH, etc.), allergen extracts (for diagnosis and treatment), antibiotics, (especially penicillin), and analgesics must be mentioned [6, 21, 24, 31, 36, 44, 48, 54, 62, 63]. Even vitamins and acetic acid can elicit anaphylactoid reactions [35].

Furthermore, additives present in drugs and injection solutions may represent the actual etiologic agent (Table 4), making it difficult to find the relevant agent by history [34, 52]. Preservatives such as sulfites may be present in antiallergic medications (e.g., β-adrenergic aerosols, corticosteroid injections, and theophylline preparations) [59]. Not only injected or ingested substances may induce anaphylactoid reactions but also airborne allergens (e.g., fish vapors in highly sensitized individuals) and contact urticariogens, giving rise to "contact anaphylaxis" [26, 46]. Special cases of anaphylaxis include anaphylactoid reactions induced by physical agents (cold, exercise, or UV irradiation) [44, 62]. Rare cases include passive transfer of IgE antibodies by blood transfusion [47] as well as an attempted suicide of a penicillin-allergic health employee [58].

In recent years an increasing number of cases have been reported in which anaphylactic symptoms occurred only after a combination of various stimuli, such as exercise

Table 4. Additives in drugs as elicitors of anaphylactoid pseudo-allergic reactions

Additives	Examples
Depot substances	In penicillins
Micelle formers	Cremophor EL in i.m. injections
Sulfites	Injections, sprays
Protein stabilizers	Caprylate in HSA
Benzyl alcohol	Injections, sterile H_2O or NaCl
Parabens	Local anesthetics
Colors	Tablets
Acetate	Dialysis

and certain foods [27]; we refer to this phenomenon as "summation anaphylaxis" and believe it to be much more frequent than is generally thought. A large number of cases with so-called idiopathic anaphylaxis [50] may fall into this group.

Pathologic Mechanisms

The classical anaphylactic reaction is mediated by *IgE antibodies* on the surface of mast cells or basophils, triggering mediator secretion after bridging with an, at least divalent, allergen [3, 5, 63]. It is still controversial as to whether other classes of cell-fixing antibodies (short-term sensitizing antibodies, e.g., IgG4) really play a role in the pathogenesis of anaphylactic reactions.

Immune-complex anaphylaxis is another mechanism leading to dramatic clinical symptoms without involvement of specific IgE antibodies [5, 17, 38, 40, 44, 53]. Clinical examples of this type of reaction occur after administration of blood or blood products; they include anaphylactic episodes in IgA-deficient individuals after plasma therapy [60], and anaphylaxis in the course of serum sickness against xenogeneic proteins [8, 41]. Severe cases of dextran shock are not pseudoallergic in origin as previously thought by many, but represent immune-complex anaphylaxis: serum samples taken immediately before the clinical reaction show extremely elevated titers of IgG antibodies against dextran (up to 1:500000) [17, 40, 43]. The elucidation of this pathologic mechanism has opened the way to a prophylactic approach according to the principle of hapten inhibition [17, 22, 29, 40].

As stated above (Fig. 1) immediate-type reactions with anaphylactoid symptoms may not only be mediated by antibodies but also by pseudoallergic mechanisms such as *direct liberation of mediator substances* (histamine is only one of these). Drugs known to induce histamine release include opioids, intravenous narcotics, colloid volume substitutes on gelatine basis, radiographic contrast media, and others [10, 11, 12, 25, 28, 42, 43, 45]. Similarly, the direct activation of the complement or other plasma protein systems (kallikrein-kinin system) may play a role in the development of anaphylactoid symptoms [2, 11, 44].

Equally, *neuropsychogenic reflex mechanisms* must be considered, especially when dealing with reactions after injection of local anesthetics [44]. In reference to psychosomatic influences one should never forget that stress itself has been shown to release vasoactive mediators, such as histamine [37, 44]. In Fig. 2 an example is shown of a patient in whom a simple bloodless dental manipulation was able to induce a significant rise in plasma histamine [44].

There is probably no single drug that is able to elicit only *one particular* type of adverse drug reaction. Penicillin is a good example of a drug that may induce almost all types of allergies and pseudoallergies in different persons and sometimes within the same individual.

Diagnoses and Differential Diagnoses

Allergy diagnosis is made on the basis of four criteria: history, skin test, in vitro techniques, and provocation tests. The clinical picture of a classical anaphylactoid

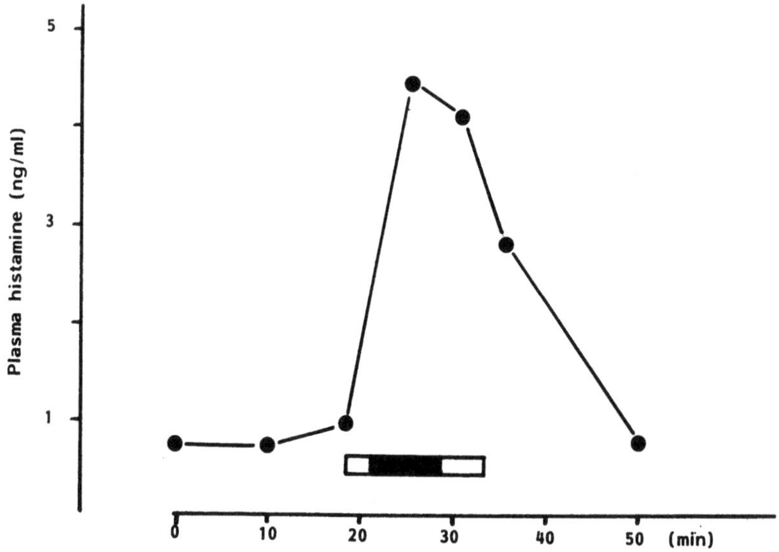

Fig. 2. Plasma histamine concentrations during dental treatment without pharmacological influence [44]. *Unshaded bar lengths,* periods of drilling; *shaded bar length,* period of sharp pain

reaction is so characteristic that there is generally no difficulty in making this diagnosis. However, under certain conditions, e. g., general anesthesia or when only some symptoms are present, made on the basis of factors listed in Table 5. Diagnoses must be a differential.

In a patient who survived an anaphylactoid reaction and who has been transferred later, it is often difficult to discover the relevant agent retrospectively. History remains the most important part of information. Unfortunately, in the most severe cases, e. g. those with loss of consciousness, or reaction under general anesthesia, information is usually insufficient. For IgE-mediated reactions skin tests may be relevant and even of predictive value. In vitro techniques such as the radio-allergo-sorbent-test (RAST) are available only for a few allergens on a routine basis (e. g., penicillin, insulin, ACTH, food allergens, Hymenoptera allergens). In special cases in vitro histamine release after stimulation of basophil leukocytes with the relevant allergen may give additional information.

Table 5. Differential diagnosis of anaphylactoid reactions

Pharmacological/toxic drug effects
Hyperventilation
Vasovagal reaction
Syncope (cardial, cerebral)
Seizure diseases
Bolus aspiration
Pulmonary embolism
Hypoglycemia
Artificial reaction (Münchhausen syndrome, hysterical reaction)

In pseudoallergic reactions skin tests are generally negative. In vitro tests are not available. Here, only specific provocation procedures will lead to a diagnosis. However, one must keep in mind that all in vivo procedures, especially provocation tests, bear the risk of a systemic and possibly life-threatening reaction and must be performed with the utmost caution. Fatal reactions after skin test procedures have been described [6, 16].

Prophylaxis

The most important rules for prophylaxis of anaphylactoid reactions are listed in Table 6. Allergen avoidance is the best means of prevention, however it is only possible on the basis of a correct diagnosis. This involves informing the patient with regard to his condition and to the nature of the eliciting agent in his environment.

When drugs with an empirically high risk of anaphylactoid reactions are indicated, so-called prophetic test procedures (allergy test without history of prior adverse reaction) may be useful in selected cases of IgE-mediated reactions (penicillin, proteins, etc.). After an injection a short observation of the patient is helpful in order to detect early anaphylactoid reactions. After oral application of the offending agent anaphylactoid reactions occur less frequently than after intravenous injection. In special cases hyposensitization with certain drugs has been tried and shown successful, e. g., in penicillin allergy, when penicillin was required as antibiotic of first choice [56] or in aspirin idiosyncrasy [55]. The induction of immunological tolerance against the xenogeneic protein has been shown to reduce the frequency of side reactions of antilymphocyte globulin therapy [8, 41, 43].

For the prevention of dextran-induced anaphylactic reactions hapten inhibition with monovalent dextran (MW 1000; Promit) injected intravenously 5 min prior to dextran infusion has considerably reduced the frequency of side effects after dextran infusion [22, 29, 40]. This principle of hapten inhibition was introduced in penicillin allergy in animal experiments; however, clinical studies have failed to introduce this as effective prophylactic regimen, mainly due to the different allergenic moieties on the penicillin molecule [63].

Table 6. Prophylaxis of anaphylactoid reactions

Correct diagnosis
Avoidance of eliciting agent
Strict indication for new drugs
"Prophetic" testing (in selected cases)
Information of the patient
Oral application of new drugs
Observation of the patient after injection
Tolerance induction (e. g., xenogeneic proteins)
Hapten inhibition (in dextran-induced anaphylaxis)
Hyposensitization (e. g., aspirin, penicillin)
Premedication with histamine H1- and H2-antagonists (e. g., radiographic contrast media, gelatine solutions, i. v. narcotics)

Table 7. Incidence of side effects (%) after prophylactic intravenous pretreatment in four groups of patients prior to infusion of 100 ml 60% meglumine diatrizoate (Urovist)

	Group I (n = 198)	Group II (n = 191)	Group III (n = 196)	Group IV (n = 194)
Pretreatment:	Prednisolone	Clemastine	Clemastine + cimetidine	Saline
Trade name:	Solu-Decortin	Tavegil	Tavegil + Tagamet	
Dose:	250 mg	0.03 mg/kg	0.03 mg/kg + 5 mg/kg[a]	5 ml 0.9%
Side effects				
Overall	18.7	18.8	16.8	19.1
Excluding "sensation of heat"	10.1	12.0	6.1*	12.9
Subjective	13.4	13.5	13.9	10.8
Objective	5.9	6.1	3.1*	9.6
Both objective and subjective	2.0	3.1	1.0*	4.6

[a] In patients with impaired creatinine clearance dose was reduced to 2 mg/kg

* $p < 0.05$

In pseudoallergic reactions due to various agents the combined application of histamine H1- and H2-antagonists has been proven successful in preventing anaphylactoid reactions [10, 25, 33, 45]. Table 7 shows the results of a prospective placebo-controlled trial in 800 patients undergoing intravenous urography: by intravenous prophylaxis with clemastine and cimetidine (group III) a significant reduction in the frequency of subjective and objective side effects compared to the placebo group was observed.

Therapy

In the treatment of anaphylactoid reactions therapeutic modalities depend upon the intensity of the reaction (see Fig. 3). The most important immediate step is introduction of an intravenous catheter and application of fluids.

There is no question that epinephrine (aqueous solution 1:1000, 0.1–0.3 ml s.c.) may act by prevention of mediator release as well as relaxation of bronchial smooth muscle in severe anaphylactoid reactions. However, in elderly patients severe cardiac arrhythmias and even ventricular fibrillation have been described after application of epinephrine [57, 64]. Some authors have seen no benefit from the application of epinephrine in the treatment of severe anaphylactoid reactions [61, 64]. In the study of Lockey et al. 18 out of 24 patients died in anaphylactic shock after immunotherapy despite epinephrine [24]. Treatment with beta-blocking agents may complicate the situation [15, 24]. However, early and sufficiently rapid volume infusion is recommended [30, 61]. Electrolytes and glucose may lead to edema, and human serum albumin seems to disappear rapidly from the circulation; these authors therefore recommend rapid infusion of dextran 70 or hydroxyethyl starch (1000 ml) [30, 44, 61].

The use of glucocorticosteroids in anaphylaxis is still controversial. Many authors believe that steroids have a too long latency in order to be effective in acute dramatic

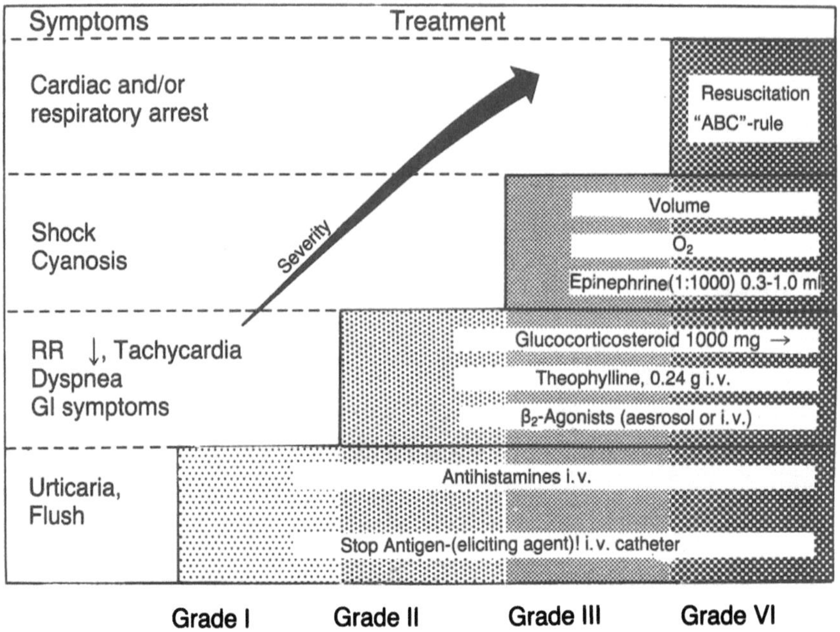

Fig. 3. Schematic diagram for immediate treatment of anaphylactoid reactions of different intensity [44]

anaphylaxis. However, steroids may well be able to suppress late-phase phenomena also observed in anaphylactoid reactions [44]. The evaluation of 19 cases with severe anaphylactoid reactions (grade IV, cardiac and/or respiratory arrest) after dextran infusion showed a clear trend toward significant benefit from immediate high-dose glucocorticosteroid treatment (Table 8 [44]). There is empirical evidence for a possible benefit from the combination of histamine H1- and H2-antagonists in the treatment of anaphylactoid reactions.

By immediate diagnosis and treatment the prognosis of anaphylactoid reactions is generally good if there are no other risk factors present. The earlier the treatment is

Table 8. Comparison of two groups of patients suffering from grade IV (cardiac arrest) anaphylactoid reactions after dextran infusion with regard to early corticosteroid application

	Patients		
	Survived (n = 12)	p	Died (n = 7)
Age (years)	38–72	NS	46–92
Amount of dextran infused (ml)	27 ± 4	NS	25 ± 5
Epinephrine given	7/12	NS	5/7
Prednisolone equivalent given immediately (mg)	1090 ± 320	< 0.01	170 ± 38
Prednisolone equivalent given over whole observation period (mg)	1173 ± 295	NS	715 ± 125

NS = not significant. From [44]

started the better the outcome which can be expected. However, fatal outcome has occurred even under the best possible conditions, in excellent and well equipped hospitals.

References

1. Ahnefeld FW (1980) Plasmaexpander in der Therapie: Nutzen und Problematik. Intensivbehandlung 49: 55
2. Arroyave CM, Tan EM (1976) Mechanism of complement activation by radiographic contrast media. Clin Exp Immunol 29: 85–89
3. Austen KF (1978) The anaphylactic syndrome. In: Samter M (ed) Immunological diseases, vol 2. Boston, Little Brown, pp 885–889
4. Barnard JH (1973) Studies of 400 hymenoptera sting deaths in the United States. J Allergy Clin Immunol 52: 259–264
5. Becker EL, Austen KF (1976) Anaphylaxis. In: Miescher PA, Müller-Eberhard HJ (eds) Textbook of immunopathology, 2nd edn. Grune and Stratton, New York, pp 117–135
6. Blanton WB, Sutphin AK (1949) Death during skin testing. Am J Med 127: 169
7. Booth PH, Patterson R (1970) Electrocardiographic changes during human anaphylaxis. JAMA 211: 627
8. Brendel W, Seifert J, Ring J (1975) Die klinische Anwendung von Antilymphozytenglobulin (ALG). Münch Med Wochenschr 117: 1361–1365
9. Delage C, Irey HC (1972) Anaphylactic deaths: a clinico-pathologic study of 43 cases. J Forensic Sci 17: 525
10. Doenicke A, Ennis M, Lorenz W (1985) Histamine release in anesthesia and surgery: a systemic approach to risk in the perioperative period. Int Anesthesiol Clin 23: 41–66
11. Endrich B, Ring J, Intaglietta M (1979) Effects of radiopaque contrast media on the microcirculation of the rabbit omentum. Radiology 132: 331–339
12. Fisher M (1977) Blood volume replacement in acute anaphylactic cardiovascular collapse related to anaesthesia. Br J Anaesth 49: 1023–1026
13. Fuchs E, Ferlinz R (1986) Allergische Krankheiten In: Wolff HR, Weihrauch TR (eds) Internistische Therapie, 6. Aufl. Urban and Schwarzenberg, München, pp 275–288
14. Gronemeyer W (1980) Noradrenalin statt Adrenalin beim anaphylaktischen Schock. Dtsch Med Wochenschr 102: 101–102
15. Hannaway PJ, Hopper GDK (1983) Severe anaphylaxis and drug induced beta-blockage. N Engl J Med 308: 1536
16. Harris MC, Shure N (1950) Sudden death due to allergy tests. J Allergy 21: 208
17. Hedin H, Richter W, Ring J (1976) Dextran-induced anaphylactoid reactions in man. Int Arch Allergy Appl Immunol 52: 145
18. Hunt KJ, Valentine MD, Sobotka AK, Benton AW, Amodio FJ, Lichtenstein LM (1978) A controlled trial of immunotherapy in insect hypersensitivity. N Engl J Med 299: 157–161
19. Kallos P, Kallos L (1980) Histamine and some other mediators of pseudo-allergic reactions. In: Dukor P et al. (eds) Pseudo-allergic reactions: involvement of drugs and chemicals. Karger, Basel, p 28
20. Kilian J (1977) Die Notfalltherapie des anaphylaktischen Schocks. Notfallmed 3: 148
21. Korenblat PE, Wedner HJ (eds) (1984) Allergy: theory and practice. Grune and Stratton, Orlando
22. Laubenthal H (1986) Dextrananaphylaxie, Pathomechanismus und Prophylaxe. Ergebnisse einer multizentrischen Studie. Springer, Berlin Heidelberg New York
23. Levi R (1972) Effects of exogenous and immunologically released histamine on the isolated heart: a quantitative comparison. J Pharmacol Exp Ther 181: 227–238
24. Lockey RF, Benedict LM, Turkeltaub TB, Bukantz SC (1987) Fatalities from immunotherapy (IT) and skin testing (ST). J Allergy Clin Immunol 79: 666–677
25. Lorenz W, Doenicke A, Dittmann I, Hug P, Schwarz B (1977) Anaphylaktoide Reaktionen nach Applikation von Blutersatzmitteln beim Menschen. Verhinderung dieser Nebenwirkung von Hämaccel durch Prämedikation mit H1- und H2-Antagonisten. Anaesthesist 26: 644–648

26. Maucher OM, Fuchs A (1983) Kontakturticaria im Epicutantest bei Pyrazolallergie. Hautarzt 34: 383–386
27. Maulitz RM, Pratt DS, Schochet AL (1979) Exercise-induced anaphylactic reaction to shellfish. J Allergy Clin Immunol 63: 433–434
28. Meßmer K, Lorenz W, Sunder-Plassmann L, Klövekorn WP, Hutzel M (1970) Histamine release as cause of acute hypotension following rapid colloid infusion. Naunyn Schmiedebergs Arch Pharmacol 267: 433–445
29. Meßmer K, Ljungström KG, Gruber UF, Richter W, Hedin H (1980) Prevention of dextran-induced anaphylactoid reactions by hapten inhibition. Lancet i: 975
30. Meßmer K (1983) Plasma substitutes and indications for their use. In: Tinker J, Rapin M (eds) Care of the critically ill patient. Springer, Berlin Heidelberg New York, pp 569–575
31. Parker CW (1972) Allergic drug responses: mechanisms and unsolved problems. CRC Crit Rev Toxicol 1: 261
32. Pavek K, Wegmann A, Nordström L, Schwander D (1982) Cardiovascular and respiratory mechanisms in anaphylactic and anaphylactoid shock reactions. Klin Wochenschr 60: 941–947
33. Philbin DM, Moss J, Akins CW (1981) The use of H1 and H2 histamine antagonists with morphine anesthesia: a double blind study. Anesthesiology 55: 292–296
34. Prenner BM, Stevens JJ (1976) Anaphylaxis after ingestion of sodium bisulphate. Ann Allergy 37: 180–182
35. Przybilla B, Ring J (1983) Anaphylaxis to ethanol and sensitization to acetic acid. Lancet i: 483
36. Przybilla B, Ring J, Grießhammer B, Braun-Falco O (1987) Schnellhyposensibilisierung mit Hymenopterengiften. Verträglichkeiten und Therapieerfolg. Dtsch Med Wochenschr 112: 416–424
37. Reimann HJ, Ring J, Ultsch B, Wendt P (1985) Intragastral provocation under endoscopic control (IPEC) in food allergy: mast cell and histamine changes in gastric mucosa. Clin Allergy 15: 195–202
38. Revenäs B, Smedegård G, Saldéen T, Fredholm B, Strandberg K (1981) Anaphylactic shock in monkeys passively sensitized with human reaginic serum (II). Acta Physiol Scand 111: 249–257
39. Richet C (1904) De l'anaphylaxie ou sensibilité croissante des organismes à des doses successives de poison. Archivio di Fisiologia 1: 129
40. Richter W, Hedin H, Ring J, Kraft D, Meßmer K (1980) Anaphylaktoide Reaktionen nach Dextran I. Immunologische Grundlagen und klinische Befunde. Allergologie 3: 51–58
41. Ring J, Seifert J, Lob G, Coulin K, Angstwurm H, Frick E, Brass B, Mertin J, Backmund H, Brendel W (1974) Intensive immunosuppression in the treatment of multiple sclerosis. Lancet ii: 1093
42. Ring J, Meßmer K (1977) Incidence and severity of anaphylactoid reactions to colloid volume substitutes. Lancet i: 466–468
43. Ring J (1978) Anaphylaktoide Reaktionen nach Infusion natürlicher und künstlicher Kolloide. Springer, Berlin Heidelberg New York
44. Ring J (1982) Angewandte Allergologie. MMW Medizin Verlag, Munich
45. Ring J, Rothenberger KH, Clauss W (1985) Prevention of anaphylactoid reactions after radiographic contrast media infusion by combined histamine H1- and H2-receptor antagonists: results of a prospective controlled trial. Int Arch Allergy Appl Immunol 78: 9–14
46. Ring J, Galosi A, Przybilla B (1986) Contact anaphylaxis from emulgade F. Contact Dermatitis 15: 49–50
47. Routledge RC, Dekretser DMH, Wadsworth LD (1976) Severe anaphylaxis due to passive sensitization by donor blood. Br Med J 1: 434
48. Schneider SB (1984) Anaphylactoid reactions. In: Korenblat PE, Wedner HJ (eds) Allergy: theory and practice. Grune and Stratton, Orlando, pp 159–170
49. Schwartz HJ, Sher PH (1984) Anaphylaxis to penicillin in a frozen dinner. Ann Allergy 53: 342–343
50. Settipane GA, Newstead GJ, Boyd GK (1972) Frequency of hymenoptera allergy in an atopic and normal population. J Allergy 50: 146–150
51. Sheffer AL, Austen KF (1980) Exercise-induced anaphylaxis. J Allergy Clin Immunol 66: 106–111
52. Simon RA (1984) Adverse reactions to drug additives. J Allergy Clin Immunol 74: 623–630

53. Smedegård G, Revenäs B, Arfors KE (1979) Anaphylaxis in the monkey: hemodynamics and blood flow distribution. Acta Physiol Scand 106: 191–198
54. Smith PL, Kagey-Sobotka A, Blecker ER, Traystman R, Kaplan AP, Gralink H, Valentine MD, Permut S, Lichtenstein LM (1980) Physiologic manifestations of human anaphylaxis. J Clin Invest 65: 1072–1080
55. Stevenson DD (1984) Diagnosis, prevention, and treatment of adverse reactions to aspirin and nonsteroidal antiinflammatory drugs. J Allergy Clin Immunol 74: 617–622
56. Sullivan T (1982) Antigen-specific desensitization of patients allergic to penicillin. J Allergy Clin Immunol 69: 500–508
57. Sullivan TJ (1982) Cardiac disorders in penicillin-induced anaphylaxis: association with intravenous epinephrine therapy. JAMA 248: 2161–2162
58. Templeton B (1965) Suicide by anaphylaxis attempted with penicillin. JAMA 192: 264
59. Twarog FJ, Leung PK (1982) Anaphylaxis to a component of isoetharine (sodium bisulphite). JAMA 248: 2030–2031
60. Vyas GN, Perkins HA, Fudenberg HH (1968) Anaphylactoid transfusion reactions associated with anti-IgA. Lancet ii: 312
61. Waldhausen E, Keser G, Marquardt B (1987) Der anaphylaktische Schock. Anaesthesist 36: 150–158
62. Wasserman SI (1983) Anaphylaxis. In: Middleton E, Reed CE, Ellis EF (eds) Allergy, 2nd ed. Mosby, St. Louis, pp 689–699
63. Weck de AL, Girard JP (1972) Specific inhibition of allergic reactions to penicillin by a monovalent hapten. Int Arch Allergy Appl Immun 42: 798
64. Wegmann A, Reuker H, Pavek K, Schwander D (1983) Katecholamintherapie und Herzrhythmusstörungen im anaphylaktischen und anaphylaktoiden Schock. Anaesthesist [Suppl] 32: 320

The Major Histocompatibility Complex and T-Lymphocyte Response*

F. H. BACH

It is the great rarity in biomedicine to find an individual who is not only an enormous contributor to medical science and practice but who also influences, in a major way, the progress in his or her field. Professor Walter Brendel is such an individual; he has made not only highly original contributions but has worked in a major way to establish the field in which he has functioned. His influence has reached far outside his own direct works, and it is in this way that he has encouraged the flourishing of basic studies.

It is an honor to be invited to contribute to this volume. I do so with admiration and respect for Professor Brendel and the "school" that he has founded. As one member of his famed Kitzbühel/Axams annual meetings, I express my gratitude for the friendship and stimulation that he has provided, both directly and indirectly. Following is an overview of the field in which I have been involved for two decades; many of the advances made by us were presented at the Brendel meetings.

Cellular Immunogenetics of HLA

The great majority of effort in defining the polymorphism of loci of the major histocompatibility complex (MHC) has focused on the use of serological reagents. I shall largely limit my discussion to HLA. Based on serological studies, we learned that there are three HLA class I loci (HLA-A, HLA-B, HLA-C) as well as several class II loci (including HLA-DR and HLA-DQ). My own laboratory has focused its studies on HLA polymorphism and isotypic complexity with T-lymphocyte reagents. Those studies were based on the mixed leukocyte culture (MLC) test which Bain et al. [1] and our laboratory [2] described in 1964, and on a series of modifications of that test including the establishment of a one-way MLC [3], the description of the primed lymphocyte typing (PLT) test [4], and cloning of T-lymphocytes [5] that recognize allodeterminants encoded by genes of the HLA complex.

It was recognized early that the genes encoding determinants recognized in MLC belong to a single locus and that this was the MHC in man [6]. The existence of the HLA-D region, in fact, was hypothesized based on results obtained using the MLC

* This is paper # 475 from the Immunobiology Research Center, Box 724 UMHC, University of Minnesota, Minneapolis, MN 55455. Work discussed herein was supported in part by NIH grants AI 17687, AI 18326, AI 19007, AI 22682.

Surgical Research:
Recent Concepts and Results
Baethmann/Messmer (Eds.)

test. Although in the great majority of cases cells of HLA identical siblings did not stimulate one another in MLC, the occasional exception to this rule suggested, as one possibility, that there were loci linked to but separate from HLA-A and HLA-B that encoded products recognized in MLC and that were responsible for stimulating the great majority of the proliferative response in MLC. This exceedingly interesting finding, that it is essentially only products of HLA that stimulate proliferative response in MLC, and that among the HLA products it is primarily the class II products that stimulate the response for allorecognition, is still not explained and remains one of the fundamental problems of cellular immunogenetics.

In an effort to unravel the complexity of the HLA complex as it relates to T-lymphocyte recognition, cellular reagents generated for use with the PLT test as well as cloned reagents derived from bulk populations that had been "sensitized" in vitro were used. It was the use of these cellular reagents, as well as homozygous typing cells (HTCs), that allowed a series of observations to be made.

The Existence of the Dw/LD Subtype Polymorphism

One of the constructs that we have investigated over the years has attempted to relate the determinants recognized by serological reagents, or the serologically defined (SD) determinants, to those determinants recognized by T-lymphocytes, or lymphocyte-defined (LD) determinants.

It was soon noted that for the class II loci and their products, a polymorphism over and above that recognized serologically can be defined with cellular reagents. Thus, for instance, individuals who type serologically as DR4 could be subdivided with HTC into five groups expressing the specificities Dw4, Dw10, Dw13, Dw14, and Dw15 [10]. This additional Dw/LD polymorphism defined with the use of HTCs was "subtypic" to the serologically defined specificity DR4, i.e., any individual expressing Dw4, Dw10 etc. expressed the SD specificity DR4 even though individuals expressing DR4 could be subdivided as just discussed.

Similar Dw/LD subtype polymorphisms could be demonstrated for other SD specificities. For instance, individuals who typed DR2 serologically could be subdivided into those expressing the LD Dw/LD specificities Dw2, Dw12, LD-MN2, and LD-5a.

In fact, the existence of LD polymorphisms within SD specificities did not apply only to the class II products. Subtype polymorphisms could be demonstrated for class I specificities such as HLA-A2. This ability of T-lymphocytes to define a more extensive polymorphism for the HLA class I and class II loci than that readily recognized serologically is important for understanding several phenomena related to HLA.

The HLA-DP Family

The existence of the *DP* loci was first recognized based on the use of cellular reagents. Even today, in fact, there are no good serological reagents defining the HLA-DP polymorphism. The six or more alleles of HLA-DP were defined using bulk PLT reagents, although a more exacting analysis has been obtained by using T-cell clones as reagents. This polymorphism thus in many ways represents a system similar to the Dw/LD subtype polymorphism that is associated, for instance, with HLA-DR4 with regard to the recognition of the polymorphism by T-lymphocytes but not readily by antibodies [11].

Associations of HLA and Disease

One of the most exciting areas of immunogenetics is based on the finding that certain HLA antigens are associated in a positive or negative manner with a number of different diseases. In some cases there are both positive and negative associations. In an attempt to evaluate whether it is the SD determinants or the LD Dw/LD subtype specificities that are associated most closely with certain diseases, we have performed extensive studies of patients with insulin-dependent diabetes (IDD). There is a strong positive association of IDD with DR3 and DR4 and a negative association with DR2. We evaluated whether one could demonstrate a subtype association for IDD for DR2 or for DR4. In both cases we found that the positive and negative associations were largely with subtypes rather than with the SD defined specificities. Among DR4 positive IDD patients there is a significantly increased frequency of the Dw/LD subtype Dw4. Among the few DR2 positive individuals who have IDD, we have found a markedly decreased frequency of Dw2 as compared with normal individuals and a significantly increased frequency of LD-MN2 as compared with normal individuals.

One possible role that HLA antigens may play in the pathogenesis of diseases is as restriction elements that determine the magnitude of the immune response to antigenic determinants that may be of importance. Given the accumulating evidence that LD allodeterminants, as defined by cellular reagents, correlate very closely with restriction elements for a number of nominal antigens, it is not surprising that the strongest correlations between HLA determinants and various diseases would be with the LD determinants rather than the SD determinants.

HLA Matching for Transplantation

Very little data is available to distinguish matching for the SD and LD determinants. It would be my assumption that the in vitro responses reflect in a significant manner at least some of the in vivo reactions that are involved in allograft rejection. To that extent, I would assume that matching for the LD determinants would be more advantageous than matching for SD determinants.

MHC Antigens and T-Lymphocyte response

There is a unique relationship between the response of T-lymphocytes and recognition of MHC-encoded molecules. For allorecognition, which is the topic reviewed here, as well as for restricted recognition of nominal antigen, the MHC-encoded molecules are a central component of the target being recognized.

In our studies of allorecognition, we noted a phenomenon that was later shown to be applicable to recognition of nominal antigen as well. Namely, a majority of the proliferating helper T-lymphocytes (Th) recognized class II alloantigens, whereas cytotoxic T-lymphocytes (Tc) recognized class I alloantigens [12]. We initially referred to the class I antigens as the SD antigens and the class II antigens as the LD antigens. The lack of absolute fidelity to this rule is demonstrated by the fact that Tc can recognize class II alloantigenic determinants, and to a lesser extent, Th can respond to class I molecules. For restricted recognition, the dichotomy appears to be more stringently followed. Although the dichotomy of recognition just mentioned is certainly not absolute, it still provides a valuable index of correlating T-lymphocyte response with a class of antigen recognized.

Although cells of each functional type studied can respond to molecules associated with each of the three presently recognized class II families (DR, DQ, and DP), there is some evidence in mouse and, to a limited extent, in man that for at least some antigens one class II product may preferentially stimulate help whereas another may stimulate "suppression". This is an enormously important point for future investigation; to the extent that the different class II molecules differentially regulate immune responsiveness, this would be an important extension of the presumed major physiological function of the MHC in immune response.

The recognition that there is differential response to class I and class II molecules by functionally disparate subpopulations of T-lymphocytes provided some of the first information that led to models of T-lymphocyte functional maturation. We suggested that it was recognition of a class I antigenic determinant that stimulated precursor Tc to mature to a "poised Tc" state in which the cells were poised to receive help. Help was, in turn, provided by class II-stimulated Th. Upon receiving help from the Th, poised Tc were able to mature to a full functional effector status [12]. Although this model has been refined by ourselves and others, the fundamental concept regarding stages through which the maturing T-lymphocyte passes, as well as the interaction between the class II responsive Th and the class I responsive Tc, appears to hold.

The model of Th-Tc collaboration (initially referred to as LD-SD collaboration) in the response to class II and class I molecules has also served as a working model for what may take place in vivo. Although for many years Tc was given the principal, if not only, role in the allograft rejection response, evidence presented a few years ago suggested that Th also play a very prominent role in rejection. Which exact mechanisms are the basis of the effects mediated by Th is not clear. Two possible roles are a delayed-type hypersensitivity response or the provision of help that is essential to allow Tc to function.

The importance of matching for class II antigens in promoting allograft survival has been demonstrated by many different centers; these findings have been critically evaluated by Professor Jon J. van Rood of Leiden, Holland, who has been a "member" of the Kitzbühel/Axams group brought together by Professor Brendel. We have suggested that the importance of class II antigens may well relate to their ability to activate Th. In the MLC, it is the degree to which Th are activated that largely determines the magnitude of the cytotoxic response that evolves and, presumably, the magnitude of a DTH-type response that would ensue. To which extent the in vitro model actually reflects what is happening in vivo must remain a point of speculation; this author, at least, adheres to the concept that "in vitro veritas".

Some Reflections

There is a very important reward for individuals participating in biomedical research, in addition to any contribution that their research may make to the overall fund of knowledge. That reward is the ability to interact with one's colleagues and friends in the discussion of results obtained and, in rare instances, to see such discussion lead to application in the clinical arena. Essential for the successful exchange of information and sketching of the frontiers to which the information may be relevant is the establishment of a forum for the fruitful exchange of ideas. That forum must combine a unique set of ingredients that are hard to define. As with the weaving of a tapestry, the threads that lead to a final effect must have the right size, the right color, and the right relationship to their neighbors. Professor Walter Brendel has achieved so very much; included in those achievements is his creation of such a forum for many individuals, including myself, for which all of us are extremely grateful. Although the tapestry is not complete, his contributions to so many aspects of the evolving picture are clearly established.

References

1. Bain B, Vas MR, Lowenstein L (1964) The development of large immature mononuclear cells in mixed leukocyte culture. Blood 23: 108–116
2. Bach FH, Hirschhorn K (1964) Lymphocyte interaction a potential in vitro histocompatibility test. Science 143: 813–814
3. Bach FH, Voynow NK (1966) One-way stimulation in mixed leucocyte cultures. Science 153: 545–547
4. Sheehy MJ, Sondel PM, Bach ML, Wank R, Bach FH (1975) HL-A LD (lymphocyte defined) typing: a rapid assay with primed lymphocytes. Science 188: 1308–1310
5. Bach FH, Inouye H, Hank JA, Alter BJ (1979) Human T lymphocyte clones reactive in primed lymphocyte typing and cytotoxicity. Nature 281: 307–309
6. Bach FH, Amos DB (1967) Hu-1: major histocompatibility locus in man. Science 156: 1506–1508
7. Amos DB, Bach FH (1968) Phenotypic expressions of the major histocompatibility locus in man (AL-A): leukocyte antigens and mixed leukocyte culture reactivity. J Exp Med 128: 623–637
8. Bach FH, Albertini RJ, Amos DB, Ceppellini R, Mattiuz PL, Miggiano VC (1969) Mixed leukocyte culture studies in families with known HL-A genotypes. Transplant Proc 1: 339–341
9. Yunis EJ, Amos DB (1971) Three closely linked genetic systems relevant to transplantation. Proc Natl Acad Sci USA 68: 3031–3035
10. Reinsmoen NL, Bach FH (1982) Five HLA-D clusters associated with HLA-DR4. Hum Immunol 4: 249–258
11. Bach FH (1985) The HLA class II genes and products: the HLA-D region. Immunol Today 6: 89–94
12. Bach FH, Bach ML, Sondel PM (1976) Differential function of major histocompatibility complex antigens in T lymphocyte activation. Nature 259: 273–281

Class II Antigens of the Human Major Histocompatibility Complex

P. A. Peterson

Introduction

Progress in the biological sciences has been remarkable during the past several decades. As the level of sophisticated knowledge expands it becomes difficult if not impossible for the individual investigator to master but a tiny segment of current biology. A consequence of this specialization is frequently the inability of scientists to communicate with colleagues in other disciplines. However, a few outstanding individuals persist in taking the renaissance approach to science. Professor Walter Brendel is the archetype for such a person. His wide interests span as diverse fields as improved surgical techniques and molecular biology of the immune system, and his Round Table discussions in the Tyrolean Alps on a variety of scientific topics have fostered an appreciation of a multidisciplinary approach to medical problems in all those individuals who have participated.

As a physiologist who early on realized the importance of clinical transplantations, Professor Walter Brendel obviously encountered the problem of graft rejection. Pioneering the use of antilymphocyte globulin as a means of suppressing graft rejections, Professor Brendel realized the importance of the major histocompatibility complex (MHC) in such events. The combined efforts of imunologists and immunogeneticists demonstrated that the human MHC represents one of the most genetically polymorphic loci hitherto identified. The genetic polymorphism as such may have represented the greatest immunological obstacle to successful transplantations. However, it was soon realized that a surprisingly large number of cells of the immune system are committed to recognizing the products of the MHC. This made it clear that MHC molecules also have central roles in physiological immune responses. Thus, the obsession of the immune system with these polymorphic proteins sets them apart from other endogenous molecules in initiating a graft rejection.

Population geneticists revealed the complexity of the human MHC by means of serological and cellular assays. A great number of alleles were identified and could be arranged into several segregant series, which today are known as *HLA-A, B, C,* and *D.* As a corollary to this work, it was observed that some alleles occurred in higher than expected frequencies in patients with certain diseases, mostly of autoimmune character. These findings have generated much speculation as to the possible causal relationship between certain allelic products and the disease etiology, but so far our knowledge is limited.

Surgical Research:
Recent Concepts and Results
Baethmann/Messmer (Eds.)

The knowledge of the molecular biology of the MHC region has expanded rapidly. Due to its obvious importance in normal immune reactions as well as in clinical transplantations, this is particularly true for the *HLA-D* region. Most of the genes and antigens of this segment of the MHC have been isolated and examined in great detail. These analyses have also given some insight into the mechanisms generating the polymorphism.

Evolution of the HLA-D Region

Molecules derived from the *HLA-D* region are called class II antigens. They are heterodimeric glycoproteins expressed on the surface of B-lymphocytes, macrophages, epidermal Langerhans cells, and, under certain circumstances, on activated T-cells and some epithelial cells. Due to their genetic polymorphism, the number of different class II antigens expressed by a single cell varies depending on whether the cell is homozygous or heterozygous as regards the *HLA-D* region. All class II molecules are composed of one α and one β chain. The *HLA-D* region contains multiple genes encoding such polypeptide chains. The α and β chains have very similar structures and are obviously evolutionarily related. Even their gross configurations suggest that the ancestral class II molecule was a homodimer. Therefore, it seems reasonable to conclude that α and β chains diverged during evolution by processes involving gene duplication and specialization. Following the emergence of genes encoding heterodimers, further duplication events gave rise to an array of genes similar to those coding for the original α and β chains. By means of a number of techniques it has been possible to demonstrate that such genes occur to a large extent as clusters in the *HLA-D* region. Thus, most if not all class II genes appear to be localized to three well-defined loci called *DP, DQ,* and *DR*.

Structure of Class II Antigen α Chains

All α chains are composed of approximately 230 amino acid residues. About 80% of the structure is expressed on the cell surface, while the remainder of the chain is equally divided between an intramembranous and a cytoplasmic portion. The surface-exposed part of the α chain appears to be folded into two discrete domains of similar sizes. Each domain contains one asparagine-linked carbohydrate moiety. The structure of the domain in closest proximity to the membrane is stabilized by a single disulfide bridge. The membrane-spanning segment of the α chain comprises hydrophobic and neutral amino acid residues surrounded by negatively and positively charged residues, as is commonly found in other transmembrane proteins. The amino acid composition of the part of the α chain which resides on the cytoplasmic side of the membrane is hydrophilic [1].

Hitherto four different types of α chains have been shown to be expressed as protein or mature mRNA. Three of the chains have clearly been defined as products of the *DP, DQ,* and *DR* loci, respectively [2], while the fourth chain may be derived from an as yet unidentified locus tentatively called *DO* [3]. The entire amino acid sequences of these chains have been elucidated from cDNA clones [4, 5], and the correctness of the identification of the chains has been verified by partial amino acid sequencing.

Comparisons of the amino acid sequences of the different chains reveal a high degree of homology. Any two sequences compared display between 50% and 60% identity. The differences occur along the whole length of the chains, although the membrane-integrated portions may exhibit as much as 80% homology, while the short cytoplasmic tails vary considerably. The N-terminal domains are slightly less homologous than the C-terminal domains. On close inspection it is obvious that short stretches of amino acid residues in any pair of α chains may show an unusually high degree of homology. However, such stretches are not conserved between three or more chains, and are therefore not informative in revealing whether any two α chains are evolutionarily particularly closely related.

Several sequences of DP α chains reveal that this polypeptide displays a low degree of genetic polymorphism [6], where only about 3% of the residues differ. The amino acid substitutions are scattered over the entire length of the α chain and no obvious clusters of replacements are discerned. The situation is dramatically different as regards the DQ α chains, which exhibit a high degree of amino acid sequence variability [5]. While the overall differences between any two DQ α chains comprise about 10% of the amino acid residues, the regional differences in the chain vary considerably. Thus, the domain in juxtaposition to the membrane, the membrane-spanning segment, and the cytoplasmic tail do not reveal any polymorphism greater than that recorded for DP α chains. Virtually all the differences between allelic DQ α chains are accordingly confined to the N-terminal domain, whose amino acid sequence varies to about 20%. This unusual distribution of the polymorphism is reminiscent of immunoglobulin variability, but is not as strictly confined to a few discrete regions of the domain, although one stretch of "hypervariability" has been identified in murine I-A α chains [7]. DO α chains are less polymorphic. Thus, the DQ α chains are unusual in terms of both magnitude and distribution of their polymorphism.

Structure of Class II Antigen β Chains

Despite the fact that four different types of α chains have been identified, only three types of β chains have been encountered. DP, DQ, and DR β chains have been structurally examined [8–10], but the reasonable assumption of the existence of a DO β chain has not yet been experimentally verified. However, a class II β chain gene has recently been isolated which may code for the elusive DO β chain (B. Servenius, in preparation).

The three types of β chains share structural features. They are all transmembrane polypeptides with a short cytoplasmic tail. Like the α chains, the predominant portion of the β chains is expressed on the surface of the cell. All human β chains seem to contain a single asparagine-linked carbohydrate moiety whose position appears invariable. The extracellular portion of the polypeptide is most likely folded into two equally large domains. Each domain is stabilized by a single disulfide bond. Sequence determinations of cDNA clones and isolated β chains have unambiguously identified the products of the *DP, DQ,* and *DR* loci. These β chains display considerable homology, and the differences between any two polypeptides are no greater than

30%–40%. Thus, β chains of different loci appear to be somewhat more closely related than the corresponding α chains [9]. The distribution of amino acid residues which differ between chains of the three loci is not confined to any particular region of the polypeptide, although the N-terminal domains are slightly more divergent than the domains closest to the membrane. The greatest identity between the chains is displayed by the membrane-integrated portions, while the cytoplasmic tails vary considerably both in amino acid sequences and length.

β Chains of all loci display extensive genetic polymorphism [11], which on the average engages approximately 10% of the polypeptide chain. The amino acid sequence variability is largely confined to the N-terminal domain [12], where 15%–20% of the residues may differ between nonallelic β chains, while available data suggest that it may be somewhat less pronounced for the DP β chains.

Class II Antigens α and β Chains Are Members of the Immunoglobulin Superfamily

Structural analyses of class II antigen α and β chains revealed their relatedness [4]. They are similarly organized in terms of extracellular domains, membrane-integrated segments, and cytoplasmic tails. In addition, both contain conspicuous disulfide bonds formed by cysteines separated from each other by approximately 60 amino acid residues. The similarities between the two types of polypeptides are strengthened by their amino acid sequences. Thus, the domains closest to the membrane display significant sequence homology, leaving little doubt that the predecessor α and β chains originated from the same ancestral gene. These portions of the polypeptides also display homology to the two subunits of class I MHC antigens. Likewise, significant homology to immunoglobulin light and heavy chains and to T-cell antigen receptor α and β chains exists. Thus, the class II antigens obviously belong to the same superfamily of proteins as several other immunologically important recognition molecules.

The amino acid sequence homology between class II antigen α and β chains and the other members of the superfamily is confined to the domains located closest to the membrane. The N-terminal domains do not exhibit statistically significant homologies to other proteins, despite the fact that the β chain domain contains an immunoglobulin-like disulfide bridge. These observations do not, of course, rule out the possibility that the N-terminal domains of both α and β chains are related to immunoglobulin constant domains in their tertiary structures. This is the case for immunoglobulin variable domains which show the basic immunoglobulin fold although their primary structures are only poorly homologous to the constant domains. Since the tertiary structure of immunoglobulin variable domains can obviously accommodate a great number of amino acid variations without this causing gross structural alterations, it is conceivable that this basic structure has been fundamental in allowing β chains and DQ α chains to accumulate mutations to establish the genetic polymorphism.

Structure of Class II α and β Genes

Several class II α and β genes have been isolated and their structures elucidated. The genes are all very similar in their exon-intron organizations [13, 14]. The α genes are composed of five exons which encode the signal sequence, the N-terminal domain, the domain in juxtaposition to the membrane, the membrane-spanning segment, and the cytoplasmic tail and the 3' untranslated region. This general outline applies to the DP, DQ, DX, DR, and DZ α genes, all of which have been sequenced.

The organization of the β genes differ from that of the α genes only as regards the exons encoding the membrane-spanning segment and the cytoplasmic tail [14, 15]. In contrast to the α chain genes, which encode these portions of the polypeptide chain in a single exon, the β genes use two or more exons for these regions. Alternate splicing also seems to occur, which may give rise to cytoplasmic tails of somewhat varying lengths. It is conceivable that the heterogeneity in the C-terminal region, which arises by structural differences in the β genes of different loci, as well as by alternate splicing, signifies discrete functional differences between the different types of β chains [16]. However, evidence to this effect is hitherto lacking.

Enumeration of Class II α and β Chain Genes

In contrast to the genes for the class I MHC antigen subunits, which reside on separate chromosomes, all class II antigen α and β chain genes seem to occur in the HLA-D region. The numbers of α and β genes discovered so far are greater than the number of polypeptide chains. Thus, six HLA-D α genes have been structurally identified, and the corresponding number of β genes is between six and nine. The uncertainty over the number of β genes is due to the fact that the *HLA-DR* locus appears to contain a haplotype-specific number of β chain genes [17]. Thus, the DR8 haplotype may comprise only one DR β chain gene, while DR4 appears to contain no less than four such genes.

The number of genes in the *DP* region is firmly established, and a molecular map of this region has been drawn. The region contains two pairs of alternating α and β genes which are clustered together within a chromosomal segment encompassing 60 kb. The two types of genes are transcribed in opposite directions. Since only one set of DP α and β chains has been observed, it is not surprising to find that one pair of α and β genes displays pseudogene characteristics. Therefore, they are unlikely to code for any polypeptides. From these observations it seems reasonable to conclude that most haplotypes will only express a single DP molecule, although it cannot be entirely ruled out that two of the *DP* genes are pseudogenes only in some haplotypes.

The *DQ* region also seems to contain two pairs of α and β genes [17]. One pair, which encode the DQ molecule, occur only 12 kb apart. The localization of the two other *DQ* genes, which have tentatively been called *DXα* and *DXβ*, has not been firmly established, but indirect evidence suggests that they are close to each other, and one may speculate that they occur in the vicinity of the expressed DQα and β genes. Sequence analyses of the DXα and β genes (A. Jonsson, unpublished observations) have not revealed any obvious characteristics that make them pseudogenes, but expressed products of these genes have not yet been identified. In contrast to the DQα and β genes proper, the DX genes exhibit a very low degree of polymorphism.

The structural similarity between the *DQ* and *DX* genes is considerably greater than, for example, the similarity between the homologous *DP* genes. While the latter are approximately 75%–80% identical, the *DQ* and *DX* genes are as similar to each other as are alleles of a single segregant series. This great similarity suggests that hybrid molecules of the types DQαDXβ and DXαDQβ may exist, provided all genes are expressed. Accordingly, each haplotype would be able to manufacture four different DQ molecules. Since both DQ α and β genes are extensively polymorphic, heterozygosity at the *DQ* locus should give rise to a minimum of four but possibly as many as 16 DQ antigens.

As noted above, the number of DR β chain genes varies with the haplotype. While DR8 and DR4 may exhibit one and four genes respectively, most DR haplotypes appear to contain three β genes. Invariably, a single DR α gene has been found. The precise location of the genes is not yet established, but preliminary evidence suggests that at least one β gene is adjacent to the DR α gene. The number of expressed β genes is not yet firmly documented. While polypeptide chain analyses have suggested that two DR β chains may be derived from a single haplotype, it is conceivable that this number will vary with the haplotype. In the DR4 haplotype at least one of the four genes is a pseudogene, as shown by sequence analysis [15]. Thus, a minimum of one and a maximum of three DR antigens may be expressed by a haplotype, and since the DR α chain is largely invariant, these numbers will of course double in heterozygous state.

The occurrence of a novel β chain gene, homologous to $A\beta_2$ of the mouse [18], was recently discovered. This gene appears to display some genetic polymorphism, but is more conserved than DQ and DR β genes. Its location and expression have not yet been examined but structural analyses suggest that it should not be grouped together with the DP, DQ, or DR β genes and may therefore be derived from a hitherto unidentified locus. It is tempting to suggest that this gene is a member of the same locus as the DZ α gene, which is most likely expressed in the form of the previously mentioned DO α chain [3, 6].

The enumeration and structural analyses of HLA-D α and β chains have revealed an unexpected complexity. It is clear that an individual heterozygous for all loci in the *D* region will express a minimum of eight different class II molecules. Depending on the degree of polymorphism of the relatively conserved genes and on which genes are expressed, the number of unique class II antigens of a heterozygous individual may in fact be as high as 30. Should hybrid molecules of the DQαDRβ type exist, this number will increase considerably.

Origin of the Class II Antigen Polymorphism

The reasons for the extensive genetic polymorphism exhibited by several genes of the MHC are enigmatic. The simplest way to account for the polymorphism is to assume that it has arisen by natural selection, i. e., that the polymorphism provides a selective advantage. This notion may gain some support from the observation that only a few of the many class I genes of the MHC are extensively polymorphic [19]. The differences in tissue distribution between polymorphic and nonpolymorphic class I genes do indeed suggest separate functions for the two types of proteins which accordingly may have provided the genes with different evolutionary constraints. The three *HLA-D* loci which contain genes whose expression has been unambiguously documented, all harbor polymorphic entities. Although it is presently not obvious why the *DQ* locus contains an extensively polymorphic α gene, in contrast to the *DP* and *DR* loci, current information does not allow a functional distinction between the three types of class II antigens. Therefore, it seems reasonable to conclude, at least provisionally, that the class II antigen polymorphism has indeed been acquired by natural selection.

The observations that the genetic polymorphism is largely confined to the exons encoding the N-terminal domains of DQ α and DP, DQ, and DR β chains raise the possibility that selective forces may operate on these exons. The variability among immunoglobulins is similarly distributed, but it is obvious that class II genes do not undergo somatic rearrangements, so other mechanisms must be responsible for the class II antigen polymorphism. Several such mechanisms can be proposed. One possibility is that sequence-specific mutagenic events occur more frequently in the polymorphic exons than in other portions of the genes [7]. Another mechanism which may account for the restricted distribution of the polymorphism is gene-conversion-like events, which may operate on the polymorphic exons with high frequency. In gene conversion events longer or shorter DNA segments are copied from one homologous gene to another [20]. Gene conversions of short DNA segments will usually increase the polymorphism. Alternatively, the conservation of other regions of the genes than the polymorphic exon may arise by gene conversions involving long DNA segments, which will homogenize the sequences.

Regardless of mechanism the genetic polymorphism is subject to evolutionary constraints operating on the class II genes and polypeptides. Such selection may be positive and favor polymorphism in one portion of the gene, or negative and conserve existing sequences in other regions. Obviously, both types of selective pressure may be operative simultaneously on discrete sections of a single exon.

Analyses of several class II β gene sequences reveal a consistent pattern in the distribution of the nucleotide substitutions, and it can be concluded that it is unlikely that the mutation rate in the polymorphic exons is significantly greater than in other regions of the genes [9]. Thus, should sequence-specific mutational mechanisms exist, their contribution to the overall polymorphism is not major. Nucleotide substitutions that give rise to amino acid replacements are, of course, considerably more frequent in the polymorphic than in the other exons. This is not necessarily due to such substitutions being favored. In fact, it seems more likely to conclude that a conservative selective pressure acts on all exons but the polymorphic ones, thereby eliminating replacement substitutions [21]. Although statistical analyses fail to support the view that the polymorphism is selected for, it should be born in mind that discrete parts of the polymorphic exons may be under positive and negative constraints which have escaped detection.

Further support for the view that it is selection, rather than specific mutational mechanisms, that is the main generator of the polymorphism was obtained by analyses of a DRβ pseudogene. Since this gene will not give rise to any translational product, it can be assumed to be relieved of most structural constraints. In keeping with this notion, all exons exhibit similar degrees of "replacement" substitutions. Thus, in the absence of a conservative selective pressure, which eliminates replacement substitutions, all exons seem to attain polymorphism to similar extents [40].

The fact that the class II antigen polymorphism may be accounted for by multiple, independent point mutations does not mean that all point mutations in a given sequence have originated within that sequence. A mutation may arise in one gene but subsequently be copied to another homologous gene by a gene-conversion-like event.

Such an event most easily explains the emergence of a mutant murine class II gene [22]. This observation strongly suggests that gene conversion or a mechanism similar to gene conversion operates on class II genes.

In conclusion, it seems reasonable to assume that different evolutionary constraints have operated on the different portions of the polymorphic class II genes. The exons encoding the N-terminal domains may have acquired amino acid replacements by selective mechanisms that either favor such replacements or at least do not impose constraints against them. Such constraints seem to be operative on the other exons. These types of selective pressures operate independently of whether substitutions occur by point mutations or by gene-conversion-like events.

Concluding Remarks

Great progress has been made in recent years in unraveling the molecular anatomy of the *HLA-D* region as regards its genes and products. It seems likely that most genes have been identified, but some may still remain undiscovered. The structures of the genes are well worked out, and the rough outline of the origin of the genetic polymorphism is being unraveled. Work in progress in several laboratories will, before too long, establish a detailed molecular map of the *HLA-D* region, and this information will most likely allow conclusions to be drawn regarding the emergence during evolution of the various *D* region loci. Future molecular analyses will undoubtedly reveal the nature and location of controlling genetic elements that confer tissue-specific expression and inducibility by γ-interferon to the class II genes.

The availability of isolated class II genes will prompt an avalanche of studies directed at the expression of transfected genes in appropriate cells. Such studies may be of great clinical importance inasmuch as the specifiities of serological and cellular reagents may be standardized. Likewise, transfected cells will allow examination of the possible existence of hybrid class II antigens. Whether DP, DQ, and DR antigens are functionally equivalent may also be approached under such simplified experimental conditions.

The precise molecular role of the class II molecules in the presentation of antigens to T-cells should be amenable to examination in view of the structural knowledge recently acquired, not only about class II antigens, but also about T-cell receptors. These and related problems will keep molecular biologists busy while, hopefully, succinct molecular concepts concerning the role of class II antigens in tolerance induction and thymus selection are being developed.

References

1. Kaufman JF, Auffray D, Korman J, Shackelford DA, Strominger J (1984) The class II molecules of the human and murine major histocompatibility complex. Cell 36: 1–13
2. Spielman R, Lee JS, Bodmer WF, Bodmer J, Trowsdale J (1984) Six HLA-D region α-chain genes on human chromosome 6: polymorphisms and associations of DC α-related sequences with DR types. Proc Natl Acad Sci USA 81: 3461–3465
3. Inoko H, Ando A, Kimura M, Ogala S, Tsuji K (1984) Isolation and characterization of the cDNA clones and the genomic clones of the HLA class II antigen heavy chains. In: Albert ED,

Baur MP, Mayr W (eds) Histocompatibility testing 1984. Springer, Berlin Heidelberg New York Tokyo, pp 559–564
4. Larhammar D, Gustafsson K, Claesson L, Bill P, Wiman K, Schenning L, Sundelin J, Widmark E, Peterson PA, Rask L (1982) Alpha chain of the HLA-DR transplantation antigen is a member of the same protein superfamily as the immunoglobulins. Cell 30: 153–161
5. Schenning L, Larhammar D, Bill P, Wiman K, Jonsson AK, Rask L, Peterson PA (1984) Both α and β chains of HLA-DC class II histocompatibility antigens display extensive polymorphism in their aminoterminal domains. EMBO J 3: 432–447
6. Trowsdale J, Young JAT, Kelly AP, Austin PJ, Carson S, Meunier H, So A, Ehrlich HA, Spielman RS, Bodmer J, Bodmer WF (1985) Structure, sequence and polymorphism in the HLA-D region. Immunol Rev 85: 5–43
7. Benoist CO, Mathis DJ, Kanter MR, Williams VE, McDevitt HO (1983) Regions of allelic hypervariability in the murine Aα immune response gene. Cell 34: 169–177
8. Larhammar D, Schenning L, Gustafsson K, Wiman K, Claesson L, Rask L, Peterson PA (1982) The complete amino acid sequence of an HLA-DR antigen-like β chain as predicted from the nucleotide sequence: Similarities with immunoglobulins and HLA-A, B, C antigens. Proc Natl Acad Sci USA 79: 3687–3691
9. Gustafsson K, Wiman K, Emmoth E, Larhammar D, Bohme J, Hyldig-Nielsen JJ, Ronne H, Peterson PA, Rask L (1984) Mutations and selection in the generation of class II histocompatibility antigen polymorphism. EMBO J 3: 1655–1661
10. Gustafsson K, Emmoth E, Widmark E, Bohme J, Peterson PA, Rask L (1984) Isolation of a cDNA clone coding for an SB β-chain. Nature 309: 76–78
11. Bohme J, Owerbach D, Denaro M, Lernmark A, Peterson PA, Rask L (1983) Human class II major histocompatibility antigen β-chains are derived from at least three loci. Nature 301: 82–84
12. Kampe O, Larhammar D, Wiman K, Schenning L, Claesson L, Gustafsson K, Paabo S, Hyldig-Nielsen JJ, Rask L, Peterson PA (1983) Molecular analyses of MHC antigens. In: Møller E, Møller G (eds) Genetics of the immune response. Plenum, New York, pp 61–87
13. Korman AJ, Auffray C, Schamboeck A, Strominger J (1982) The amino acid sequence and gene organization of the heavy chain of the HLA-DR antigen: homology to immunoglobulins. Proc Natl Acad Sci USA 79: 6013–6017
14. Larhammar D, Hyldig-Nielsen JJ, Servenius B, Andersson G, Rask L, Peterson PA (1983) Exon-intron organization and complete nucleotide sequence of a human major histocompatibility antigen DC β gene. Proc Natl Acad Sci USA 80: 7313–7317
15. Larhammar D, Servenius B, Rask L, Peterson PA (1985) Characterization of an HLA DRβ pseudogene. Proc Natl Acad Sci USA 82: 1475–1479
16. Peterson PA, Andersson G, Bill P, Bohme J, Denaro M, Emmoth E, Gustafsson K, Hammerling U, Hyldig-Nielsen JJ, Jonsson AK, Kalm B, Larhammar D, Schenning L, Servenius B, Widmark E, Rask L (1983) Features of class I and II antigens of the major histocompatibility complex at the DNA and protein level. Prog Immunol 5: 171–186
17. Bohme J, Andersson M, Andersson G, Møller E, Peterson PA, Rask L (1985) HLA-DR β genes vary in number between different specificities, whereas the number of DQ β genes is constant. J Immunol 135: 2149–2155
18. Larhammar D, Hammerling U, Denaro M, Lund T, Flavell R, Rask L, Peterson PA (1983) Structure of the murine immune response I-A_α locus: sequence of the I-A_β gene and an adjacent β-chain second domain exon. Cell 34: 179–188
19. Steinmetz M, Hood L (1983) Genes of the major histocompatibility complex in mouse and man. Science 222: 727–733
20. Jackson AJ, Fink GR (1981) Gene conversion between duplicated genetic elements in yeast. Nature 292: 306–310
21. Rask L, Gustafsson K, Larhammar D, Ronne H, Peterson PA (1985) Generation of class II antigen polymorphism. Immunol Rev 84: 113–133
22. McIntyre KR, Seidman JG (1984) Nucleotide sequence of mutant I-A_β^{bm12} gene is evidence for genetic exchange between mouse immune response genes. Nature 308: 551–553

Subject Index

MIX
Papier aus verantwortungsvollen Quellen
Paper from responsible sources
FSC® C105338

If you have any concerns about our products,
you can contact us on
ProductSafety@springernature.com

In case Publisher is established outside the EU,
the EU authorized representative is:
Springer Nature Customer Service Center GmbH
Europaplatz 3, 69115 Heidelberg, Germany

Printed by Libri Plureos GmbH
in Hamburg, Germany